INFANTICIDE

Psychosocial and Legal
Perspectives on Mothers Who Kill

INFANTICIDE

Psychosocial and Legal Perspectives on Mothers Who Kill

Edited by

Margaret G. Spinelli, M.D.

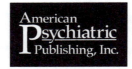

American
Psychiatric
Publishing, Inc.

Washington, DC
London, England

Note: The authors have worked to ensure that all information in this book is accurate at the time of publication and consistent with general psychiatric and medical standards, and that information concerning drug dosages, schedules, and routes of administration is accurate at the time of publication and consistent with standards set by the U.S. Food and Drug Administration and the general medical community. As medical research and practice continue to advance, however, therapeutic standards may change. Moreover, specific situations may require a specific therapeutic response not included in this book. For these reasons and because human and mechanical errors sometimes occur, we recommend that readers follow the advice of physicians directly involved in their care or the care of a member of their family.

Manufactured in the United States of America on acid-free paper
07 06 05 04 03   5 4 3 2 1
First Edition

Typeset in Adobe's Berling Roman and Cantoria

American Psychiatric Publishing, Inc.
1400 K Street, N.W.
Washington, DC 20005
www.appi.org

Library of Congress Cataloging-in-Publication Data
Infanticide : psychosocial and legal perspectives on mothers who kill /
edited by Margaret G. Spinelli.—1st ed.
    p. ; cm.
    Includes bibliographical references and index.
    ISBN 1-58562-097-1 (alk. paper)
    1. Infanticide—Psychological aspects. 2. Infanticide—Social aspects.
3. Women murderers. 4. Mothers—Psychology. 5. Postpartum
depression. I. Spinelli, Margaret G., 1947–
    [DNLM: 1. Infanticide—psychology. 2. Depression, Postpartum—
psychology. 3. Infanticide—legislation & jurisprudence. 4. Mothers—
psychology. W 867 I437 2002]
RG852 .I53 2002
364.15′23′0852—dc21   2002071116

British Library Cataloguing in Publication Data
A CIP record is available from the British Library.

To Erik, Keith, Bob, and Phil,
for their belief in my journey

In memory of
Professor Ramesh "Channi" Kumar

Contents

Contributors. xi

Introduction xv
Margaret G. Spinelli, M.D.

Acknowledgments xxiii

Part I
Epidemiology and Historical Legal Statutes

Chapter 1
A Brief History of Infanticide and the Law. 3
Michelle Oberman, J.D., M.P.H.

Chapter 2
Epidemiology of Infanticide 19
Mary Overpeck, Dr.P.H.

Part II
Biopsychosocial and Cultural Perspectives on Infanticide

Chapter 3
Postpartum Disorders: Phenomenology, Treatment Approaches,
and Relationship to Infanticide. 35
Katherine L. Wisner, M.D., M.S., Barbara L. Gracious, M.D.,
Catherine M. Piontek, M.D., Kathleen Peindl, Ph.D., and
James M. Perel, Ph.D.

Chapter 4
Neurohormonal Aspects of Postpartum Depression and Psychosis... 61
Deborah Sichel, M.D.

Chapter 5
Denial of Pregnancy..................................... 81
Laura J. Miller, M.D.

Chapter 6
Neonaticide: A Systematic Investigation of 17 Cases 105
Margaret G. Spinelli, M.D.

Chapter 7
Culture, Scarcity, and Maternal Thinking.................. 119
Nancy Scheper-Hughes, Ph.D.

Part III
Contemporary Legislation

Chapter 8
Criminal Defense in Cases of Infanticide and Neonaticide........ 133
Judith Macfarlane, J.D.

Chapter 9
Medical and Legal Dilemmas of Postpartum Psychiatric Disorders... 167
Cheryl L. Meyer, Ph.D., J.D., and Margaret G. Spinelli, M.D.

Chapter 10
Infanticide in Britain.................................... 185
Maureen N. Marks, D.Phil., C.Psychol., A.F.B.P.S.

Part IV
Treatment and Prevention

Chapter 11
How Could Anyone Do That?: A Therapist's Struggle With
Countertransference...................................... 201
Anonymous

Chapter 12

The Mother-Infant Relationship: From Normality to Pathology. . . . 209
Pamela Meersand, Ph.D., and Wendy Turchin, M.D.

Chapter 13

The Promise of Saved Lives: Recognition, Prevention, and
Rehabilitation. 235
Margaret G. Spinelli, M.D.

Index 257

Contributors

Barbara L. Gracious, M.D.
Assistant Professor of Psychiatry, University of Rochester Medical Center, Strong Memorial Hospital, Rochester, New York

Judith Macfarlane, J.D.
Practicing Attorney, Human Services Division, The City of New York Office of the General Counsel, Legal and Government Affairs Division, New York, New York

Maureen N. Marks, D.Phil., C.Psychol., A.F.B.P.S.
Senior Lecturer, Sections of Perinatal Psychiatry and Psychotherapy, Institute of Psychiatry; Consultant Adult Psychotherapist, Perinatal Services, South London and Maudsley NHS Trust, Institute of Psychiatry, London, England

Pamela Meersand, Ph.D.
Assistant Professor of Psychology, Columbia University; Director, Therapeutic Nursery, The New York Presbyterian Hospital; Faculty Member, The Parent-Infant Program of the Institute for Psychoanalytic Training and Research, Columbia University, New York, New York

Cheryl L. Meyer, Ph.D., J.D.
Associate Professor of Law and Psychology, Wright State University School of Professional Psychology, Dayton, Ohio

Laura J. Miller, M.D.
Associate Professor of Psychiatry, Chief of Women's Services Division, University of Illinois at Chicago, Chicago, Illinois

Michelle Oberman, J.D., M.P.H.
Professor of Law, DePaul University College of Law, Chicago, Illinois

Mary Overpeck, Dr.P.H.
Epidemiologist, U.S. Maternal and Child Health Bureau, Rockville, Maryland

Kathleen Peindl, Ph.D.
Assistant Professor of Psychiatry, Thomas Jefferson University, Philadelphia, Pennsylvania

James M. Perel, Ph.D.
Professor of Psychiatry and Pharmacology, University of Pittsburgh Medical Center, Western Psychiatric Institute and Clinic, Pittsburgh, Pennsylvania

Catherine M. Piontek, M.D.
Assistant Professor of Psychiatry and Human Behavior, and Obstetrics and Gynecology, Thomas Jefferson University, Philadelphia, Pennsylvania

Nancy Scheper-Hughes, Ph.D.
Professor of Medical Anthropology; former Chair, Department of Anthropology; Director, Graduate Program in Critical Studies in Medicine, Science, and the Body, University of California at Berkeley, Berkeley, California

Debra Sichel, M.D.
Instructor, Harvard University Medical College; Director of Helsia Women's Health Center, Boston, Massachusetts

Margaret G. Spinelli, M.D.
Assistant Professor of Psychiatry, Columbia University College of Physicians and Surgeons; Director, Maternal Mental Health Program, and Research Psychiatrist, New York State Psychiatric Institute, New York, New York

Wendy Turchin, M.D.
Assistant Professor of Psychiatry, Cornell University; Director, Pediatric Mental Health, The New York Presbyterian Hospital; Faculty Member, The Parent-Infant Program of the Institute for Psychoanalytic Training and Research, Columbia University, New York, New York

Katherine L. Wisner, M.D., M.S.
Professor of Psychiatry, Obstetrics and Gynecology and Pediatrics, Women's Behavioral HealthCARE, University of Pittsburgh Medical Center, Western Psychiatric Institute and Clinic, Pittsburgh, Pennsylvania

Introduction

Margaret G. Spinelli, M.D.

The infant's life is a vulnerable thing and depends to a great extent
on the mother's good will. Sara Ruddick . . . has captured the contradictions well in noting that mothers, while so totally in control of the
lives and well being of their infants and small babies, are themselves under the dominion and control of others. Simultaneously powerful
and powerless, it is no wonder that artists, scholars, and psychoanalysts can never seem to agree whether "mother" was the primary
agent or the primary *victim* of various domestic tragedies. And so
myths of a savagely protective "maternal instinct" compete at various
times and places with the myth of the equally powerful, devouring,
"infanticidal" mother.

Nancy Scheper-Hughes (1992)

Maternal infanticide, or the murder of a child in the first year of life
by its mother, is a subject both compelling and repulsive. The killing of
an innocent elicits sorrow, anger, and horror. It is a crime. It demands retribution. That is the law.

Yet the perpetrator of this act is often a victim too, and that recognition makes for a more paradoxical response. On one hand is the image of
a defenseless infant, killed by the person on whom he or she depended
for survival. On the other is the image of a mother, insane, isolated and
imprisoned for a crime unthinkable to many. These competing images
elicit ambivalence, if not outrage.

Such contradictions are a theme of this book, the production of which
was motivated by the dearth of up-to-date, research-based literature on this
tragic cause of infant deaths. As I introduce this subject, I ask the reader to

share in a difficult task: to reach beyond rage, to stretch the limits of compassion and enter the minds of mothers who kill their babies. I do so in the hope that advancing the knowledge base and stimulating inquiry in this neglected area of maternal-infant research will save young lives.

The paucity of research-related reports on this tragic and arguably preventable cause of infant mortality demands action. Thus, my initial goal in compiling the existing knowledge base is to provide a framework within which can be designed research strategies for early identification and treatment of women at risk of committing infanticide and for prevention of maternal infanticide.

My second—and more practical and immediate—goal is to assist mental health and law practitioners who participate in the court cases of women accused of infanticide. Scant literature is available for the mental health professional who is facing the challenges of the criminal court system or for the attorney who must understand the implications of psychiatric diagnoses as defenses for infanticide and neonaticide. I hope this book can serve as a preliminary resource.

Historically, society and the law have treated infanticide with ambivalence (Lagaipa 1990; Oberman 1996). In Biblical times, infanticide was sanctioned as a method of human sacrifice and population control. In the early seventeenth century, infant murder became so prevalent that laws were enacted and severe punishments, including execution, were imposed on mothers (especially unmarried women) who killed their babies. In 1647, Russia assumed a more humane position, and by 1881, all European states except the United Kingdom had followed suit. In 1922, Britain passed the Infanticide Act (amended and expanded in 1938), changing the relevant charge from murder to manslaughter and proscribing sentences of probation and mandatory psychiatric treatment for women found guilty. Canada has almost identical legislation. At present, the infanticide laws in most countries allow for lenient sentencing and psychiatric treatment.

In contrast, a woman convicted of infanticide in the United States may face a long prison sentence or even the death penalty. Because of the scarcity of psychiatric treatment in our overcrowded prison system, these women serve their time and exit the system in their childbearing years with the same psychopathology that brought them into it in the first place.

This work was in the early phase of production when the nation was riveted by the news that Andrea Yates drowned her five children (ages 6 months to 7 years) in the bathtub of her Houston, Texas, home (CourtTV 2002). Perhaps no other case demonstrates the paucity of medical and legal understanding of postpartum psychosis and associated infanticide than that of *Yates v. Texas*. The tragedy of the Yates family parallels the theme of this book.

Andrea Pia Yates was a registered nurse who became a stay-at-home mom who home-schooled her children. She was a champion swimmer, high school valedictorian, and a devoted and loving mother. Although she was consistently pregnant and /or breast feeding over the past 7 years, she cared for her bedridden father as well as her own growing family: Noah 7, John 5, Paul 3, Luke 2, and Mary 6 months.

Mrs. Yates also had a history of psychiatric illness. She blocked her thoughts when she felt Satan's presence and "heard Satan's voice" tell her to "pick up the knife and stab the child" after Noah's birth in 1994. She told no one because she feared Satan would hear her and harm her children. She also worried that some of her doctors might be Satan or be influenced by Satan. Two suicide attempts after her fourth pregnancy were driven by attempts to resist Satanic voices commanding her to kill her infant.

Six months after the birth of her fifth child, her family recognized that Andrea Yates appeared "catatonic." In the month before she killed her children, her friend noticed that she walked around the house like a "caged animal."

After two psychiatric hospitalizations, Andrea Yates continued to deteriorate. When her psychiatrist discontinued her antipsychotic medication 2 weeks before the tragedy, she became floridly psychotic. Cartoon characters called her a bad mother. She was no longer able to resist the commanding voices in her head. Satan directed her to kill her children to save them from the fires and turmoil of hell.

Yates was charged with capital murder with possible penalty of death. She requested a razor to shave her head and reveal the "mark of the beast— 666" that she believed was on her scalp. "I am Satan," she said.

It took the jury 3½ hours to return a guilty verdict. The prosecution sought the death penalty. After 35 minutes of deliberation, the jury selected life in prison.

My personal impetus for embarking on this book grew from my experience as a perinatal psychiatrist who has had professional involvement in infanticide cases in the judicial system. The scarcity of contemporary research and literature on childbirth-related psychiatric diagnoses available to mental health and legal professionals leaves room for great doubt that the system is functioning justly or effectively or humanely. And because diagnostic guidelines for postpartum disorders are limited, decisions about guilt, sentencing, and potential for treatment often rest in the hands of the judicial community. The existing literature does not support alternatives to assist the court in this process.

In a court of law, expert witness testimony must be founded on scientific standards that are recognized in the professional psychiatric community. Yet the defenses available for women alleged to have committed infanticide are limited to early and outdated literature. Motivated by a desire to address the lack of current and usable resources, I began this project by focusing on the psychiatric and legal implications of infanticide.

As work progressed, a panoply of contributors with expertise in infanticide—clinicians, scholars, academicians, researchers, clinical and forensic psychiatrists and psychologists, pediatric psychoanalysts, attorneys, an anthropologist, and an epidemiologist—expanded my early vision of this book. Together, they have painted a broader and far richer picture: They have provided a preliminary biopsychosocial and legal model of maternal infanticide. They have explored the unique biological roles of women and examined their combined psychosocial, psychodynamic, and caregiving roles. They have suggested directions and described strategies for research, treatment, and prevention of infanticide.

The first part of the book introduces historical and epidemiological data. Michelle Oberman, who is a researcher and academician in the fields of law, public health, and infanticide, describes historical legal statutes of infanticide and the evolution of contemporary legislation. She presents a compelling discussion of the contrasting legal views of infanticide in the United States, United Kingdom, and other Western countries. Professor Oberman and Cheryl Meyer have amassed and classified the largest database of female perpetrators of infanticide in the United States. Drawing from hundreds of cases, Professor Oberman provides an overview of a new typology and associated characteristics in mothers who kill (Meyer and Oberman 2001).

Mary Overpeck, an epidemiologist, describes the most recent statistics on maternal infanticide and calls attention to the problems of underreporting and the lack of available documentation. Professor Overpeck identifies problems of ascertainment, particularly in early neonatal deaths, and describes future methods of investigation to facilitate description of risk as well as improved prevention.

The five chapters that make up the book's second part illustrate the biopsychosocial and cultural underpinnings of infanticide. The authors explore clinical diagnosis, symptom recognition, risk factors, and biological precipitants as well as alternative motives such as cultural infanticide.

Chapter 3 was developed to assist the attorney or the mental health professional in understanding the implications of postpartum psychiatric illness as they relate to infanticide. It is a comprehensive review of psychiatric disorders associated with childbirth written by an international perinatal expert and researcher, Katherine Wisner, and her colleagues. Dr. Wisner and her colleagues provide a review of the most recent literature on differential diagnoses, etiology, evaluation, and state-of-the-art treatment on childbirth-associated psychiatric illness. They emphasize and illustrate a sensitive and thorough inquiry into infanticidal ideation.

In Chapter 4, Debra Sichel, a perinatal psychiatrist and clinician, provides the most recent data and clinical applications of underlying physiological mechanisms associated with childbirth. Dr. Sichel emphasizes neurohormonal mechanisms of the acute hormone withdrawal state as the initial etiological trigger affecting brain chemistry and mental status changes associated with delivery.

Chapters 5 and 6 examine neonaticide, or child murder within 24 hours of birth—a topic that is often sensationalized in news media coverage. In Chapter 5, Laura Miller shares her expertise in the psychopathology of pregnancy denial—which often precipitates neonaticide—and distinguishes three types of denial and potential sequelae. In Chapter 6, I describe the first systematic evaluation of the cases of 17 women alleged to have committed neonaticide. I also identify a prodrome of similar phenomenology, psychopathology, presentation, and family history in a subset of neonaticidal mothers.

Chapter 7 illuminates how economic and cultural realities can contribute to the prevalence and even acceptance of maternal infanticide. In this chapter, Nancy Scheper-Hughes, former chair of the Department of Anthropology at the University of California, Berkeley, recounts her experience on the Alto do Cruzeiro (Hill of the Crucifix), the shantytown region of Northeastern Brazil. Professor Scheper-Hughes invites us into a culture in which the high expectation of death produces patterns of nurturing that differentiate those infants thought of as "thrivers" from those thought of as born "already wanting to die." The survivors and keepers are nurtured, while the stigmatized or "doomed" infants are allowed to die "of neglect"—"angels . . . freely offered up to Jesus and His Mother" in order to preserve the limited resources for stronger, older children and working adults.

Contemporary legislation is the central theme of the third part. Chapter 8 is authored by practicing attorney Judith MacFarlane, who describes the present standard for the insanity defense in the United States and its relevance to infanticide and neonaticide. This chapter is an excellent resource for the attorney or the expert psychiatric witness who is preparing for an infanticide or neonaticide case in the criminal court system. In Chapter 9, law professor and psychologist Cheryl Meyers and I discuss the American criminal and civil courts' discrepant treatment of postpartum psychiatric disorders. We contrast the admissibility of postpartum syndromes on women's behalf in the civil courts (as in child custody suits) with their inadmissibility in criminal cases. In Chapter 10, Maureen Marks, lecturer in psychiatry at the Institute of Psychiatry at the Maudsley Hospital in England, describes current controversies over England's Infanticide Act and discusses that country's strategies for preventing and treating postpartum disorders through services such as health visits to the home and inpatient mother and baby units.

The final chapters focus on clinical experiences with mothers as perpetrators, mothers and infants at risk, and early treatment and prevention. In Chapter 11, a perinatal expert, psychotherapist, and faculty member of a major academic institution anonymously describes a 2-year psychodynamic treatment of a woman awaiting trial for neonaticide after a denied pregnancy associated with rape. This therapist describes initial negative countertransference reactions, the limitations on dynamic work against the backdrop of an impending murder trial, the risk of decompensation, "timely decisions to support rather than confront defenses," and termination issues at the time of the patient's incarceration.

The closing chapters explore pregnancy and early parenting as the peak time for prevention and intervention. In Chapter 12, two child psychoanalysts, Pamela Meersand and Wendy Turchin, focus on normal mother-infant attachment as baseline in an attempt to understand the pathological changes that occur when bonding fails. They emphasize early intervention through evaluation of mothers-at-risk and mother-infant psychotherapy. My epilogue on prevention (Chapter 13) suggests that the foregoing body of knowledge may be used as a stepping-off point for desperately needed inquiry into the neglected area of maternal infanticide. I emphasize early identification of mothers at risk and prevention of pathological sequelae.

A theme conspicuously absent from this book is paternal infanticide and filicide (murder of a child under 5 years of age). Although parents are the most likely perpetrators of infanticide, little information on paternal filicide exists in the literature (Marks and Kumar 1993). The existing literature on infanticide by fathers consists of small-sample case studies of male perpetrators in various settings (Campion et al. 1998; Cordier 1983; Kaye et al. 1990; Marleau et al. 1999; Martin 1984). Only four cases of paternal neonaticide have been reported in the literature (Kaye et al. 1990).

Although infanticide may be viewed as an act of child abuse (Lowenstein 1997), and males are responsible for half of these crimes, child abuse by fathers is a neglected area of study. Of 66 studies of child abuse published in the literature over 5 years, 28 included only mothers; 2 included fathers, and the 36 remaining articles neglected to mention sex differences (Martin 1984). Haskett et al. (1996) reviewed 126 articles of maltreatment from 1989 through 1994; males were included in fewer than half (47.7%) of 77 reviewed articles. Only 3 studies included males, yet 40 involved female participants.

Reports suggest that men are more likely to use violence as a method of murder and more likely to receive longer prison sentences than are women (Marks and Kumar 1993). At least one report suggests that men are more likely to kill spouses along with children (Byard et al. 1999). In general, the treatment resources for abusing men are inadequate, and therefore there is little or no potential for prevention.

Sex differences in reporting are not easily explained, especially since the subject of infanticide is generally underrepresented in the literature. One factor may be that childbirth is universally identified as a time of vulnerability for women. Postpartum disorders affect 10%–15% of new mothers. Kendell et al. (1987) demonstrated that the peak lifetime prevalence for psychiatric disorders and hospital admissions for women occur in the first 3 months after childbirth, the identical time frame for the occurrence of 50% of infanticides. Why do we continue to neglect this field of research?

Whether the cause of maternal infanticide is postpartum psychiatric illness, dissociative disorder and denial of pregnancy, substance abuse, child neglect, or child abuse, women at risk of committing infanticide are presenting to us in antepartum, postpartum, and well-baby clinics, hospitals, and other settings. Absent research-based information on the temporal relationship between childbirth and infanticide, and a clinical framework for understanding the diagnosis and phenomenology that underlie infanticide, we are, in all likelihood, missing the signs of potential tragedy.

I offer this book as a springboard and inspiration for research aimed at classifying infanticide according to the biopsychosocial model of psychiatry and contemporary diagnostic criteria. Therein lies the hope of prevention and the promise of saved lives.

References

Byard RW, Knight D, James RA: Murder-suicides involving children: a 29-year study. American Journal of Forensic Medicine and Pathology 20:323–327, 1999

Campion JF, Cravens JM, Covan F: A study of filicidal men. Am J Psychiatry 145: 1141–1144, 1998

Cordier J: The child, privileged victim of crimes of passion. Victimology 8(1–2): 131–136, 1983

CourtTV: Texas mom drowns kids. Available at http://www.courttv>com/trials/ yates. Accessed March 2002.

Haskett ME, Marziano B, Dover ER: Absence of males in maltreatment research: a survey of recent literature. Child Abuse Negl 20:1175–1182, 1996

Kaye NS, Borenstein NM, Donnelly SM: Families, murder, and insanity: a psychiatric review of paternal neonaticide. Journal of Forensic Sciences 35:133–139, 1990

Kendell RE, Chalmers JC, Platz C: Epidemiology of puerperal psychoses. Br J Psychiatry 150:662–673, 1987

Lagaipa SJ: Suffer the little children: the ancient practice of infanticide as a modern moral dilemma. Issues Compr Pediatr Nurs 13:241–251, 1990

Lowenstein LF: Infanticide—a crime of desperation. Criminologist 21(2):81–92, 1997

Marks MN, Kumar R: Infanticide in England and Wales, 1982–1988. Med Sci Law 33:329–339, 1993

Marleau JD, Poulin B. Webanck T, et al: Paternal filicide: a study of 10 men. Can J Psychiatry 44:57–63, 1999

Martin JA: Neglected fathers: limitations in diagnostic and treatment resources for violent men. Child Abuse Negl 8:387–392, 1984

Meyer CL, Oberman M: Mothers Who Kill Their Children. New York, New York University Press, 2001

Oberman M: Mothers who kill: coming to terms with modern American infanticide. American Criminal Law Review 34:1–110, 1996

Ruddick S: Maternal Thinking: Toward a Politics of Peace. Boston, MA, Beacon, 1989

Scheper-Hughes N: Death Without Weeping: The Violence of Everyday Life in Brazil. Berkeley, University of California Press, 1992

Acknowledgments

This book would not have come together without the contributions, assistance, encouragement, patience, and good humor of many people. To start, I am grateful to my colleagues Drs. Katherine Wisner, Jean Endicott, and Debra Sichel, each of whom is a dedicated, internationally known expert in the field of women's mental health. I deeply value their friendship and their encouragement and support of this project.

I next want to acknowledge Professor Ian Brockington for his scholarly contributions to our field, Dr. Richard Brown for his confidence in my endeavor, attorney Michael Dowd for his dedication to defending those in need, and the late Dr. Susan Hickman for her pioneering work with young mothers.

I remain always grateful to Drs. Joanne Woodle and Orli Etingin, to Mary Hanrahan, and to the Boorman and Tomei families.

I am thankful to the faculty of the Columbia Psychoanalytic Center for Training and Research for giving me the opportunity to study and to appreciate the analytic significance of this project.

My heartfelt appreciation goes to the distinguished authors who contributed chapters to this book. They have brought considerable insight and expertise to this project, and I thank them for giving of their time and talent.

I also value the efforts of the members of Depression after Delivery, Postpartum Support International, and the Marcé Society for the Prevention and Treatment of Postpartum Disorders. Their courageous work to assist mothers and families affected by postpartum mental illness is inspiring.

I thank Dr. Carol Nadelson, former editor-in-chief of American Psychiatric Press, who proposed this book and helped make it a reality; her successor, Dr. Robert Hales, who took it to completion; Madeline Beusse, who edited portions of the book; Suzy Blumenthal, for her assistance; and the staff at American Psychiatric Publishing, for their patience and cooperation.

I want to recognize the sorrow and the courage of the women and families whose stories of childbirth-related mental illness are recounted in or helped shape this book. Their experiences broadened the contributing authors' and this editor's understanding of postpartum mental illness and infanticide. By sharing their stories with us, the people directly affected by postpartum psychiatric illnesses suggest and illuminate the path for professional progress toward treatment and prevention.

Finally, I hope this book in some way honors the memory of the late Professor Ramesh (Channi) Kumar, who headed the Department of Perinatal Psychiatry and the Mother-Baby Unit at the Maudsley and Royal Bethlem Hospitals, the Institute of Psychiatry, in London, England. "Channi," as friends and colleagues knew him, possessed not only great integrity but also enthusiasm and energy that attracted professionals from around the world to the field of mother-infant mental health. He was a kind physician who loved his patients and dedicated his life to mothers and infants everywhere. For those of us who were graced by his presence, he remains a vital source of inspiration.

This work was supported by a National Institute of Mental Health Research Scientist Development Award for Clinicians (Grant #1K20 MH 01276-01).

Part **I**

Epidemiology and Historical Legal Statutes

Chapter *1*

A Brief History of Infanticide and the Law

Michelle Oberman, J.D., M.P.H.

Submitted to Samuel Bard, M.D., president[,] and the trustees and professors of the College of Physicians and Surgeons of the University of the State of New York:

The science of Medical Jurisprudence, of which the subject of the following Dissertation (Infanticide) form[s] an important branch, lays claim to the attention of every one who feels any concern in the pure administration of justice. To the Physician, it recommends itself consideration even still more interesting. . . . In most criminal trials for poisoning, drowning, infanticide etc., the testimony of the Medical witness must necessarily in a great measure decide the fate of the accused. It cannot, therefore[,] but be obvious how useful and even indispensably necessary it is for him to possess an intimate acquaintance with a branch of knowledge whose object it is to supply him with the means for forming just inductions and correct decisions whenever he may be called into a court of justice or before a coroner's inquest.

Inaugural dissertation on infanticide, publicly defended for the degree of Doctor of Medicine by John B. Beck, A.M., sixth day of April, 1817

Portions of this chapter are reprinted from Meyer CL, Oberman M: *Mothers Who Kill Their Children: Understanding the Acts of Moms from Susan Smith to the "Prom Mom."* New York, New York University Press, 2001. Copyright 2001, New York University Press. Used with permission of New York University Press.

Infanticide is not a random, unpredictable crime. Instead, a quick survey of history reveals that it is deeply embedded in and responsive to the societies in which it occurs. The crime of infanticide, or child murder in the first year of life, is committed by mothers who cannot parent their child under the circumstances dictated by their unique position in place and time. The factors in such circumstances vary from poverty to stigma to dowry, but the extent to which infanticide is a reflection of the norms governing motherhood is a constant that links these seemingly disparate acts.

One seeking to make sense of the persistence of infanticide in contemporary society would do well to understand the manner in which cultural norms have shaped this crime throughout history. This same history also reveals the seemingly inconsistent and even incoherent manner in which societies have responded to infanticide. However, as a result of viewing together both the persistence and consistency of infanticide and the societal responses to it, we are afforded a perspective that permits us to reconcile the act of infanticide with the body of laws that govern infanticide in societies throughout the contemporary world.

Toward that end, I provide here a brief chronological review of the sociocultural imperatives underlying the crime of infanticide in various cultures. The aim is not to provide a comprehensive record of the crime of infanticide, but rather to illustrate the intricate relationship between a society's construction of parenthood and mothering and its experience of infanticide. Special attention is paid to the manner in which distinct societies have understood, rationalized, and punished infanticide.

Infanticide in Ancient Cultures

Although little is known about actual infanticidal practices in ancient cultures, such as which parents killed their children and under what circumstances, archeological evidence suggests that infant sacrifice was commonplace among early people, particularly insofar as it enabled them to control population growth and to minimize the strain placed on society by sickly newborns (Langer 1974; Moseley 1986).

Records from the Babylonian and Chaldean civilizations, dating from approximately 4000 to 2000 B.C., constitute the earliest written historical references to infanticide. But perhaps the richest historical records of infanticide in ancient cultures emanate from ancient Greece and Rome. It seems clear that infanticide was widely practiced in these societies, with the reasons used to justify these actions ranging from population control to eugenics to illegitimacy. Ancient Greco-Roman literature routinely refers to the exposure of unwanted newborns. Exposure helped to prevent overpopulation, and, because those exposed often were either sickly or disabled, the practice was viewed as eugenic in nature (Moseley 1986). Under Roman law, infanticide became less of a civic virtue or imperative than it was a private matter. Fathers were given the absolute legal authority to govern all matters falling within their "domestic" purview (Moseley 1986).

Infanticide also was common to non-Western ancient cultures. For example, female infanticide was a common practice in early Muslim and pre-Islamic culture in seventh-century Arabia. Scholars attribute this to the status of women as "property" in that society (Chaudhry 1997). In addition, some speculate that in order to spare a female child a life of misery, mothers frequently disposed of their female babies (Chaudhry 1997).

The advent of Islamic rule called for the abolition of female infanticide. Nonetheless, there is little reason to believe that call was heeded. Over the ensuing centuries, the traditional Indian dowry system, requiring that a woman's family make a sizeable gift to the groom's family upon marriage, constituted a powerful incentive to avoid having female offspring (Chaudhry 1997). Despite efforts to reform or even abolish the dowry system, it is entrenched in Indian culture. As such, even today, the birth of a daughter automatically triggers the pressure of saving a suitable dowry. If a family cannot provide a suitable dowry, it risks social ostracism. Among poor rural families, the persistence of female infanticide and sex-selective abortions of healthy female fetuses is attributable to this fear (Bumiller 1990).

Traditional Chinese culture also reveals a long history of female infanticide. Female children have long been regarded as less valuable, as Confucian doctrine does not permit women to carry on the family's name or otherwise honor the family's ancestors (Lee 1997). As such, daughters from both poor and rich families are vulnerable to infanticide (Kellum 1974; Langer 1974; Lee 1998; Moseley 1986; Trexler 1973).

This traditional limit on women's value was compounded by the Chinese adoption, during the Qing dynasty of the eighteenth and nineteenth centuries, of the practice of giving a dowry to the groom's family upon the marriage of a daughter. This practice, at first confined to the wealthy classes, served to enhance the preference for sons among wealthy families and caused a shocking increase in female infanticide among the dynastic families. Over time, it spread so extensively that estimates suggest a full 10% of daughters born into Qing dynasty families were killed at birth. As in India, the practice of female infanticide continues in contemporary China. In 1979, China implemented a policy of one child per family in an effort to stem rapid population growth. This policy triggered a dramatic rise in the abandonment and infanticide of baby girls as well as a rise in the abortion of female fetuses (Greenhalgh and Li 1995). The customs favoring sons are so deeply entrenched that female infanticide persists, in spite of the Chinese government's attempt to reform the underlying cultural norms and laws thought to contribute to son preference (Mathew 1997).

Infanticide in Medieval Judeo-Christian Society

In 318 A.D., when the Roman Empire converted to Christianity, Constantine declared an end to *patria potens*, the absolute right of the father over his children, and infanticide was declared to be a crime. Yet, all indications are that infanticide remained commonplace throughout early Christian society (Langer 1974; Moseley 1986). Vital records, kept by churches throughout Europe during the Middle Ages, show ample evidence of sex-selective infanticide. Additional evidence of the prevalence of infanticide emerges from occasional references to the crime in medieval handbooks of penance. These describe the sin of overlying a child (i.e., lying on top of the child and suffocating him or her); this sin is included in a list of the venial or minor sins, such as failing to be a good samaritan or quarreling with one's wife (Kellum 1974). From the ninth to the fifteenth century, the standard penance for overlying was 3 years, with 1 of these on bread and water, compared with 5 years, with 3 on bread and water, for the accidental killing of an adult. Scholars consider this casual mention and lenient treatment of infanticide to be evidence of its relatively commonplace nature (Moseley 1986).

Infanticide in early Judeo-Christian Europe was associated with the familiar factors of poverty and scarce familial resources. In addition, Christianity brought with it a new set of pressures that encouraged infanticide. Specifically, the Catholic Church's profound religious and cultural hostility to nonmarital sex and childbearing became an additional factor associated with infanticide. The Catholic Church dictated that a child born to an unmarried woman was to be deemed "illegitimate" (Deuteronomy 23:2). As a result of the church's condemnation of nonmarital sexual relations, medieval society virtually disregarded the illegitimate child. Illegitimate children were "deprived . . . of the ordinary rights of man" (Satava 1996). But it was not only the children who were stigmatized by illegitimacy. Unmarried mothers suffered considerable social approbation for bearing a child out of wedlock, regardless of how they came to be impregnated (Mendlowicz et al. 1998).

Sixteenth- and seventeenth-century European society penalized sexual offenses such as bastardy and fornication. The penalties for these crimes were particularly harsh in England. For example, in 1576 Parliament passed a "poor law" that punished impoverished parents of bastard children. These laws punished, through public whipping and/or imprisonment, mothers who refused to identify the men who fathered their illegitimate children (Hoffer and Hull 1981).

Fear of punishment under these laws created an obvious incentive to conceal a sexual affair as well as a resulting pregnancy. This incentive was particularly intense for unmarried women whose jobs were jeopardized as a result of a pregnancy. For example, the commonplace nature of sexual harassment against women employed as domestic servants fostered a perverse and tragic link between sexuality, pregnancy, and infanticide. (Kellett 1992).

The link between illegitimacy and infanticide during this era in European society was so widely acknowledged that, to a large extent, infanticide was considered a crime committed exclusively by unmarried women. In fact, the earliest criminal laws pertaining to infanticide refer solely to the crime of "bastardy infanticide"—infanticide committed by an unmarried woman (An Act to Prevent the Destroying and Murthering of Bastard Children 1623). The punishment for this crime ranged from burial alive to drowning and decapitation (Moseley 1986). Interestingly, during the witchcraft inquisition, the crime of infanticide was widely attributed to witches, and the gruesome punishments meted out to supposed witches also were received by those convicted of infanticide (Trexler 1973). Because of the law's focus on "bastardy," married women generally were not convicted of infanticide (Moseley 1986).

Infanticide and British Legal History: A Case Study in Ambivalence

An overview of British legal history for the 300 years between 1623 and 1922 provides a vivid illustration of that society's ambivalence in responding to the crime of infanticide. In 1623, Parliament passed a law making it a capital offense to conceal the birth of an illegitimate child—whether still- or liveborn—by a secret disposition of its body (Hoffer and Hull 1981). This law essentially reversed the presumption of innocence, requiring that unless a defendant could produce an eyewitness to testify that the baby was stillborn, the jury must find that she murdered the child (Oberman 1996). Obviously, few women could meet this test, as it is hard to imagine that a woman inclined to hide her illegitimate pregnancy would choose to have someone witness the birth. Nonetheless, given the high infant mortality rates of that era, it is inevitable that the law had the effect of condemning to die a large number of women who had attempted to conceal their pregnancies and then either miscarried or gave birth to stillborn fetuses (Backhouse 1984).

In its first years of operation, this law generated a tremendously high number of convictions. Indeed, two historians of the era suggest a 225% increase in the rates of infanticide indictments in the 28 years following its passage (Hoffer and Hull 1981). Nonetheless, there is no evidence to suggest that the law had any deterrent effect on the crime of infanticide. Instead, after several decades of enforcement of the Jacobean law, juries began refusing to convict these women by adopting several widely accepted defenses to the crime (e.g., a woman could defend herself by showing she had linen for the baby, which was taken to mean that she wanted it to survive) (Hoffer and Hull 1981). As a result, by the early 1700s, British conviction rates for infanticide reverted to the relatively low rates seen in the early 1600s, prior to the law's passage (Hoffer and Hull 1981).

Finally, in 1830, Parliament passed a new infanticide statute requiring that the prosecution in an infanticide case prove that the baby had been born alive (43 Geo ch 5853 [Eng 1803]). In the event that the state could not prove this, the woman received a maximum sentence of 2 years for the crime of concealing the birth of an illegitimate child. If convicted of infanticide, however, the woman was sentenced to death. As a result, this lesser offense became the overwhelming preference of juries in infanticide trials, and "courts regularly returned verdicts of not guilty despite overwhelming evidence to the contrary" (Backhouse 1984).

Twentieth-Century Responses to Infanticide: The Medical Model

Until the start of the twentieth century, societal responses to infanticide indicate that it generally was viewed as a crime committed by desperate and/or immoral women. The twentieth century introduced a dramatic new perspective on the crime—that of illness (see Chapter 3: "Postpartum Disorders"). Two late-nineteenth-century French psychiatrists, Jean-Etienne Esquirol and Victor Louis Marcé, first posited the notion that there might be a causal relationship between pregnancy, childbirth, and subsequent maternal mental illness (Mendlowicz et al. 1998). Others quickly adopted their research, and almost immediately people around the world began to associate infanticide with mental illness. Nowhere was this vision more powerfully embraced than in England, where the infanticide statutes of 1922 and 1938, taking into account the impact of pregnancy and birth on the mother's mental status, recognized infanticide as a distinct form of homicide.

The British Infanticide Act of 1922 (amended and expanded in 1938) requires that mothers who can show that they suffered from a postpartum mental "disturbance" be charged with manslaughter rather than murder (Infanticide Act 1938) (see Chapter 10: "Infanticide in Britain"). As this is relatively easy to demonstrate, the vast majority of women convicted of infanticide receive sentences associated with manslaughter, most commonly probation, and are required to undergo counseling rather than to serve time in prison (N. Walker 1968).

The British statute has been replicated in slightly varying forms in at least 22 nations around the world (Oberman 1996). Many nations have statutes specific to infanticide; all but one of these make infanticide a less severe crime than ordinary homicide (Oberman 1996).

Americans have been far less sanguine with regard to the adoption of a medical model for understanding infanticide. To date, there are no statutes (federal or state) governing infanticide. Nor do American medical experts agree about the nature of postpartum mental disorders and their capacity to cause infanticide (American Psychiatric Association 1994). The result is that U.S. law governing infanticide is remarkably inconsistent. The only "medical" explanation for infanticide on which medical experts in the United States and around the world agree is the relatively rare disorder known as *postpartum psychosis*. Postpartum psychosis is characterized by a dramatic break with reality, accompanied by hallucinations or delusions (see Chapter 3). Women who kill their infants during an episode of postpartum psychosis tend to manifest these symptoms at an extreme level.

Consider Sheryl Massip, a California woman who was convicted of killing her 6-week-old son. At her 1987 murder trial, the prosecution proved that she threw her son into oncoming traffic, picked him up, and carried him to her garage, where she hit him over the head with a blunt object and then killed him by running him over with her car (Lichtblau 1990). As is typical of other cases of postpartum psychosis–related infanticide, Massip continued to display severely disordered thinking after she killed her child. She told investigators that a black object with orange hair and white gloves, who "wasn't really a person," had kidnapped the baby (Lichtblau 1990).

Postpartum psychosis presents unique problems for the criminal justice system because it is brief in duration and because, even if the condition is untreated, symptoms may disappear within several months of onset (O'Hara 1987). For example, by the time of her trial, Massip was no longer psychotic. Nonetheless, the jury was troubled by the notion that she could simply go free, after having killed her son. It therefore convicted Massip of second-degree murder and sentenced her to prison. Two months later, the judge overturned the verdict, acquitting Massip on the grounds that she was insane at the time of the murder. Because she was no longer insane, the judge allowed Massip to go free ("A Mother Tells Why She Killed Her Son" 1994).

Contemporary Responses to Infanticide in the United States

Despite the medical community's growing acceptance of postpartum psychosis, it is clear that this disorder explains only a very small minority of the infanticides that occur annually in the United States and elsewhere. Indeed, when one examines the body of contemporary cases involving mothers who kill their children, it is evident that none of the excuses of generations past—poverty, stigma, disability, or mental illness—fully explain the persistence of infanticide. Some speculate that the only women who commit infanticide are those who are either insane or simply evil.

For example, Linda Chavez, president of a Washington-based think tank, refers to women who commit infanticide as "monster-women" and suggests that welfare policy may be linked to infanticide (Chavez 1995). In support of her point, she quoted then U.S. Representative Newt Gingrich, who asserted in response to a particularly gruesome murder case that "[w]elfare policy has created 'a drug addicted underclass with no sense of humanity, no sense of civilization and no sense of the rules of life'" (Chavez 1995). Contrast these remarks with those of psychiatrist Park Elliott Dietz, who theorizes that "[n]o amount of stress alone can account for women killing their children. . . . It doesn't come from who you hang out with, what your opportunities in life are or how much money you have. It comes from something being wrong with the person" (quoted in Smith 1991).

My research, which involved culling and sorting hundreds of contemporary accounts of infanticide from the media and legal databases, suggests that neither of these explanations adequately accounts for the persistence of infanticide (Meyer and Oberman 2001). Instead, one finds five broad categories of contemporary infanticide cases (Table 1–1), all of which are responsive to the societal construction of and constraints on mothering.

Table 1–1. Contemporary typology for infanticide/filicide

Type of infanticide	Maternal characteristics	Other characteristics
Neonaticide	Young or immature Emotionally isolated from partner Limited potential for economic independence	Pregnancy concealed or denied No prenatal care Unattended birth
Assisted/coerced	Limited economic independence Limited social support Psychological profile: "battered woman"	Violent and/or abusive male partner
Neglect-related	Limited economic means Burdened with parenting Overwhelmed by economic obligations Inattentive or distracted parenting	Completely accidental death
Abuse-related		Chronic child abuse Lack of parental impulse control Death unintentional Especially high risk for abuse at mealtimes and bedtimes

Mental illness–related	Acute: postpartum-onset depression or psychosis
	   Socially isolated
	   Alone with the baby
	   Guilt over inability to cope
	Chronic: schizophrenia; lifelong depression and psychosis
	   Socially isolated
	   Incapable of parenting without assistance
		High expectations of mother's capacity to parent
		
		Child protection agency errors often a major factor
		Placing children with ill mothers
		Suicidal women: may be trying to protect their children by taking them with them "to heaven"

Neonaticide

Neonaticide, or the killing of one's offspring within the first 24 hours of life, is a crime that typically involves young women who determine, correctly or not, that they would be completely cut off from their social support network were they to disclose their pregnancies. Subsequent psychiatric evaluation of these girls reveals that many suffer from severe dissociative states associated with a history of early abuse and chaotic family life (Spinelli 2001). For various reasons, including religion, culture, money, ambivalence, and immaturity, these girls are unable or unwilling to pursue the alternatives of abortion or adoption. Denial of their pregnancy is so profound that, day after day, they ignore the impending birth of their child.

Assisted/Coerced Infanticide

A second category of infanticide involves women who kill their infants or children in *conjunction with their male partners*. These cases predominantly involve women whose intimate partners are violent and abusive. Often, the women are themselves caught in the cycle of an abusive relationship and are unable to act to protect themselves or their children. Their behavior may be readily understood through the lens of research on battered women, which provides ample description of the fears that trap women in abusive relationships (L. E. Walker 1979).

Neglect-Related Infanticide

A third category of infanticide cases involves mothers whose infants die as a result of *neglect* (Meyer and Oberman 2001). In these cases, the child's death is, for the most part, due to the mother's having been distracted. For example, many contemporary cases involve babies who die when their mothers are taking care of other tasks—tasks that frequently are also related to parenting. A common example is a baby who is left in the bathtub or in the care of a still-young older sibling while the mother is in the kitchen cooking.

It is critical to note the way in which the societal construction of motherhood shapes our response to these crimes. In the past, these deaths might have been viewed as tragic accidents. Today, they are homicides. Mothering has thus become more than simply a full-time job. According to the unwritten rules that govern the role of mother, one must be constantly vigilant, losing all thought of self-interest. Here again, it seems absurd to explain these women's actions by terming them either insane or evil. Indeed, an attempt to do so eclipses important insights about the circumstances that give rise to these children's deaths.

The two remaining categories of infanticide—those related to *child abuse* and those growing out of *mental illness*—illustrate the devastating results of a system that relies on a single individual to parent under the unwritten rules that govern the role of mother. To be sure, some women can parent under extremely challenging circumstances, because their support networks and coping skills are sufficiently strong. Others, however, are not prepared for this task.

Abuse-Related Infanticide

Another category of infanticide cases involves women whose abuse of their child leads to his or her death. Often these women abuse their children with some regularity, and the deaths of these children occur during efforts to discipline that go awry (Meyer and Oberman 2001). Although cases of chronic child abuse carry with them a unique horror, even among infanticide cases, it is important to note that there are regular, even predictable, patterns to these children's deaths. Indeed, epidemiologists have demonstrated the specific hours during each day when children are most at risk of death by homicide (Chew et al. 1999). These periods coincide with mealtimes and bedtimes, events that often are, even in stable, loving households, accompanied by stress, arguments, and the need to discipline (Chew et al. 1999). As such, one might temper the inclination to dismiss these mothers as simply evil and, instead, observe that women who kill their children in abuse-related infanticides are affected by the extraordinarily demanding tasks associated with child care. Seen from this angle, many of the abuse-related cases seem to involve mothers who lacked the impulse control of their peers, but the impulse that motivated these killings is surprisingly commonplace.

Mental Illness–Related Infanticide

The final category of infanticide cases involves women with severe mental illness, whether acute or chronic, who clearly are not prepared for the task of mothering. A significant depressive or psychotic episode may render a woman unable to generate the continual flow of selfless compassion and patience that children demand. Likewise, a woman with a chronic mental impairment may be constitutionally incapable of meeting the demands of parenting in isolation, without external support. Tragically, there are numerous infanticide cases involving severely impaired women who were expected to care for their children, essentially alone ("Abandoned to Her Fate" 1995; "Report of the Independent Committee" 1993).

Infanticidal Jurisprudence in the United States

Because the United States lacks a statute such as England's that treats infanticide cases alike on the basis of an explicit justification for mitigating the severity of this crime, each case tends to be viewed on its own merits. The result has been a tendency to treat each infanticide case as exceptional rather than to recognize the profound similarities that underlie the many contemporary infanticide cases. Often, the media seem to play a powerful role in dictating the defendant's blameworthiness and even in determining the resolution of these cases (Meyer and Oberman 2001).

The result is that U.S. infanticide jurisprudence is incoherent and often arbitrary. Sentences range wildly, with women convicted of substantially equivalent crimes, such as neonaticide, receiving sentences that vary from probation with counseling to life imprisonment (Oberman 1996). The fact that the United States lacks a statute to dictate an appropriate punishment for infanticide need not imply that we must tolerate this level of randomness in resolving these cases. Judges and juries faced with infanticide cases must take into consideration the extent to which a given individual is morally blameworthy.

The central task of the criminal justice system in punishing infanticide cases is to ascertain the purposes to be served by punishing these women. There are three basic justifications for punishment: deterrence (both general and specific), retribution, and rehabilitation. *General deterrence* refers to the notion that punishing a given defendant will serve to deter others who might be contemplating committing the same crime. Given all that we know about the crime of infanticide, this rationale for punishment seems almost absurd. The mothers who commit infanticide seem relatively desperate, and there is little reason to believe that they spend time contemplating the potential consequences of their acts. Instead, infanticide seems for the most part to be a spontaneous crime, reflecting a loss of control rather than a cool-headed calculation.

Specific deterrence endorses the punishment of an individual who has committed a crime on the grounds that this will deter that individual from committing the same crime again in the future. When applied to certain categories of infanticide, this argument may have some merit. One might argue, for example, that the mother whose child is killed after prolonged abuse must be punished in order to ensure that she understands the limits the law places on disciplining children. On closer examination, though, specific deterrence has limited relevance to many of the other categories of infanticide. For instance, the woman with either acute or chronic mental illness at the time she killed her child does not need the law to deter from killing again in the future. On the contrary, she is much more likely to need treatment for her condition.

The second major justification for punishment is *retribution*. This ancient rationale is predicated on society's right to punish one who unjustifiably harms another. Struck by the need to cry out against the deaths of these innocent children, it is obvious why society might be inclined to invoke this rationale in punishing infanticide. To the extent that retribution is justifiable, there must be clearly delineated lines of blame. This is precisely not the case with infanticide, though, as it so often seems difficult to allocate blame to a single individual. Instead, these cases often leave one with a sense that there might be more than one blameworthy party.

Consider the following case illustration, introduced earlier: In the weeks preceding her son's death, numerous others were aware of Sheryl Massip's deteriorating condition. Her lawyer noted that

> [f]or two weeks, Sheryl Massip's family recognized something was wrong with her. Her husband . . . sent her away to her mother's home to spend a night, to get some rest, because they thought that would solve the problem. She came back, he sent her away again. On . . . the Monday before she killed her child, she came home from spending the night with her mother, and she went to the doctor and said, "Doctor, what's wrong with me? I'm hallucinating. I can't sleep. Something is wrong with me. Help me." He looked at her and said, "Oh, you're just suffering from baby blues," [and] gave her a couple of Mellarils. ("A Mother Tells Why She Killed Her Son" 1994)

There is no doubt that during her psychotic episode, Massip was incapable of caring for her son. Her family and her physician all were on notice that she was in crisis, and all attempted to comfort her. Nonetheless, none of them took the time to evaluate in a serious manner the gap between her present abilities and the caregiving tasks she was required to perform when left alone with her child. Had any one of these three people recognized her needs, they could readily have identified a course of action that would have saved her son's life.

The final justification for punishment is that it is necessary in order to *rehabilitate* the individual defendant. In view of the overcrowded and underfunded conditions that prevail in U.S. prisons, it is difficult for anyone to argue that a woman who commits infanticide is likely to be rehabilitated for society by virtue of incarceration. Indeed, the sort of treatment that these women are likely to need—mental health services, parenting classes, substance abuse treatment—are in particularly scarce supply in women's prisons. A woman is much more likely to find these services outside of prison, and a judge can most certainly require a woman to obtain any or all of these services as a condition of probation. In essence, this is the British legal system's approach to punishment for this crime. Its experience of 80 years of using probation in lieu of incarceration suggests that probation is at least as effective at preventing or deterring infanticide as is incarceration, and it is considerably more efficient and cost-effective (Edwards 1986; Wilczynski 1991).

Conclusion

In considering how society should best respond to a woman who has committed infanticide, the key question to ask is why we are punishing this woman and what we seek to gain by virtue of this punishment. At times, what we gain by punishing her may be no more than an opportunity to vent our rage at a life so needlessly lost. At those times, it is imperative to consider the underlying policies that have contributed to that lost life. This is not to say that those who commit infanticide are blameless, but rather that, as seen against the backdrop of the construction of motherhood, on some occasions this terrible crime may be all but inevitable. The task, then, in a civilized and compassionate society, is to determine how to deal justly with those who kill their children and, more importantly, how to mobilize all of our resources to prevent these needless deaths in the future.

References

Abandoned to her fate: neighbors, teachers, and the authorities all knew Elisa Izqierdo was being abused but somehow nobody managed to stop it. Time, December 11, 1995, p 32

An act to prevent the destroying and murthering of bastard children, 21 James I, C27 (Eng), 1623

American Psychiatric Association: Diagnostic and Statistical Manual of Mental Disorders, 4th Edition. Washington, DC, American Psychiatric Association, 1994

Backhouse C: Desperate women and compassionate courts: infanticide in nineteenth century Canada. University of Toronto Law Journal 34:447–478, 1984

Bumiller E: Vivid description of the persistence of female infanticide in contemporary India, in May You Be the Mother of 1000 Sons: A Journey Among the Women of India. New York, Fawcett Columbine, 1990, pp 104–124

Chaudhry Z: The myth of misogyny. Albany Law Review 61:513, 1997

Chavez L: The tragic story of Medea still lives. The Denver Post, December 3, 1995, E4

Chew K, McCleary R, Lew M, et al: Epidemiology of child homicide: California, 1981–1990. Homicide Studies 2:78–85, 1999

Edwards SM: Neither mad nor bad: the female violent offender reassessed. Women's Studies International Forum 9:79–87, 1986

Greenhalgh S, Li J: Engendering reproductive policy and practice in peasant China: for a feminist demography of reproduction. Signs 20:601–641, 1995

Hoffer PC, Hull NEH: Murdering Mothers: Infanticide in England and New England, 1558–1803. New York, New York University Press, 1981, p 13

Infanticide Act, 2 Geo 6, ch 36 (Eng 1938)

Kellett R: Infanticide and child destruction—the historical, legal and pathological aspects. Forensic Science International 53:1–28, 1992

Kellum BA: Infanticide in England in the later middle ages. History of Childhood Quarterly 1:367–388, 1974

Langer WL: Infanticide; a historical survey. History of Childhood Quarterly 1: 353–365, 1974

Lee JA: Family law of the two Chinas. Cardozo Journal of International Comparative Law 5:217–247, 1997

Lee J: 6.3 brides for seven brothers (one quarter of humanity: Malthusian mythology and Chinese reality 1700–2000). The Economist, December 19, 1998, pp 56–58

Lichtblau E: Appeal argued in postpartum case. Los Angeles Times, May 24, 1990, B1

Mathew P: Case note: Applicant A v. minister for immigration and ethnic affairs: the high court and "particular social groups": lessons for the future. Melbourne Univeristy Law Review 21:277–330, 1997

Mendlowicz MV, Rapaport MH, Mecler K, et al: A case-control study on the socio-demographic characteristics of 52 neonaticidal mothers. Int J Law Psychiatry 52:209–218, 1998

Meyer C, Oberman M: Mothers Who Kill Their Children: Understanding the Acts of Moms From Susan Smith to the "Prom Mom." New York, New York University Press, 2001

Moseley KL: The history of infanticide in Western society. Issues Law Med 1:346–357, 1986

A mother tells why she killed her son. Larry King Live (CNN television broadcast), L King interviewing M Grimes, criminal defense attorney for Sheryl Massip, November 17, 1994

Oberman M: Mothers who kill: coming to terms with modern American infanticide. American Criminal Law Review 34:1–109, 1996

O'Hara MW: Postpartum "blues," depression and psychosis: a review. J Psychosom Obstet Gynaecol 7:205–227, 1987

Report of the independent committee to inquire into practices, processes, and proceedings in juvenile court as they relate to the Joseph Wallace cases, Cook County, Illinois, October 1, 1993

Satava SE: Discrimination against the unacknowledged illegitimate child and the wrongful death statute. Capital University Law Review 25:933–991, 1996

Smith L: Experts seek reasons behind irrational crime. The Los Angeles Times, October 15, 1991, A25

Spinelli MG: A systematic investigation of 16 cases of neonaticide. Am J Psychiatry 158:811–813, 2001

Stuart Bastard Neonaticide Act, 21 James I, c 27 (Eng 1624)

Trexler R: Infanticide in Florence: new sources and first results. History of Childhood Quarterly 1:100–102, 1973

Walker LE: The Battered Woman. New York, Harper & Row, 1979

Walker N: Crime and Insanity in England, Vol 1. New York, Columbia University Press, 1968, pp 128–132

Wilczynski A: Images of women who kill their infants: the "mad and the bad." Women and Criminal Justice 2:71–88, 1991

Chapter 2

Epidemiology of Infanticide

Mary Overpeck, Dr.P.H.

The child shall be registered immediately after birth and shall have the right from birth to a name.

Article 7, United Nations Convention on the
Rights of a Child (1989); quoted in Scheper-Hughes 1992

Infanticides resulting from maternal behavior may be among the least well documented deaths in the United States. Problems inherent in reporting systems and the nature of the deaths limit our knowledge about prevalence and the relationship of perpetrators. One study of infants dying before their first birthday based on nationally available death certificate records found that nearly one infant is killed every day (Overpeck et al. 1998). However, the prevalence in the United States may be double that number (Herman-Giddens et al. 1999; McClain et al. 1993). Estimates made by McAllen and Herman-Giddens on the basis of in-depth inter-agency record reviews in North Carolina and Missouri projected underascertainment of fatalities of young children due to child abuse and neglect in the United States (Ewigman et al. 1986; Herman-Giddens et al. 1999). These and other state studies found that prevalence counts of infanticides and other child fatalities from abuse or neglect based on only death certificates were seriously lacking (California Department of Justice 1997).

Moreover, perpetrator identity is limited on death certificates and other records. Only one cause of death on certificates addresses childhood battering and maltreatment and provides codes to designate the relationship of the perpetrator, including "a parent." More than 90% of infant deaths assigned this classification between 1983 and 1997 were left with the relationship "unspecified" (Centers for Disease Control and Prevention 2000; Overpeck et al. 1998).

Perpetrators

What do we know about perpetrators of infanticide? Special studies have been required to describe perpetrator identity and circumstances of deaths among infants and young children. Such studies are usually completed at local levels or as part of clinical case studies. Reviews of traumatic deaths among young children indicate that most infant homicides are carried out by parents or stepparents, and a slight majority are attributable to males (Christoffel 1990; Jason 1983; Kunz and Bahr 1996; National Center on Child Abuse and Neglect 1997). Some state and local studies have found that mothers are the perpetrators in the majority of cases only for homicides during the first week of life (Jason et al. 1983; Kunz and Bahr 1996; Sorenson and Peterson 1994). These early deaths for whom the mother may be responsible are the primary focus of concern in this chapter. However, such cases may be the least likely to be reflected in our official data systems.

The Bureau of Justice Statistics (2000) of the U.S. Department of Justice has compiled national-level information on perpetrators in cases for which police reports have been filed. Again, these data show that the majority of perpetrators are males who are related to the infants and young children. However, perpetrator relationship for deaths occurring in the first week or months of life was not specified for infants killed before their first birthday.

Police reports are not filed in all cases examined by medical examiners or coroners who complete death certificates, even when a determination has been made that homicide was the cause (Inter-Agency Council on Child Abuse and Neglect 1998). Therefore, prevalence estimates based on police or legal system reports tend to show fewer infanticides than do counts from state or local vital statistics agencies.

Reporting of Infant Deaths

At the national level, we rely on death certificates submitted by state vital statistics agencies for annual total counts by cause and age at death (Kowaleski 1997; Rosenberg and Kochanek 1995). *Infant death* most frequently refers to deaths occurring prior to the first 12 months of life

(Hartford 1992; United Nations 1955). Infant deaths may be further categorized as *neonatal* (under 28 days of age) and *postneonatal* (28 days through 11 months of age). Neonatal deaths are further categorized as *late* (7–28 days of age) and *early* (under 7 days of age).

Cause of Death

Cause of death on certificates is specified by medical examiners or coroners according to the *International Classification of Diseases*, Ninth Revision (ICD-9; World Health Organization 1977). Classification is generally organized as due to a natural, a traumatic, or an unknown cause. Infanticides are classified as part of traumatic deaths according to external cause codes (E codes), which describe the mechanism of death, such as suffocation or blunt-force trauma (National Center for Health Statistics 1987). These external causes are further classified by intent.

The category *traumatic deaths* includes deaths due to suffocation or asphyxiation as well as fatal injury due to being struck, shaken, dropped, burned, drowned, poisoned, and so forth (World Health Organization 1977). It also includes deaths from neglect, abandonment, and extreme exposures. For deaths from external causes, the medical examiner or coroner may designate a death as intentional, as unintentional, or as due to undetermined intent. The last designation is supposed to be used only if the examiner is unwilling to classify a death as unintentional because of the suspicious nature of the death but does not expect to have enough information to classify it as intentional. Table 2–1 shows the distribution of infant injury deaths classified as intentional or due to undetermined but suspicious intent from 1990 through 1997. The latter deaths—those classified as due to undetermined intent—represent about 4% of all injury deaths to infants.

About one-third of the deaths resulted from battering or other maltreatment. The next primary cause is from assault (28%), with no indication of the means used to assault the infant. About 13% were killed by suffocation or strangulation. Drowning, criminal neglect, and firearms each accounted for about 3%–4%. The homicides do not include deaths from abandonment, neglect, or exposure classified as unintentional (60 cases from 1990 through 1997).

If further investigation is to be done because cause or intent is not clear, the examiner may classify the finding as "pending" at the time the certificate is originally filed. In this case, intent, and possibly even cause, may be left unspecified on the certificate. Any subsequent legal findings to determine intent may differ from the designation on the certificate. Although the certificate should be amended in the state vital statistics

Table 2–1. Infant injury deaths classified by intent and cause of homicides: United States, 1990–1997

Cause of homicides (E codes for intentional and undetermined intent)	Number	Proportion, %
Total	3,077	100.0
Battering, other maltreatment (E967, E987)[a]	1,054	31.3
Assault, unspecified means (E968.9, E988.9)	859	27.9
Suffocation/strangulation (E963, E983)	387	12.6
Drowning (E964, E984)	118	3.8
Criminal neglect (E968.4)[a]	96	3.1
Firearms (E965, E985)	90	2.9
Arson (E968.0, E988.1)	39	1.3
Cuts and stabbing (E966, E986)	39	1.3
Other specified causes	395	12.8

[a]Classification not used for deaths from undetermined intent. Sixty additional deaths not included were classified as due to unintentional neglect and abandonment (ICD code E904).
Source. Centers for Disease Control and Prevention WONDER compressed mortality files for 1990–1997.

agencies, state files submitted for annual national statistics on cause of death may not include amendments because of the time required for investigations and amendments (Overpeck et al. 2002).

Cases for which a cause is not shown in the national data also have higher proportions of infant deaths occurring soon after delivery when compared with other "unexpected" infant deaths, which include deaths from sudden infant death syndrome (SIDS) and traumatic causes. Deaths from natural causes, including prematurity, should be classified elsewhere. From 1990 through 1997, 14% of deaths from unknown causes happened during the first day and week of life (10% and 4%, respectively), compared with 4% of deaths classified as unintentional injury (2% and 2%, respectively) or less than 1% of SIDS deaths (Centers for Disease Control and Prevention 2000).

From 1990 through 1997, 6,686 infant deaths were classified with unknown cause, a number comparable to the number of unintentional injury fatalities (6,853) and more than twice the number of fatalities classified as intentional or suspicious (3,007). The proportion and number of infant deaths in the first day and week of life classified with unknown cause are higher than the proportion and number of those classified as intentional or suspicious. It is apparent from the relatively high proportion of neonatal deaths with unknown causes that national and state statistics are missing probable homicides or other traumatic deaths that meet the pattern consistent with deaths related to maternal behavior proximal to time of birth. Also, an analysis of linked birth and death certificates available since 1983 (Overpeck et al. 2002) found that for deaths of unknown cause occurring in the first weeks of life, compared with later deaths, it was less likely that birth certificates were available for linkage.

Age at Death

An analysis of risk factors for probable homicides during the first year of life from 1983 through 1991 did not specifically address infants killed proximal to the time of birth, partly because it was based on deaths for which birth certificates could be found to provide additional risk factor information (Overpeck et al. 1998, 1999b). These linked certificates represented 98% of all recorded deaths. Even so, the analysis showed that among infant deaths classified as intentional or due to suspicious intent, one-fourth of the infants were dead by the end of the second month of life, and one-half were dead by the fourth month (National Center for Health Statistics 1988–1999).

A more recent review of all traumatic infant deaths from 1990 through 1997 from intentional or suspicious but undetermined circumstances (probable homicides), as classified by medical examiners or coroners, showed that 8% of the infants died in the first day, and an additional 2% died during the first week (Centers for Disease Control and Prevention 2000) (Figure 2–1). About 15% of probable infant homicides occurring before the first year of life occurred during the first month.

These data support concerns that many of the deaths around the time of delivery involve infants whose mothers deliver outside of hospitals. The study of data available on birth certificates since 1989 and linked to death certificates for 1989–1991 and 1995–1996 provides better information on births occurring in clinical settings with assistance from trained birth attendants (Overpeck et al. 2002). In the 5 years of data available from linked files, 5% of homicides involved infants not delivered in clinical settings (hospitals, doctor offices, or clinics) and delivered without a trained birth attendant (doctor, nurse-midwife, or other midwife). About 90% of deaths of infants who were not delivered in clinical settings or by trained attendants occurred during the first week of life, and about two-thirds occurred in the first day. Since unattended births are less likely to have a birth certificate issued, many deaths during the first day and week of life are probably unattended and possibly hidden.

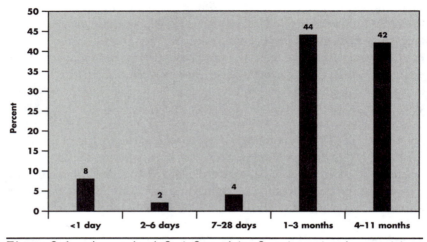

Figure 2–1. Age at death for infants dying from intentional or suspicious causes, United States, 1990–1997.

Source. Centers for Disease Control and Prevention WONDER compressed mortality file for 2000.

Risk Factors for Infanticide

The analysis of risk factors associated with infant homicides from 1983 through 1991 discussed in the previous section used linked death and birth certificates to provide information about maternal, infant, and, to a lesser extent, paternal characteristics (Overpeck et al. 1998). For that study, 2,776 probable homicides were identified from the ICD-9 coding of cause of death and intent. Available birth certificate variables were reviewed on the basis of suggestive findings from earlier state-level and clinical studies or from elevated relative risks. The maternal and infant factors predictive of homicide finally were selected on the basis of increased relative risks and adequate numbers for stable estimates. Availability of a large national database allowed assessment of the magnitude of the problem and implications for public health interventions.

The infants at highest risk were the second or subsequent children born to mothers younger than 17 years (relative risk [RR] = 10.9) or mothers aged 17–19 years (RR = 9.3) (both comparisons with firstborn children of mothers aged 25 years or older). Similar risks were evident for second or subsequent children born to mothers aged 17–19 years (RR = 9.3). These infants at highest risk represented 17% of U.S. infant homicide victims. The combined effects of maternal age and birth order as the highest risk factor were consistent for blacks and whites.

Other separate risk factors included maternal age younger than 15 years (RR = 6.8; comparison with mothers 25 years or older) and no prenatal care (RR = 10.4; comparison with care begun in the first or second month of pregnancy). Of all infants whose mothers had no prenatal care, almost 15% were at highest risk (5.8% of mothers were younger than 17 years, and 8.8% were aged 17–19 years with two or more children). Of the highest risk mothers, 11% had no prenatal care.

Maternal education at time of birth also was a risk factor for infant homicide. Infants whose mothers did not complete high school were greater than eight times more likely to be killed than those whose mothers completed 16 or more years of school. However, the relationship between maternal education and infant homicide is confounded by age, since many mothers younger than 17 years have not yet had the opportunity to complete 12 years of education. Births to mothers younger than 17 years accounted for about one-fifth of all homicides among infants whose mothers did not complete 12 years of education. After mothers younger than 17 years who had not had a chance to complete high school were excluded, maternal education of less than 12 years was still a high risk factor (RR = 8.0; comparison with mothers with 16 or more years of school). A similar comparison was made after mothers aged 19 years or younger were excluded, because childbearing could have delayed the completion of their education. For infants of mothers aged 20 years or older who did not complete high school, the relative risk of homicide was seven times greater than that for mothers who had 16 or more years of school.

Paternal factors were not addressed in this study on infant homicide because so much information on fathers was missing on birth certificates linked to homicide death cases. A review of later data through 1996 showed that about 40% of homicide cases with linked certificates were missing any information on fathers, compared with only 13% of all birth certificates. This lack of information is probably indicative of some of the strongest underlying risk factors for infant homicide that are not measured on birth and death certificates. Lack of data on fathers probably indicates unstable supportive relationships, particularly when the mothers are very young. Since studies of perpetrators have indicated that males, and particularly related males, are responsible in the majority of cases, the role and preparedness of other household members as infant caregivers require further exploration.

Getting Better Information

Why is the prevalence of infanticide underestimated? What are the issues surrounding the measurement of early neonatal deaths? Since the phenomenon of maternal infanticide is the concern addressed in this chapter, and because mothers are more likely to be perpetrators only in the first week of life, ascertainment of these early neonatal deaths requires some emphasis.

Problems in Ascertainment for Early Neonatal Deaths

When an infant body is found with signs that death occurred in proximity to the period of delivery, the question may be raised about whether the delivery resulted in a live birth. If after an autopsy or other examination the examiner decides that there were signs consistent with life, a death certificate would be issued (Hartford 1992; Kowaleski 1997). If the examiner decides that there are not signs of a live birth, a fetal death registration is completed. This may be particularly problematic for premature births prior to 28 weeks of gestation, when life outside the uterus would be difficult without clinical intervention. It may also be difficult in cases in which the body has deteriorated considerably prior to examination.

Fetal death registrations historically have been required in most states for gestations of at least 20 weeks or when weight is more than 500 grams. Registration requirements are changing because of our technological capability to save infants delivered at less than 500 grams, but the issue of probable viability without clinical intervention is most important to examiners for bodies retrieved without knowledge of maternal health care status (Kowaleski 1997; National Center for Health Statistics 1978). Therefore, it is important to consider that a number of pregnancy outcomes could be classified as either live births or fetal deaths when the mother did not deliver in a clinical setting (hospitals, centers, clinics or offices) or with a trained attendant such as a doctor, nurse-midwife, or other midwife.

Preliminary analysis of linked birth and death certificates for 1989–1991 and 1995–1996 shows that about 8% of infants dying from infanticide were not delivered in clinical settings, compared with less than 1% of total live births. About 5% of infants killed in the first year of life were not delivered by trained attendants, compared with 1% of all live births. This information is not available for death certificates for which no corresponding birth certificate could be found for linkage.

Perinatal deaths (including both fetal and infant deaths) should be considered when addressing the problems of "hidden pregnancies." One perinatal mortality definition that includes only early neonatal births (<7 days of age) and fetal deaths for gestations at more than 28 weeks' duration might be appropriate for reviewing potential prevalence of such deliveries (Hoyert 1995). Fetal death registrations have generally not been reviewed for causes related to traumatic deaths, including abandonment or neglect.

Natural causes associated with prematurity or extremely short gestational age are the leading cause of infant death, particularly in the first day or week of life (Hoyert 1995). This may be a factor in the determination that an infant "lived"—the requirement for a decision by a medical examiner or coroner to issue a death certificate. Even when this determination is made for extremely premature deliveries, classification of cause of death may be difficult, resulting in ambiguity in measurement of probable homicides occurring during the early neonatal period (Overpeck et al. 1999a).

Underestimation of Prevalence

The state studies of prevalence tracked the possible sources of underascertainment by reviewing records from vital statistics, medical examiner or coroner records, law enforcement files, and social service registries (California Department of Justice 1997; Ewigman 1986; Herman-Giddens et al. 1999). The discrepancies found among state-level data sources may have resulted from 1) inability to report, such as when an infant disappears but no body is found or there is disagreement as to whether to designate the death as a homicide; 2) failure of involved agencies to properly categorize or code information; and/or 3) inadequate gathering of case information for drawing accurate conclusions (California Department of Justice 1997).

The California report was performed by comparing information from different agencies about circumstances of unexpected childhood deaths (California Department of Justice 1997). The formation of such interagency teams to review these deaths is relatively recent (Durfee et al. 1992). Most states now have authorizing legislation for child fatality review teams, although many of these teams do not perform statewide reviews, nor do they necessarily review all unexpected deaths.

Infanticides also may be attributed to SIDS or unintentional injury deaths in a small proportion of cases. With the decrease in SIDS deaths associated with changes in sleep position in recent years, the American Academy of Pediatrics suggests that the proportion of SIDS deaths attributable to infanticide may be increasing (American Academy of Pediatrics 2000). Some researchers have estimated that child abuse and neglect was involved in 5%–20% of SIDS cases (Emery 1993; Ewigman et al. 1986), while others disagree (O'Halloran et al. 1998). Ewigman et al. (1986) concluded that child abuse and neglect in children under age 5 years may have been involved in 7%–27% of injury deaths reported from 1983 through 1986 in Missouri as unintentional and in at least 5% of deaths attributed to SIDS.

In addition, traumatic deaths classified as due to an undetermined but suspicious intent on death certificates because intentionality could not be determined are frequently ignored in prevalence estimates and homicide studies. Yet, careful review of such cases indicates that they always should be considered (Christoffel et al. 1985; Sorenson and Peterson 1994; Sorenson et al. 1997). Fatalities classified with undetermined intent had risk profiles that more closely resemble profiles for intentional deaths than profiles for unintentional deaths (Overpeck et al. 1999a). Fatalities with undetermined intent had larger relative risks in the highest risk categories than did either intentional or unintentional injuries. Elevated risks occurred for infants of mothers with the least education, no prenatal care, young maternal age, and single marital status, as well as for infants who are second or later born, premature, black, or American Indian.

Conclusion

Risk profiles and prevalence issues are relevant only when they assist in targeting highest risk mothers and families for interventions that assist communities in prevention of traumatic fatalities or nonfatal child abuse and neglect. For some traumatic deaths, the issue of intent may be problematic, particularly when the events occur during moments of distraction or high emotion or under the influence of alcohol or other drugs (Overpeck and McLoughlin 1999). We do not have a source of information that sufficiently describes the circumstances of birth and death in enough cases to include familial and personal attributes as risk factors for deaths perpetrated by mothers. However, intent may be peripheral to both the act and the injury mechanism for purposes of interventions in high-risk cases. Interventions that address multiple risk factors should be made early in pregnancy, or even before conception. We need to replicate research on interventions that address social support, the caregiving environment, and behavior modification (Committee on the Assessment of Family Violence Interventions 1998). These interventions include a delay between conceptions to better space childbearing, completion of maternal education, and reduction in drug and alcohol abuse.

Obviously, knowledge of the etiology of deaths resulting from maternal behavior, based on our current sources of information, is limited, particularly for those infants dying in proximity to delivery. Wissau (1998) suggested that postpartum depression must be considered in cases in which the mother is responsible for infant deaths. The issues surrounding infant deaths occurring in the first weeks of life is discussed thoroughly in this volume.

The American Academy of Pediatrics (1999) has called for improved comprehensive death investigation of sudden, unexpected deaths in order to provide proper death certification for children. The Academy emphasizes the continuing need for careful, timely review of deaths attributable to SIDS and trauma by appropriately constituted review teams. Better dissemination of information about circumstances around fatalities from child death review investigations should improve the official reporting and description of risk factors and thereby facilitate development of better interventions to prevent infanticide.

References

American Academy of Pediatrics, Committee on Child Abuse and Neglect and Committee on Community Health Services: Investigation and review of unexpected infant and child deaths. Pediatrics 104:1158–1160, 1999

American Academy of Pediatrics, Task Force on Infant Sleep Position and Sudden Infant Death Syndrome: Changing concepts of sudden infant death syndrome: implications for infant sleeping environment and sleep position. Pediatrics 105:650–656, 2000

Blaffer-Hrdy S: Mother Nature: A History of Mothers, Infants, and Natural Selection. New York, Pantheon, 1999, pp 288–317

Bureau of Justice Statistics: Homicide Trends in the U.S (NCJ Publ No 179767). Washington, DC, U.S. Dept of Justice, 2000. Available at: www.ojp.usdoj.gov/bjs/homicide

California Department of Justice, State Child Death Review Board: Child Deaths in California, 1992–1995. Sacramento, California Department of Justice, 1997

Centers for Disease Control and Prevention: WONDER Compressed Mortality Files, 2000. Available at: www.cdc.gov/wonder

Christoffel KK: Violent death and injury in US children and adolescents. Am J Dis Child 144:697–706, 1990

Christoffel KK, Zieserl E, Chiaramonte J: Should child abuse and neglect be considered when a child dies unexpectedly? Am J Dis Child 139:876–880, 1985

Committee on the Assessment of Family Violence Interventions: Violence in Families: Assessing Prevention and Treatment Programs. Washington, DC, National Academy Press, 1998, pp 220–223

Durfee MJ, Gellert GA, Tilton-Durfee D: Origins and clinical relevance of child death review teams. JAMA 267:3172–3175, 1992

Emery JL: Child abuse, sudden infant death syndrome, and unexpected death. Am J Dis Child 147:1097–1100, 1993

Ewigman B, Kivlahan C, Land G: The Missouri Child Fatality Study: underreporting of maltreatment fatalities among children younger than five years of age, 1983 through 1986. Pediatrics 91:330–337, 1986

Hartford RB: Definitions, standards, data quality, and comparability, in Perinatal and Infant Mortality, Vol 3. Hyattsville, MD, National Center for Health Statistics, 1992, Section II, pp 12–16

Herman-Giddens ME, Brown G, Verbiest S, et al: Underascertainment of child abuse mortality in the United States. JAMA 282:463–467, 1999

Hopwood JS: Child murder and insanity. Journal of Mental Sciences 73:95–108, 1927

Hoyert DL: Perinatal mortality in the United States, 1985–91. Vital Health Stat 20(26), 1995

Inter-Agency Council on Child Abuse and Neglect: Child Death Review Team Report for 1998. El Monte, CA, Los Angeles County Inter-Agency Council on Child Abuse and Neglect, 1998, p 83

Jason J: Fatal child abuse in Georgia: the epidemiology of severe physical child abuse. Child Abuse Negl 7:1–9, 1983

Jason J, Guilliland JC, Tyler CW: Homicide as a cause of pediatric mortality in the United States. Pediatrics 72:191–197, 1983

Kowaleski J: State Definitions and Reporting Requirements for Live Births, Fetal Deaths, and Induced Terminations of Pregnancy, 1997 Revision. Hyattsville, MD, National Center for Health Statistics, 1997

Kunz J, Bahr S: A profile of parental homicide against children. Journal of Family Violence 11:347–362, 1996

McClain PW, Sacks JJ, Froehlke RG, et al: Estimates of fatal child abuse and neglect, United States, 1979–88. Pediatrics 91:338–343, 1993

National Center for Health Statistics: Model State Vital Statistics Act and Model State Vital Statistics Regulations. Washington, DC, National Center for Health Statistics, 1978

National Center for Health Statistics: Medical Examiners' and Coroners' Handbook on Death Registration and Fetal Death Reporting (DHHS Publ PHS 87-1110). Hyattsville, MD, National Center for Health Statistics, 1987

National Center for Health Statistics: Linked Birth/Infant Death Data Set: Public Use Data File Documentation for 1983 to 1991 and 1995 to 1996. Hyattsville, MD, U.S. Public Health Service, 1988–1999

National Center on Child Abuse and Neglect: Child Maltreatment 1995: Reports From the States to the National Center on Child Abuse and Neglect. Washington, DC, U.S. Department of Health and Human Services, 1997, pp 2–9

O'Halloran RL, Ferratta F, Harris M, et al: Child abuse reports in families with sudden infant death syndrome. Am J Forensic Med Pathol 19:57–62, 1998

Overpeck MD, McLoughlin E: Did that injury happen on purpose? Does intent really matter? Inj Prev 5:11–12, 1999

Overpeck MD, Brenner RA, Trumble AC, et al: Risk factors for infant homicide in the United States. N Engl J Med 339:1211–1216, 1998

Overpeck MD, Brenner RA, Trumble AC, et al: Infant injury deaths with unknown intent: what else do we know? Inj Prev 5:272–275, 1999a

Overpeck MD, Trumble AC, Berendes HW, et al: Risk factors for infant homicide (letter). N Engl J Med 340:895–897, 1999b

Overpeck MD, Brenner RA, Cosgrove C, et al: National underascertainment of sudden unexpected infant deaths associated with deaths of unknown cause. Pediatrics 109:274–283, 2002

Rosenberg HM, Kochanek KD: The death certificate as a source of injury data, in Proceedings of the International Collaborative Effort on Injury Statistics, Vol 1 (DHHS Publ No PHS 95-1252). Hyattsville, MD, National Center for Health Statistics, 1995, Chapter 8, pp 1–17

Scheper-Hughes N: Death Without Weeping: The Violence of Everyday Life in Brazil. Berkeley, University of California Press, 1992, p 286

Sorenson SB, Peterson JG: Traumatic child death and documented maltreatment history, Los Angeles. Am J Public Health 84:623–627, 1994

Sorenson SB, Shen H, Kraus JF: Undetermined manner of death: a comparison with unintentional injury, suicide, and homicide death. Evaluation Review 21: 43–57, 1997

United Nations: Handbook of Vital Statistics Methods. New York, United Nations, 1955

Wissau LS: Infanticide (editorial). N Engl J Med 339:1239–1241, 1998

World Health Organization: World Health Classification: Manual of the International Statistical Classification of Diseases, Injuries, and Causes of Death, Ninth Revision. Geneva, World Health Organization, 1977

Part **II**

Biopsychosocial and Cultural Perspectives on Infanticide

Chapter 3

Postpartum Disorders

Phenomenology, Treatment Approaches, and Relationship to Infanticide

Katherine L. Wisner, M.D., M.S.
Barbara L. Gracious, M.D.
Catherine M. Piontek, M.D.
Kathleen Peindl, Ph.D.
James M. Perel, Ph.D.

The type of insanity most commonly observed amongst these lunatic criminals is delusional mania. As a rule they are demonstrative and noisy, obscene in language, degraded in behavior, and subject to outbursts of paroxysmal violence. . . . The maniacal affection is often associated with delusions of suspicion and persecution and with aural and visual hallucinations; perversions of the sense of smell and taste . . .

[It seems evident,] from a study of the Broadmoar cases, that infanticide occurs much more frequently in connection with the insanity of lactation. . . . In such a condition those in attendance would naturally remove the child and guard against the contingency of danger.

These tragedies are frequently preventable. Although the patient is, as a rule, sanely conscious of many things and usually coherent, it

This work was supported by National Institute of Mental Health grants (MH-57102 and MH-60335) to Dr. Wisner and a Psychopharmacology Core Center grant (MH-30915) to Dr. Perel.

begins to dawn on the friends that the mind is gradually giving way, yet owing to some perverse reasoning they defer placing her under asylum care and treatment, even if the woman herself begs to be safeguarded.

John Baker, M.D. (1902)

P ostpartum mood disorders are common and are seen frequently by health care professionals who serve women of childbearing age. In a prospective study, O'Hara et al. (1984, 1990) found that 12% of postpartum women had illnesses that fulfilled Research Diagnostic Criteria (RDC; Spitzer and Endicott 1978) for major or minor depression, both of which require impairment in usual function. Cox and colleagues (1993) found a clustering of new cases in a sample of women within 5 weeks after childbirth when compared with a control sample of nonchildbearing women. We (Wisner et al. 1993) studied a large sample of women who presented to an urban psychiatric hospital over a 2½-year period. We categorized women as having childbearing-related–onset episodes (occurring during pregnancy or within 3 months of birth or termination) or non-childbearing-related episodes. The proportion of women with childbearing-related–onset illness among women aged 15–44 years was 9%. When the sample was restricted to women who had ever experienced a pregnancy, one of seven women (14%) who sought care was experiencing an episode related to childbearing. Women incur major risk for psychiatric morbidity along with the responsibility for childbearing.

The ratio of the number of psychiatric hospital admissions immediately after childbirth to the number before birth is a measure of the relative risk for serious psychiatric episodes associated with childbirth in a population. The relative risk for hospitalization within 90 days of birth is 3.8; within 30 days of birth it is 6.0. The comparable risk figures for first-time mothers are even higher: 5.8 and 10.9 within 90 and 30 days, respectively (Kendell et al. 1987). Women are more vulnerable to psychosis in the postbirth period than at any other time during the female life cycle. In the first 30 days after birth, a woman is 21.7 times more likely to develop psychosis than in the 2-year period prior to childbirth. If she has not had a child before, she is 35 times more likely to develop psychosis (Kendell et al. 1987). The magnitude of these relative risks demonstrates that postpartum psychiatric morbidity is a major public health problem.

Recognition and treatment of maternal psychiatric disorders must become a priority on the public health agenda if we are to achieve the goal of reducing the risk of maternal morbidity and infanticide. In this chapter, we review information about postpartum disorders and present cases to illustrate symptom presentations. Our objective in this chapter is to integrate the research literature with our clinical experience in the hope that clinical care and public health policy for childbearing women will be improved and that further research will be stimulated.

Epidemiology and Nosology

We begin with a discussion of a basic question: what are postpartum disorders? The answer is far from simple. Historically, postpartum depression and psychosis were differentiated by the predominance of depressive or psychotic features and by symptom severity. However, current conceptualizations dictate that depression and psychoses are distinct psychiatric illnesses, not merely different severity levels of the same disorder. We will analyze the two components of the question: first, what does the term *postpartum* mean, and second, what specific disorders occur in the postpartum period?

An international meeting was held in Satra Bruk, Sweden, in 1999 to review issues related to the classification of postpartum disorders (Elliott 2000). Both epidemiological studies and clinical experience were reviewed. Epidemiologists have defined the duration of postpartum on the basis of judgments about the break point between increased risk for psychiatric illness postbirth and baseline risk for psychiatric episodes in women of childbearing age. Paffenbarger and McCabe (1966) found an "explosive peak" of psychiatric admissions in the first month postpartum. Kendell and colleagues (1976, 1981, 1987) extensively investigated the association between childbirth and psychiatric contact in a population of women. They linked birth and psychiatric registries for contacts 2 years before and after a birth and found a significant peak in the rate of contact for both depressive and psychotic illnesses in the 90-day period after childbirth. Although it fell rapidly thereafter, the rate of admission remained significantly higher throughout the 2-year postpartum period than it had been before birth.

Serious postpartum disorders have a rapid onset and progression of symptoms. Rapidity of onset is supported by data from the work of Kendell et al. (1987). In a sample of 111 women with symptoms beginning in the first 90 days postbirth, onset was distributed as follows: 49% of the sample within 7 days, 79% within 30 days, and 94% within 60 days. Data from our studies confirmed our clinical suspicion that decompensation after initial symptoms also was rapid. Mothers' responses to Schedule for

Affective Disorders and Schizophrenia (SADS; Endicott and Spitzer 1978) interview item #215 (length of time from first sign of development of the major syndrome to gross impairment in social or occupational functioning) were reviewed. Times to decompensation were as follows: <2 days ($n = 18$, 47%), 2 days to <1 week ($n = 4$, 11%), 1 week to <2 weeks ($n = 2$, 5%), 2 weeks to <1 month ($n = 3$, 8%), 1 month to <2 months ($n = 4$, 11%), and >2 months ($n = 7$, 18%).

The two major international psychiatric diagnostic systems vary in their definitions of postpartum. The International Classification of Diseases (ICD-10; World Health Organization 1992) permits designation as mental and physical disorders associated with the puerperium only if the disorders have onset within the first 6 weeks after birth and do not meet criteria for disorders classified elsewhere (Elliott 2000). The current version of the *Diagnostic and Statistical Manual of Mental Disorders*, DSM-IV-TR (American Psychiatric Association 2000), allows the designation with postpartum onset to be made as specifier for a limited number of diagnoses that begin within the first 4 weeks postpartum.

In summary, the time definition of postpartum can be set at 90 days according to epidemiological studies, 6 weeks by ICD-10, and 4 weeks by DSM-IV-TR. However, the Satra Bruk group noted that international investigators use definitions of up to 1 year postpartum, particularly if services for new mothers are tied to the definition. The conclusion of the Satra Bruk group was that research into the etiological significance of birth to psychiatric episodes would be aided by systematic recording of specific time of onset or exacerbation after birth for a variety of disorders. The term *postpartum onset* may be an appropriate specifier for multiple diagnoses. For example, the postpartum period is a high-risk time for the first lifetime onset of anxiety disorders such as panic disorder (Sholomskas et al. 1993; Wisner et al. 1996b) and obsessive-compulsive disorder (Sichel et al. 1993; Williams and Koran 1997). A new multiaxial profile for postpartum disorders was suggested as a research endeavor (Guedeney 2000). The system is a descriptive scheme that emphasizes the importance of context, dyadic processes, and familial system function and child temperament and development.

These classification systems set the stage for the second question: what are the types of psychiatric episodes that occur in the postpartum period? The majority of serious illnesses that begin in the postpartum period are mood disorders (Kendell et al. 1976, 1981, 1987). Of 120 women admitted within 90 days of birth, 80% received diagnoses of mood disorders. In these studies, 38% of the women had major depression, 17% had minor depression, 18% had mania, 4% had schizoaffective mania and 3% had schizoaffective depression, 3% had schizophrenia, 11% had unspecified functional psychosis, and 6% had personality disorders or other illnesses. Among women with a previous history of admission for psychiatric illness, the highest risk for another postpartum admission was for women with bipolar disorder (manic depression): 21.4% of deliveries to women with bipolar disorder were followed by another admission, as compared with 13.3% of deliveries to women who had experienced major depression.

Episodes of psychosis with acute postpartum onset are also predominantly mood disorders. Brockington et al. (1981) found that 91% of women with postpartum psychosis had mood disorders as defined by RDC. In a group of women who were treated preventively in the postpartum period with lithium, Stewart et al. (1991) found that 91% had conditions that met the RDC for mood disorders. Benvenuti et al. (1992) found that 90% of a sample of 30 psychotic women had illnesses that fit DSM-III-R criteria for mood disorders. An interesting observation is the high frequency of bipolar and cyclical schizoaffective episodes that occurred in these samples. The frequencies of bipolar plus schizoaffective disorder in these studies were, respectively, 51% (Brockington et al. 1981), 63% (Stewart et al. 1991), 57% (Benvenuti et al. 1992), and 72% (Wisner et al. 1995).

Conversely, 40%–70% of women with established bipolar disorder will have a recurrent episode postbirth (Bratfos and Haug 1986; Reich and Winokur 1970; vanGent and Verhoeven 1992). In a family psychiatric history investigation, Whalley and colleagues (1982) tested the hypothesis that postpartum psychosis is genetically related to manic-depressive disorder. The investigators found no evidence of a genetic distinction between postpartum psychosis and bipolar disorder. Considering the findings above and our clinical experience, we concluded that any acute-onset psychosis in the postpartum period should be considered bipolar disorder and treated as such until proven otherwise (Wisner et al. 1995).

Clinical Phenomenology

The symptoms of postpartum major depression are the same as those of major depression that occur at other points in women's lives (Cooper et al. 1988; Wisner et al. 1994). According to DSM-IV-TR (American Psychiatric Association 2000), major depression is defined by the presence of at least five of the symptoms listed in Table 3–1, one of which must be either 1) depressed mood or 2) loss of interest or pleasure. The remainder of the symptoms characterize the physiological rhythm disruptions that occur in depression, such as sleep and appetite dysregulation. Symptoms

Table 3–1. Symptoms of major depression

(1) Depressed mood (often accompanied by anxiety)
(2) Markedly diminished interest or pleasure in activities
(3) Appetite disturbance (usually loss of appetite with weight loss beyond expectation postbirth)
(4) Sleep disturbance (most often insomnia and frequent awakenings even when the baby sleeps)
(5) Physical agitation (more commonly) or retardation
(6) Fatigue, decreased energy
(7) Feelings of worthlessness or excessive or inappropriate guilt
(8) Decreased concentration or ability to make decisions
(9) Recurrent thoughts of death or suicidal ideation

Source.   Adapted from American Psychiatric Association 2000.

must be present for most of the day nearly every day for 2 weeks. The symptoms must result in a change from the previous level of functioning and produce significant impairment or distress.

Many of our depressed patients also have described obsessional thoughts. According to DSM-IV-TR, obsessions are recurrent and persistent thoughts, impulses, or images that are experienced as intrusive and inappropriate and cause marked anxiety or distress; they are not simply excessive worries about real-life events, such as ruminations. The person attempts to ignore or suppress obsessions or tries to neutralize them with some other thought or action. For example, some mothers have obsessional thoughts about stabbing their children, and they dispose of every sharp object in the house. By definition, obsessions are not psychotic symptoms, because the person recognizes that the thoughts, impulses, or images are a product of her own mind (not imposed by an external force, as might occur as a symptom of psychosis). Additionally, the obsessional visual images are brief and are perceived as being in the mind as opposed to in the environment, as in an hallucination. For example, one of our patients described horrifying images of herself and her newborn in a casket.

We hypothesized that these thoughts were more common in postpartum depression than in non-childbearing-related depression (Wisner et al. 1999b). We compared the rates, severity, and type of obsessional thoughts and compulsions in women with postpartum major depression with those in women with nonpostpartum major depression. We found that almost half our sample of depressed women endorsed obsessional thoughts in the context of major depression. Contrary to our hypothesis, the intensity of obsessions and compulsions did not differ between the two groups. However, our clinical observation that the character of the obsessional thoughts differed was supported. Women with postpartum depression had significantly more aggressive obsessional thoughts. These women had violent thoughts (put the baby in the microwave, drown the baby, stab the baby with a knife) that they found abhorrent. It is tempting to speculate that these thoughts, which are violent thoughts specific to the baby, may be the result of dysregulated serotonin function in the postpartum period (Wisner et al. 1999b).

Postpartum depression also must be distinguished from the "baby blues," which are very common and occur in 50%–80% of women. Symptoms, which peak on days 4–5 postpartum, consist of a mild mood disturbance without the pervasive dysphoria characteristic of major depression. The blues are transient, resolve by 10 days postpartum, and typically do not require treatment. However, early onset of postpartum depression can be difficult to distinguish from the blues, and careful follow-up of the course of the episode will establish the diagnosis.

Postpartum psychotic disorders can present a diagnostic challenge. Hallucinations or delusions are required for the diagnosis of a psychotic process. The symptoms can be fluctuating and variable in type and intensity. Patients have various levels of awareness and insight into their psychopathology, which affects willingness to reveal symptoms.

Postpartum psychoses have been reported to differ from other psychotic episodes because of alterations in cognition and confusion (Brockington et al. 1981; Platz and Kendell 1988; Protheroe 1969; Wisner et al. 1994). Brockington et al. (1981) compared psychoses that began within 2 weeks of childbirth with episodes of psychosis that occurred in women of the same age in the same hospital. There were significant differences in three areas: increased manic symptoms, absence of schizophrenic symptoms, and marked confusion in the puerperal group. The confused, delirium-like, disorganized clinical picture of postpartum psychosis has been observed and reported repeatedly (Brockington et al. 1981; Hamilton 1982). We (Wisner et al. 1994) compared women who had childbearing-related psychoses and women with non-childbearing-related psychoses. Our most dramatic finding was from our factor analysis: the childbearing psychotic women had a high score on the factor we named "cognitive disorganization/psychosis," which contained the following symptoms: thought disorganization, bizarre behavior, lack of insight, delusions of reference, persecution, jealousy, grandiosity, suspiciousness, impaired sensorium/orientation, and self-neglect. These women displayed prominent symptoms of cognitive impairment and bizarre behavior. The clinical picture of women with postpartum psychosis was that of an acute-onset illness that suggested a delirium to physicians, as evidenced by cognitive examinations (such as drawings of clock faces and figures) and extensive laboratory evaluations. Women with postpartum psychosis also had more unusual psychotic symptoms, such as tactile, olfactory, and visual hallucinations.

We (Wisner et al. 1994) speculated that sleep deprivation, which is often extreme during labor and postbirth, might be responsible for this cognitive disorganization. The disorganized state induced by the disruption of circadian rhythms that sleep deprivation causes (Ehlers et al. 1988) may play an etiological role in disorganized mood states in vulnerable women. Sleep deprivation creates a risk for hypomanic or manic states in women with bipolar disorder. Strouse et al. (1992) used partial sleep deprivation as a treatment for three women with postpartum psychotic depression. All three women switched from disorganized depressed states into activated manic or hypomanic states.

Herzog and Detre (1976) suggested that qualitative differences may exist between postpartum and other psychoses because of the powerful influence of childbirth and motherhood on thought content. Protheroe (1969) noted that guilt that involves the child, spouse, or patient is the most frequent content of delusional thought in women with postpartum psychotic depression. Common themes were feelings of inability to care for the new child or not having enough love for either the baby or the husband. Guilt feelings over infanticidal thoughts were also common.

> The patient, a 22-year-old white married woman, was about 4 months postpartum when her family found her wading in a lake with her infant in January in the Midwest. Several relatives had been committed to long-term mental health facilities, so the family was very reluctant to bring the new mother for psychiatric assessment because they thought she would be institutionalized. On examination, the patient laughed about how hot it was and how she enjoyed the beautiful sunshine. She called the examiner "sister golden-hair" and stated that she intended to walk into the lake again to purify herself. The patient invited the examiner to accompany her so she could purify the examiner and rid her of sins. She denied any intent to harm her baby, but she believed that the infant also needed to be purified in the lake. She endorsed all symptoms of depression and was disoriented to time and place. Her family described several periods during which she was grandiose, loud and verbose, and extremely physically active. Her husband was dismayed by the constant sexual demands she made during those times.

Particularly for disorganized patients, input from the family about behavior is essential for proper diagnosis and management. Postpartum psychosis can be the first manifestation of psychiatric disorder in women. Acute-onset postpartum psychosis is usually bipolar disorder, as in the case above, in which the patient exhibited ultra-rapid cycling between depressed and manic phases with psychotic features. The symptoms can be misinterpreted by family, friends, and health care professionals as postbirth adaptation or the common "baby blues." In this case, the family was adamant about caring for the patient at home. They developed a 24-hour family observation plan for the mother, and family members provided care for the baby (who was developing well). The woman eventually made a full recovery after treatment with lithium and psychotherapy.

> The patient, a 30-year-old surgical nurse, had delivered her infant at the hospital where she worked. The day after birth, she developed her first manic episode with psychotic features. She was grandiose a few hours after the birth and told the lactation consultant that she did not need any help with breast-feeding because she was an expert in the physiology of lactation. The ward staff found her scrubbing the bathroom walls in an energized frenzy. When they asked about perineal pain, she exclaimed that she had cured herself. She refused to stop cleaning the bathroom and insisted they bring more cleaning supplies. When the nursing staff presented a description of their colleague's behavior to the resident physician, he commented that she probably was "just excited about having her first baby." A few hours later, the patient left the maternity ward and ran through the halls to the emergency room in her hospital gown. She danced in the middle of the emergency room and demanded that all the patients gather around her so that she could cure them of their pain. When another nurse tried to escort her back to the maternity ward, the patient kicked her repeatedly. The patient shouted rapidly several times that she was "Mother Mary" and that she had the power to cure. She was restrained and admitted to the psychiatric unit involuntarily.

Training in the recognition and initial management of postpartum psychosis must become a standard component in the education of maternity service professionals to promote safety and prompt intervention.

> A 19-year-old mother was evaluated after an attempted infanticide [Wisner et al. 1996a]. The mother had symptoms of anxiety and depression after the birth of her child. At her postpartum obstetrical checkup, the patient's husband told the physician that his wife seemed depressed. The husband stated that the physician told him his wife had the baby blues and that she would feel better when she resumed her usual activities. When the baby was about 2 months old, the mother pointed a gun at her infant. Although several family members urged her (and her husband) to seek a psychiatric evaluation, she refused because she did not want to be separated from her infant. Her husband insisted that his wife "just do her job and take care of the baby." The next day the mother became convinced that someone was going to rape and torture herself and the baby girl. She attempted to poison the infant with a toxic chemical and made a near-fatal suicide attempt by stabbing.

This type of delusional altruistic homicide (and associated parental suicide attempt) to save mother and infant "from a fate worse than death" was described in a review of filicides (Resnick 1969). Resnick was discouraged by the observation that 40% of the perpetrators of filicide had seen either psychiatrists or physicians just prior to the tragedy. Sensitive direct questions about thoughts of harm to the infant, as well as harm to self, are imperative in the examination. We inquire as follows: "Some women who have a new baby have thoughts such as wishing the baby were dead or about harming the baby; has this happened to you?" It is important to explore the answer to questions about harm to self or infant carefully. Some women respond that the baby was unplanned and become tearful about being overwhelmed in caring for the infant but deny any psychotic symptoms or intent to harm the infant. The risk is much less than with someone who has a psychosis into which the infant has been incorporated (see case example below). Other women speak of a specific episode (often at night) when the baby has been crying and the mother is distressed that nothing seems to comfort the child. The mother thinks of putting something over the baby's mouth to muffle the crying but does not act on this thought, has no intent to harm, and has no psychotic symptoms. Again, the risk in this situation is minimal. Some women who have nonpsychotic depression have no hope for the future and express thoughts that the baby (and sometimes themselves) would be better off dead, but they deny intent to harm.

Women with severe depression are often presumed to have psychosis despite lack of specific psychotic symptoms. Another example of misinterpretation of symptoms as psychotic occurs with obsessional thoughts, which are by definition nonpsychotic, ego-dystonic (not consistent with the sense of self) intrusive thoughts. As discussed earlier, aggressive obsessional thoughts are common in women with postpartum depression. Obsessional thoughts are not associated with increased risk of harm to the infant unless other factors are present, such as coexisting psychosis or behavior that presents other risks (e.g., severe depression that results in caregiving failure).

A 38-year-old woman who was 6 weeks postpartum presented to our women's specialty program because she felt that "something was wrong." She was an attorney who was well-dressed, relaxed, and eloquent during the examination. She readily admitted to all symptoms of major depression. When asked about thoughts of harming her baby, she said that she would not harm the infant, but that there was a "dark shadow" within her that came out and tried to hurt the baby. She explained that she walked on the porch all day (in winter) with the baby and her 2-year-old son to keep the dark shadow from coming out. The day before her appointment, she explained that the dark shadow came out and forced her hands to try to suffocate her baby. She was convinced she would have killed the infant if her crying son had not pulled on her pant leg and brought her back under control (which banished the dark shadow). She stated that the dark shadow was a black silhouette that takes over her body movements. She refused admission and was involuntarily committed. Her husband was angry and defiant about the forced admission until she told him about the dark shadow, at which point he burst into tears of disbelief.

A woman's general appearance and superficial conversation cannot be used to establish the absence of psychosis. Questions about hallucinations and delusional thought content must be asked sensitively and directly when a woman responds positively to the question about infant harm, as in this case.

Biological Considerations

Postpartum depression occurs in the context of a physiological milieu that is distinct from any other in a woman's life (see Chapter 4: "Neurohormonal Aspects of Postpartum Depression and Psychosis"). Although it is widely believed that there is a hormonal contribution to the etiology of postpartum depression (Epperson et al. 1999), only one comprehensive study of hormone concentrations in postpartum women has been published (O'Hara et al. 1991). Women who developed postpartum depression, compared with nondepressed subjects, had significantly lower estradiol levels at 2 days postpartum and a trend toward lower mean estradiol levels. Following this line of reasoning, Gregoire et al. (1996) compared estradiol with placebo for the treatment of postpartum depression. 17-β-Estradiol 200 μg/day was delivered by transdermal patch. The estradiol-treated group showed a 50% reduction in depression scores in the first month of treatment (see Chapter 4).

Cizza et al. (1997) proposed that the efficacy of estradiol in treating postpartum depression is through normalization of corticotropin-releasing hormone (CRH) secretion. During pregnancy, free CRH levels are elevated because of placental production of CRH, decreased levels of CRH-binding protein, and elevated serum estradiol levels. At delivery, these sources of stimulation are removed. Coupled with postpartum estrogen deficiency, a state of hypoactivation occurs. In one study, women who became depressed postpartum, compared with nondepressed women, had more severe and prolonged blunting of the mean plasma adrenocorticotropic hormone (ACTH) response to CRH (12 weeks postpartum) stimulation (Magiakou et al. 1996). After birth, the hypothalamic-pituitary-adrenal (HPA) axis depends on hypothalamic CRH secretion to maintain its activity. The promoter of the CRH gene contains estrogen receptor–binding elements that are activated by estradiol therapy.

Bloch et al. (2000) published data that provide direct evidence of the role of reproductive hormones in the development of postpartum depression. These investigators simulated the withdrawal of hormones at birth by inducing a hypogonadal state in nonpregnant women with leuprolide, adding back supraphysiological doses of estradiol and progesterone for 8 weeks, then withdrawing both steroids under double-blind conditions. Five of the eight women with a history of postpartum depression and none of the eight women without a history of postpartum or other depressive episodes developed significant mood symptoms (see Chapter 4). The investigators suggested that women with a history of postpartum depression are differentially sensitive to the mood-destabilizing effects of withdrawal from gonadal steroids at birth.

Biological factors are also believed to contribute to the etiology of postpartum psychosis (Epperson et al. 1999; Wisner and Stowe 1997). Estrogen has direct and indirect effects on mesolimbic and mesostriatal dopamine activity that are dose- and time-dependent (Van Hartesveldt and Joyce 1986). Interesting case reports support the importance of estrogen withdrawal and neurotransmitter system recovery following parturition in the development of psychotic symptoms. Mallett et al. (1989) described a male transsexual who developed psychosis after estrogen withdrawal. Hopker and Brockington (1991) studied a woman who developed postpartum psychosis after two pregnancies and also after the removal of a hydatidiform mole.

Additional clinical studies and observations implicate the role of gonadal hormones, altered neurotransmitter receptor sensitivity, and the rate at which these systems recover to prepregnancy states in postpartum psychosis. Case reports of the induction of manic symptoms after treatment with bromocriptine, a dopamine agonist historically used to terminate lactation, support the hypothesis of altered dopaminergic system sensitivity (Brockington and Meakin 1994; Fisher et al. 1991; Iffy et al. 1989). Brockington et al. (1988) and others have reported the phenomenon of premenstrual psychotic relapse in women with postpartum psychosis, which suggests a role for progesterone in its development or recurrence. Brockington et al. (1990) also presented the case histories of four women who had a history of postpartum psychosis with recurrent episodes late in pregnancy (>36 weeks' gestation). Serum levels of progesterone decreases during late pregnancy prior to the onset of labor (Turnbull et al. 1974). These clinical data underscore the contribution of alterations in gonadal hormones and potential long-term sensitivity alterations associated with pregnancy in the etiology of postpartum psychosis.

The mean corrected and ionized serum calcium values of women with postpartum psychosis were reported to be significantly higher than those of a control group of women who were psychiatric patients or psychiatrically healthy postpartum women (Riley and Watt 1985). This finding was shown only for women who had no personal or family history of psychiatric illness. During treatment, the fall in ionized serum calcium levels correlated positively and significantly with the improvement in symptoms. The authors concluded that a subgroup of women (about one-third of their sample) appeared to have a disorder of calcium homeostasis. To our knowledge, this interesting work has not been replicated.

Evaluation and Treatment

What is the appropriate medical evaluation for a woman who presents with a postpartum-onset disorder? The emergence of an episode of mood disorder or a psychotic episode in the postpartum period dictates that medical causes of altered neurological status be investigated. Women with postpartum major depression should receive a complete review of systems, medical history, and general physical examination and history so that organic contributions to the mood disorder can be assessed. The use of prescribed medication (particularly pain medication) and over-the-counter medication, as well as use of drugs and alcohol, must be assessed. Thyroid studies should be obtained to rule out postpartum thyroiditis, as should a hemoglobin count to rule out severe anemia. For postpartum psychosis, we obtain a serum calcium level to rule out hypercalcemia, as described by Riley and Watt (1985).

O'Hara et al. (2000) found that interpersonal psychotherapy (IPT) modified for treatment in the postpartum period was effective in treating women with depression. The wait-list control subjects (who remained depressed across time) also responded comparably to IPT when it was implemented after the waiting period. This research group has collected information about the subsequent functioning of offspring when mothers are effectively treated for postpartum depression, which, when published, will be an enormous contribution to the literature.

There are very few systematic data regarding the pharmacological treatment of depression related to childbearing (Table 3–2). Dean and Kendell (1981) observed that fewer women with postpartum depression responded to tricyclic antidepressants (TCAs) than did nonpostpartum depressed women.

In the only controlled study, and the only one to compare a form of therapy with medication, Appleby et al. (1997) found that both fluoxetine and cognitive-behavioral counseling were effective treatments for postpartum depression. Women were randomized to four groups: fluoxetine

Table 3–2.   Treatment for postpartum depression

Study	Treatment	Dosage, mg/day	Dosage range, mg/day
Appleby et al. 1997	Fluoxetine (plus 1 or 6 sessions of CBT)	20	NA (set dose)
O'Hara et al. 2000	IPT	12 weeks	
Stowe et al. 1995	Sertraline	108 ± 37	50–100
Wisner et al. 1999a	TCAs		Nortriptyline: 60–125 Desipramine: 200 Imipramine: 250
	SSRIs		Sertraline: 100–200 Fluoxetine: 20–40 Paroxetine: 30

Note.   CBT = cognitive-behavioral therapy; IPT = interpersonal psychotherapy; NA = not applicable; SSRI = selective serotonin reuptake inhibitor; TCA = tricyclic antidepressant.

20 mg/day or placebo plus one or six sessions of counseling. Significant improvement was seen in all four groups. The improvement in the women who received fluoxetine was significantly greater than that in the women who received placebo. The improvement after six sessions of counseling was significantly greater than that after a single session. There was no additive benefit observed in the women who received both treatments.

Stowe et al. (1995) completed an open-label study of the serotonin selective reuptake inhibitor (SSRI) sertraline in 26 women with postpartum depression. The moderately depressed women were treated with sertraline at a dosages of 50–200 mg/day. Of the 21 women who completed the 8-week study, 20 (95%) demonstrated a response (>50% reduction in initial depression score). These data suggest that women with postpartum depression may be particularly responsive to SSRIs.

Naturalistic data from our tertiary care clinic support the finding that SSRIs are superior to TCAs for the treatment of postpartum depression (Wisner et al. 1999a). The difference in proportions of response was small (0.2), as would be expected from a comparison of two drugs, both of which are significantly more effective than placebo. We are conducting a randomized clinical trial to test the comparative efficacy of an SSRI and a TCA for postpartum depression and to identify predictors of response to each class of drug.

Selection of treatment options for women with postpartum depression is based on the past response to treatment (if any), severity of the episode, presence of breast-feeding, and patient preference. Psychotherapy may be used for mild to moderately severe postpartum depression and is typically combined with medication in treating women with impairing physiological symptoms, such as sleep continuity disturbance and loss of appetite. Past successful treatment with a specific antidepressant strongly dictates the choice of that agent. If the patient has not had drug treatment, the first-line medication choice is an SSRI. These medications generally have low rates of serious side effects and are not toxic in overdose. The objective of antidepressant treatment is to eradicate the symptoms listed in Table 3–1. Full remission with return of the patient's previous functional level is the goal of therapy. Use of sedatives alone for symptoms only, such as sleep disturbance, is not effective for treating the full syndrome of depression.

A unique aspect of the treatment of women with postpartum depression is exposure of infants to drugs during lactation. The approach to studying risk to infants when lactating mothers take antidepressants has been serum level monitoring in mother and nursing infant. The majority of mother-infant serum levels have been published for the SSRIs sertraline, paroxetine, and fluoxetine and for the TCA nortriptyline.

In a review, Wisner et al. (1996c) found that TCAs and their metabolites typically were not found in quantifiable amounts in nurslings. On the basis of infant serum level data and no reported adverse effects, use of the tricyclic drugs amitriptyline, nortriptyline (Wisner et al. 1997), desipramine, or clomipramine was recommended for the treatment of breast-feeding women with depression. There was no evidence of accumulation of tricyclics in infant sera when sampling was repeated. The collective data on serum levels suggested that infants older than 10 weeks were at low risk for adverse effects from TCAs. The only reported adverse outcome for a TCA occurred in a nursing infant whose mother was taking doxepin. The 8-week-old infant developed sedation and respiratory depression due to elevated doxepin metabolite.

Several studies about SSRIs during lactation have been published. Epperson and colleagues (2001) studied the serum levels of two newborns and two infants whose lactating mothers took sertraline at a dosage of 50 or 100 mg/day. All infant serum levels were less than 2.5 ng/mL of sertraline or 5 ng/mL of its metabolite. This group also evaluated the functional effects of these nonquantifiable levels of sertraline in infants by assessing platelet serotonin. In humans, platelet and neuronal serotonin transporters are identical, and animal studies have shown that SSRIs cause similar central and peripheral blockade. In the mothers, the expected marked decline in platelet serotonin levels was observed after treatment, whereas minimal change in these levels was seen in the infants exposed to sertraline through breast milk.

Stowe et al. (1997) determined the serum concentrations of sertraline and its metabolite in 11 mother-infant pairs. Eight infants had nonquantifiable concentrations of sertraline, and the other three had levels of 3 ng/mL or lower. The authors frequently found low levels of the metabolite N-desmethylsertraline in infant sera, with five samples being nonquantifiable and nine having levels of 10 ng/mL or lower. Wisner et al. (1998) studied serum levels in nine mother-infant pairs. Sertraline levels were less than 2 ng/mL in seven of nine infants and 2.9 ng/mL in one. N-Desmethylsertraline levels were 6 ng/mL or lower in seven of nine infants. None of the infants exposed to sertraline during breast-feeding developed adverse effects.

Similar data have been published for paroxetine in mothers and breast-fed infants (Hendrick et al. 2001; Misri et al. 2000; Stowe et al. 2000); no quantifiable concentrations of paroxetine were found in the infant sera (i.e., <2 ng/mL). Paroxetine does not have an active metabolite.

Colic and serum levels similar to those observed in adults were described in a 6-week-old breast-fed infant (Lester et al. 1993) and an additional two infants (Kristenson et al. 1999) whose mothers were treated with fluoxetine. Unlike the TCAs, fluoxetine and its metabolite norfluoxetine have very long half-lives (84 and 146 hours, respectively). Therefore, continuous exposure through breast milk carries the potential to promote newborn serum level development. Kim et al. (1997) reported maternal and nursling fluoxetine and norfluoxetine serum levels from six pairs. The mothers had been treated with fluoxetine for 3–4 weeks. There were no detectable levels of either compound in four of the six serum samples from infants aged more than 2.5 months. In the other two infants, norfluoxetine (but not fluoxetine) was detected at levels that were 36% and 3% of maternal levels. The authors concluded that norfluoxetine was detected in the younger infants because of slow neonatal elimination. The variability noted in this study has been reflected in the literature, with some infants of fluoxetine-treated lactating mothers having no apparent difficulties (Taddio 1996).

Breast-feeding during antidepressant therapy is a case-specific risk-benefit decision, and the available data are generally favorable, particularly for nortriptyline and sertraline. Obtaining a baseline of the infant's behavior prior to treatment of the mother helps to avoid interpretation of typical behavior as new problems. We always advise the mothers to observe the infants for any new rash, since infants can be allergic to minute amounts of any allergen, such as small amounts of drug in breast milk. The importance of parental caregiving, which may be compromised by depression, must be weighed heavily in the decision-making process. Consultation with the infant's pediatrician is standard procedure in our clinic.

Postpartum depression is a model of psychiatric illness that provides an ideal opportunity for prevention because 1) its onset is preceded by a clear marker (birth), 2) there is a defined period of risk for illness onset, and 3) mothers at high risk (those who have had major depression) are identifiable (Wisner et al. 2001). There are few controlled data to guide clinicians who must respond to women who are understandably fearful of postpartum depression. Prophylactic provision of medication postbirth should be considered; however, the TCA nortriptyline does not confer protective efficacy when compared with placebo, and the risk for recurrence is about 25% (Wisner et al. 2001). The postpartum treatment plan should include, at a minimum, monitoring for depression recurrence with a plan for rapid intervention and consideration of starting the drug to which the patient responded or an SSRI.

There is little information about the treatment of psychosis in the puerperal period. Dean and Kendell (1981) reported no difference between puerperal and control cases of manic disorder with respect to the type of treatment received or to hospital length of stay. Since postpartum psychosis usually represents bipolar spectrum disorders (Brockington et al. 1981; Kendell et al. 1987; Wisner et al. 1995), mood stabilizers, such as lithium or valproate, should be strongly considered in the pharmacological treatment of women with postpartum psychosis. Electroconvulsive therapy is also an excellent choice. In our experience, use of typical antipsychotic medications alone yields only a partial response in women with postpartum psychosis. The role of newer atypical antipsychotics, which have some place in the treatment of mania, has not been explored in postpartum psychosis.

Ahokas et al. (2000) found that 10 women with ICD-10 postpartum psychosis had baseline serum estrogen levels that were lower than the threshold value for gonadal failure. During the first week of sublingual 17-β-estradiol treatment, psychiatric symptoms diminished significantly. Until the end of the second week of treatment, serum estradiol concentrations progressively rose to near the values normally found during the follicular phase, and patients dramatically improved. Reversal of symptoms in all patients by treating documented estrogen deficiency suggested that estradiol plays a role in the pathophysiology of postpartum psychosis and may be therapeutic in this condition. There was a rebound of psychotic symptoms in one patient who discontinued estrogen treatment. This intriguing study compels replication.

Prevention of recurrent postpartum psychosis has also been investigated. Dean et al. (1989) found a 50% recurrence rate with later births among women with a history of nonpostpartum as well as postpartum episodes, compared with a 36% rate among women with only postpartum episodes. Promising data from uncontrolled open trials by Stewart et al. (1991) and Austin (1992) showed that administration of lithium in the immediate postpartum period prevented recurrent psychosis. Stewart et al. (1991) treated 21 women with lithium and averted recurrent psychotic episodes in 19 patients. This 10% recurrence rate is less than the risk defined by other studies (20%–50%). Austin (1992) studied 17 pregnant women with a prior episode of postpartum psychosis. Of 9 women who received lithium prophylaxis, 2 experienced postpartum mania; in contrast, 6 of 8 women who were not receiving medication experienced manic episodes. Cohen et al. (1995) reported that lithium prevented postpartum episodes in women with bipolar disorder.

Estrogen has been administered to women with previous histories of puerperal psychosis, and a diminished rate of relapse has been reported (Bower and Altschule 1956). Hamilton (1982) reported anecdotally that 40 patients who had been given a mixture of estrogen and testosterone at delivery to suppress lactation did not experience a recurrence of postpartum psychosis (see Chapter 4). Sichel et al. (1995) studied seven women with histories of postpartum psychosis and four with postpartum major depression (see Chapter 4). They were treated immediately after delivery with estrogen, which was tapered gradually. None of the women had histories of nonpostpartum affective illness, and all women were affectively well through the current pregnancy and at delivery. Despite the high risk for recurrent illness, only one woman developed relapse of postpartum affective illness. This low rate of relapse suggested that estrogen may treat a postpartum withdrawal state that drives acute postpartum psychosis.

When treating postpartum psychosis, the clinician must evaluate the mother's commitment to breast-feeding. The risk of induction of maternal mania or hypomania because of sleep deprivation due to infant care must be considered. However, many women are adamant about breast-feeding their infants, and the clinician must take their preference into account when selecting drugs. A partner or family member who is willing to bottle-feed the baby at night is not available to all women. The American Academy of Pediatrics Committee on Drugs (1994) considers carbamazepine and valproate, but not lithium, to be compatible with use during breast-feeding. Carbamazepine has been associated with transient hepatic toxicity and cholestatic hepatitis (Frey et al. 1990; Merlob et al. 1992) in neonates exposed during both pregnancy and breast-feeding. The infant of a woman who was treated during breast-feeding developed a carbamazepine level that was 15% and 20% of the total and free maternal levels, respectively (Wisner and Perel 1998). Our group (Piontek et al. 2000) reported serum levels from six mothers who took valproate during breast-feeding. The mothers were not exposed during pregnancy. The women developed levels ranging from 39 to 79 µg/mL. Infant serum levels were low (0.7 to 1.5 µg/mL). No adverse clinical effects were observed in the infants. Chaudron and Jefferson (2000) have written an excellent review of issues related to treating lactating women with bipolar disorder.

Effects of Maternal Mental Illness on Offspring

What are the mechanisms by which postpartum psychosis can lead to infanticide? The processes through which children are affected by parental illness are complex (Rutter and Quinton 1984). Genetic factors that increase vulnerability to affective disorder in the offspring contribute. Although some children are resilient, the risk of diagnosable psychiatric disorder in the offspring of parents with depression and bipolar disorder is higher than in children of non–psychiatrically ill mothers (Weissman et al. 1984). Environmental factors that are correlated with parental psychiatric illness, such as violence, hostility, irritability, and involvement in parental delusions, are also important predictors of poor outcome (Rutter and Quinton 1984). Children of psychiatrically disturbed parents have difficulty establishing secure relationships with their mother, have less adaptive coping skills, are less competent socially, and are more likely to be abused (Cohler and Musick 1985). Indirect effects of parental mental illness, such as family disruption, placement out of the home, impaired caregiving skills, and neglect, affect child development. Other correlates of parental mental illness, such as marital discord, low socioeconomic status, poor nutrition, and inadequate medical care, interact to contribute to increased childhood risk.

DaSilva and Johnstone (1981) reassessed 47 women who had developed severe postpartum disorders of mixed diagnostic type over a period of 1–6 years. They found 2 cases of maternal suicide, 10 cases of episodes of self-injury, 2 cases of impaired health in the child that was secondary to neglect, and 6 cases of infant injury due to abuse. Twenty percent of the mothers were unable to be the primary caregiver for their children. These findings are less favorable than those of Protheroe (1969), who found a favorable outcome in 74% of the cases.

The total dependence of the newborn on the caregiver creates a number of risks. Infanticide by poisoning or force has been discussed earlier in this chapter. However, infanticide by starvation has also been described (Meade and Brissie 1985). The serious cognitive disorganization in women with postpartum psychosis can lead to failure to provide the vulnerable newborn with life-sustaining needs, such as adequate fluid and nutritional intake, appropriate environmental temperatures, safety, and emergency medical care. Examples are failure to seek medical care for otitis media that becomes complicated by fatal sepsis, or leaving an infant in a place accessible to a hostile pet.

Conclusion

How can we reduce the risk of infanticide? The answer to this question has multiple levels of response. Improved awareness by both health care professionals and childbearing women must be promoted through education. Unfortunately, media attention often focuses on the negative outcome (infanticide) rather than on early identification, prevention, treatment, and research. Childbirth education classes are incomplete without information for expectant mothers about postpartum psychiatric illnesses. A formal educational module to include in all programs for maternity care professionals must be developed, piloted, and included as part of specialty certification. Prevention strategies should be offered to women at risk for postpartum decompensation. Women with a previous episode of postpartum depression or psychosis and women with bipolar disorder are at significant risk for recurrence after another birth. At a minimum, postpartum monitoring for the emergence of symptoms should be a collaborative plan between the physician and the patient's family.

Because postpartum depression is common in the general population of new mothers, screening to identify cases for early intervention is another important public health goal. Most screening studies have been done in the United Kingdom with the Edinburgh Postnatal Depression Scale (EPDS; Cox et al. 1987), a 10-item self-report questionnaire. We had the opportunity to assess the EPDS as a screening tool for identification of postpartum depression. We found that a score of greater than 10 on the EPDS was a strong and consistent indicator that women had postpartum depression—a finding similar to those from studies in Europe (Murray and Carothers 1990; Wickberg and Hwang 1996). Our data strongly suggest that the EPDS can be used as an effective screen for postpartum depression.

We now have tools for screening postpartum depression, and demonstration projects can be implemented to determine the feasibility of proceeding to nationwide screening programs. Because pediatricians have more contact than most physicians with new mothers, they are particularly important members of any screening strategy (Seidman 1998).

Aggressive treatment for women who develop the disorder with a thoughtful plan for family monitoring of the infant for safety or alternative care while the mother recovers is imperative. Inpatient hospitalization in Europe and other countries often includes both mother and infant as a dyadic target for therapy, but such services have been rare experiments in America (Wisner et al. 1996a). Multi-site randomized clinical trial investigations of therapeutic interventions for women with postpartum disorders would be a major contribution to the field. Exciting research possibilities also exist to improve care for women with postpartum disorders. Replication of European and Scandinavian studies suggesting that estrogen may be both a preventive and an acute therapy for postpartum depression and psychosis is critical. Investigation of the relationship between the massive hormonal stimulation during pregnancy and the acute postpartum withdrawal state on psychiatric symptoms holds promise for understanding the etiology of postpartum and other depressions in women.

Finally, we know little about how a woman's symptoms vary across her reproductive lifetime, and research information is needed for improved longitudinal disease management. If a woman has a postpartum-onset depression or psychosis, what mood changes can she expect as she begins her menstrual cycles postpartum? What if she takes or abruptly stops oral contraceptive therapy? Clearly she needs to be educated about the risks and prophylactic options following another pregnancy and about the likelihood that she will experience other episodes. What is the most effective educational strategy for such preparation of women and their families? If a hysterectomy is necessary at a later point in her life, should she consider preventive therapy? What can she expect during the menopausal transition? Postpartum disorders are tragedies for women who suffer them and for their families, and assisting women in using the experience to improve outcomes over the long term is a highly desirable goal.

In his report on mental health issued in 1999, Surgeon General David Satcher emphasized that mental health is fundamental to all health and that education of the public about mental health is crucial (U.S. Department of Health and Human Services 1999). The last decade of research and policy development is cause for optimism about improving the mental health of childbearing women. Our ability to provide data and assist women with decisions about management of mood disorder during childbearing has increased dramatically. With these successes come new challenges. Let us prepare to take advantage of the great potential for advancement in the care of childbearing women with depression.

References

Ahokas A, Aito M, Rimon R: Positive treatment effect of estradiol in postpartum psychosis: a pilot study. J Clin Psychiatry 61:166–169, 2000

American Academy of Pediatrics, Committee on Drugs: The transfer of drugs and other chemicals into human milk. Pediatrics 93:137–150, 1994

American Psychiatric Association: Diagnostic and Statistical Manual of Mental Disorders, 4th Edition, Text Revision. Washington, DC, American Psychiatric Association, 2000

Appleby L, Warner R, Whitton A, et al: A controlled study of fluoxetine and cognitive-behavioural counselling in the treatment of postnatal depression. BMJ 314:932–936, 1997

Austin M-VP: Puerperal affective psychosis: is there a case for lithium prophylaxis? Br J Psychiatry 161:692–694, 1992

Benvenuti P, Cabras PL, Servi P, et al: Puerperal psychoses: a clinical case study with follow-up. J Affect Disord 26:25–30, 1992

Bloch M, Schmidt PJ, Danaceau M, et al: Effects of gonadal steroids in women with a history of postpartum depression. Am J Psychiatry 157:924–930, 2000

Bower WH, Altschule MD: Use of progesterone in the treatment of post-partum psychosis. N Engl J Med 254:157–160, 1956

Bratfos O, Haug JO: Puerperal affective illness in manic depressive females. Acta Psychiatr Scand 41:285–294, 1986

Brockington IF, Meakin CJ: Clinical clues to the aetiology of puerperal psychosis. Prog Neuropsychopharmacol Biol Psychiatry 18:417–429, 1994

Brockington IF, Cernik AF, Schofield EM, et al: Puerperal psychosis, phenomena and diagnosis. Arch Gen Psychiatry 38:829–833, 1981

Brockington IF, Margison FR, Schofield EM, et al: The clinical picture of the depressed form of puerperal psychosis. J Affect Disord 15:29–37, 1988

Brockington IF, Oates M, Rose G: Prepartum psychosis. J Affect Disord 19:31–35, 1990

Chaudron LH, Jefferson JW: Mood stabilizers during breastfeeding: a review. J Clin Psychiatry 61:79–90, 2000

Cizza G, Gold PW, Chrousos GP: High-dose transdermal estrogen, corticotropin-releasing hormone, and postnatal depression (letter). J Clin Endocrinol Metab 82:704, 1997

Cohen LS, Sichel D, Robertson LM, et al: Postpartum prophylaxis for women with bipolar disorder. Am J Psychiatry 152:1641–1645, 1995

Cohler BJ, Musick JS: Psychopathology of parenthood: implications for mental health of children. Infant Mental Health Journal 4:140–164, 1985

Cooper PJ, Campbell E, Day A, et al: Non-psychotic disorder after childbirth: a prospective study of prevalence, incidence, course, and nature. Br J Psychiatry 152:799–806, 1988

Cox JL, Holden JM, Sagovsky R: Detection of postnatal depression: development of the 10-item Edinburgh Postnatal Depression Scale. Br J Psychiatry 150:782–786, 1987

Cox JL, Murray D, Chapman G: A controlled pilot study of the onset, duration and prevalence of postnatal depression. Br J Psychiatry 163:27–31, 1993

DaSilva L, Johnstone EC: A follow-up study of severe puerperal psychiatric illness. Br J Psychiatry 139:346–354, 1981

Dean C, Kendell RE: The symptomatology of puerperal illnesses. Br J Psychiatry 139:128–135, 1981

Dean C, Williams RJ, Brockington IF: Is puerperal psychosis the same as bipolar manic-depressive disorder? A family study. Psychol Med 19:637–647, 1989

Ehlers CL, Frank E, Kupfer DJ: Social zeitgebers and biological rhythms. Arch Gen Psychiatry 45:948–952, 1988

Elliott S: Report on the Satra Bruk Workshop on Classification of Postnatal Mental Disorders, November 7–10, 1999. Archives of Women's Mental Health 3:27–33, 2000

Endicott J, Spitzer RL: A diagnostic interview: the Schedule for Affective Disorders and Schizophrenia. Arch Gen Psychiatry 35:837–844, 1978

Epperson CN, Wisner KL, Yamamoto B: Gonadal steroids in the treatment of mood disorders. Psychosom Med 61:676–687, 1999

Epperson CN, Czarkowski KA, Ward-O'Brien D, et al: Maternal sertraline treatment and serotonin transport in breast-feeding mother-infant pairs. Am J Psychiatry 158:1631–1637, 2001

Fisher G, Pelonero AL, Ferguson C: Mania precipitated by prednisone and bromocriptine (letter). Gen Hosp Psychiatry 13:345–346, 1991.

Frey B, Schubiger G, Musy JP: Transient cholestatic hepatitis in a neonate associated with carbamazepine exposure during pregnancy and breastfeeding. Eur J Pediatr 150:136–138, 1990

Gregoire AJP, Kumar R, Everitt B, et al: Transdermal oestrogen for treatment of severe postnatal depression. Lancet 347:930–933, 1996

Guedeney N: Appendix: Satra Bruk multiaxial descriptive profiles for perinatal mental health disorders. Archives of Women's Mental Health 3:32–33, 2000

Hamilton JA: The identity of postpartum psychosis, in Motherhood and Mental Illness. Edited by Brockington IF, Kumar R. London, Academic Press, 1982, pp 1–17

Hendrick V, Fukuchi A, Altshuler L, et al: Use of sertraline, paroxetine and fluvoxamine by nursing women. Br J Psychiatry 179:163–166, 2001

Herzog A, Detre T: Psychotic reactions associated with childbirth. Diseases of the Nervous System 37(4):229–235, 1976

Hopker SW, Brockington IF: Psychosis following hydatidiform mole in a patient with recurrent puerperal psychosis. Br J Psychiatry 158:122–123, 1991

Iffy L, Lindenthal J, Azodi Z, et al: Puerperal psychosis following ablaction with bromocriptine. Med Law 8:171–174, 1989

Kendell RE, Wainwright S, Hailey A, et al: The influence of childbirth on psychiatric morbidity. Psychol Med 6:297–302, 1976

Kendell RE, Rennie D, Clarke JA, et al: The social and obstetric correlates of psychiatric admission in the puerperium. Psychol Med 11:341–350, 1981

Kendell RE, Chalmers JC, Platz C: Epidemiology of puerperal pyschoses. Br J Psychiatry 150:662–673, 1987

Kim J, Misri S, Riggs KW, et al: Stereoselective excretion of fluoxetine and nor-fluoxetine in breast milk and neonatal exposure, in 1997 New Research Program and Abstracts, American Psychiatric Association, 150th Annual Meeting,. San Diego, CA, May 17–22, 1997. Washington, DC, American Psychiatric Association, 1997, #221

Kristenson JH, Ilett KF, Hackett LP, et al: Distribution and excretion of fluoxetine and norfluoxetine in human milk. Br J Clin Pharmacol 48:521–527, 1999

Lester BM, Cucca J, Andreozzi L, et al: Possible association between fluoxetine hydrochloride and colic in an infant. J Am Acad Child Adolesc Psychiatry 32:1253–1255, 1993

Magiakou MA, Mastorakos G, Rabin D, et al: Hypothalamic corticotropin-releasing hormone suppression during the postpartum period: implications for the increase of psychiatric manifestations in this period. J Clin Endocrinol Metab 76:260–262, 1996

Mallett P, Marshall EJ, Blacker CVR: Puerperal psychosis following male-to-female sex reassignment? Br J Psychiatry 155:257–259, 1989

Meade JL, Brissie RM: Infanticide by starvation: calculation of caloric deficit to determine degree of deprivation. J Forensic Sci 30:1263–1268, 1985

Merlob P, Mor N, Litwin A: Transient hepatic dysfunction in an infant of an epileptic mother treated with carbamazepine during pregnancy and breastfeeding. Ann Pharmacother 26:1563–1565, 1992

Misri S, Kim J, Riggs KW, et al: Paroxetine levels in postpartum depressed women, breast milk, and infant serum. J Clin Psychiatry 61:828–832, 2000

Murray L, Carothers AD: Validation of the Edinburgh Postnatal Depression Scale on a community sample. Br J Psychiatry 157:288–290, 1990

O'Hara MW, Neunaber DJ, Zekoski EM: Prospective study of postpartum depression: prevalence, course, and predictive factors. J Abnorm Psychol 93:158–171, 1984

O'Hara MW, Zekoski EM, Phillipps LH, et al: A controlled prospective study of postpartum mood disorders: comparison of childbearing and nonchildbearing women. J Abnorm Psychol 99:3–15, 1990

O'Hara MW, Schlechte JA, Lewis DA, et al: Controlled prospective study of postpartum mood disorders: psychological, environmental, and hormonal variables. J Abnorm Psychol 100:63–73, 1991

O'Hara MW, Stuart S, Gorman LL, et al: Efficacy of interpersonal psychotherapy for postpartum depression. Arch Gen Psychiatry 57:1039–1045, 2000

Paffenbarger RS, McCabe LJ: The effect of obstetric and perinatal events on risk of mental illness in women of childbearing age. Am J Public Health 56:400–407, 1966

Piontek CM, Baab S, Peindl KS, et al: Serum valproate levels in breastfeeding mother-infant pairs. J Clin Psychiatry 61:170–172, 2000

Platz C, Kendell RE: A matched-control follow-up and family study of "puerperal psychoses." Br J Psychiatry 153:90–94, 1988

Protheroe C: Puerperal psychoses: a long term study 1927–1961. Br J Psychiatry 115:9–30, 1969.

Reich T, Winokur G: Postpartum psychosis in patients with manic depressive disease. J Nerv Ment Dis 151:60–68, 1970

Resnick PJ: Child murder by parents: a psychiatric review of filicide. Am J Psychiatry 126:325–334, 1969

Riley DM, Watt DC: Hypercalcemia in the etiology of puerperal psychosis. Biol Psychiatry 20:479–488, 1985

Rutter M, Quinton D: Parental psychiatric disorder: effects on children. Psychol Med 14:853–880, 1984

Seidman D: Postpartum psychiatric illness: the role of the pediatrician. Pediatr Rev 19:128–131, 1998

Sholomskas DE, Wickamaratne PJ, Dogolo L, et al: Postpartum onset of panic disorder: a coincidental event? J Clin Psychiatry 54:476–480, 1993

Sichel DA, Cohen LS, Rosenbaum JF, et al: Postpartum onset of obsessive compulsive disorder. Psychosomatics 34:277–279, 1993

Sichel DA, Cohen LS, Robertson LM, et al: Prophylactic estrogen in recurrent postpartum affective disorder. Biol Psychiatry 38:814–818, 1995

Spitzer RL, Endicott J: Research diagnostic criteria: rationale and reliability. Arch Gen Psychiatry 35:773–782, 1978

Stewart DE, Klompenhouwer JL, Kendell RE, et al: Prophylactic lithium in puerperal psychosis: the experience of three centers. Br J Psychiatry 158:393–397, 1991

Stowe ZN, Casarella J, Landry J, et al: Sertraline in the treatment of women with postpartum depression. Depression 3:49–55, 1995

Stowe ZN, Owens MJ, Landry JC, et al: Sertraline and desmethylsertraline in human breast milk and nursing infants. Am J Psychiatry 154:1255–1260, 1997

Stowe ZN, Cohen LS, Hostetter A, et al: Paroxetine in human breast milk and nursing infants. Am J Psychiatry 157:185–189, 2000

Strouse TB, Szuba MP, Baxter LR: Response to sleep deprivation in three women with postpartum psychosis. J Clin Psychiatry 53:204–206, 1992

Taddio A, Ito S, Koren G, et al: Excretion of fluoxetine and its metabolite norfluoxetine in human breast milk. J Clin Pharmacol 36:42–47, 1996

Turnbull AC, Patten PT, Flint AP, et al: Significant fall in progesterone and rise in oestradiol levels in human peripheral plasma before onset of labour. Lancet 1:101–103, 1974

U.S. Department of Health and Human Services: Mental Health: A Report of the Surgeon General—Executive Summary. Rockville, MD, Substance Abuse and Mental Health Services Administration, Center for Mental Health Services/National Institutes of Health, National Institute of Mental Health, 1999

vanGent EM, Verhoeven WMA: Bipolar illness, lithium prophylaxis and pregnancy. Pharmacopsychiatry 25:187–191, 1992

Van Hartesveldt C, Joyce JN: Effects of estrogen on the basal ganglia. Neurosci Biobehav Rev 10:1–14, 1986

Weissman MM, Leckman JF, Merikangas KR, et al: Depression and anxiety disorders in parents and children: results from the Yale Family Study. Arch Gen Psychiatry 41:845–852, 1984

Whalley LJ, Roberts DF, Wentzel J, et al: Genetic factors in puerperal affective psychosis. Acta Psychiatr Scand 65:180–193, 1982

Wickberg B, Hwang CP: The Edinburgh Postnatal Depression Scale: validation on a Swedish community sample. Acta Psychiatr Scand 94:181–184, 1996

Williams KE, Koran LM: Obsessive-compulsive disorder in pregnancy, the puerperium, and the premenstruum. J Clin Psychiatry 58:330–334, 1997

Wisner KL, Stowe ZN: Psychobiology of postpartum mood disorders: brain, behavior and reproductive function. Semin Reprod Endocrinol 15:77–90, 1997

Wisner KL, Perel JM: Serum levels of valproate and carbamazepine in breastfeeding mother-infant pairs. J Clin Psychopharmacol 18:167–169, 1998

Wisner KL, Peindl KS, Hanusa BH: Relationship of psychiatric illness to childbearing status: a hospital-based epidemiologic study. J Affect Disord 28:39–50, 1993

Wisner KL, Peindl KS, Hanusa BH: Symptomatology of affective and psychotic illnesses related to childbearing. J Affect Disord 30:77–87, 1994

Wisner KL, Peindl KS, Hanusa BH: Psychiatric illness in women with young children. J Affect Disord 34:1–11, 1995

Wisner KL, Jennings KD, Conley B: Clinical consequences of the nonavailability of joint-admission mother-baby units. Int J Psychiatry Med 26:479–493, 1996a

Wisner KL, Peindl KS, Hanusa BH: Effects of childbearing on the natural history of panic disorder with comorbid mood disorder. J Affect Disord 41:173–180, 1996b

Wisner KL, Perel JM, Findling RL: Antidepressant treatment during breastfeeding. Am J Psychiatry 153:1132–1137, 1996c

Wisner KL, Perel JM, Findling RL, et al: Nortriptyline and its hydroxymetabolites in breastfeeding mother and newborns. Psychopharmacol Bull 33:249–251, 1997

Wisner KL, Perel JM, Blumer J: Serum sertraline and N-desmethylsertraline levels in breast-feeding mother-infant pairs. Am J Psychiatry 155:690–692, 1998

Wisner KL, Peindl KS, Gigliotti T: Tricyclics vs SSRIs for depression. Archives of Women's Mental Health 1:189–191, 1999a

Wisner KL, Peindl KS, Gigliotti T, et al: Obsessions and compulsions in women with postpartum depression. J Clin Psychiatry 60:176–180, 1999b

Wisner KL, Perel JM, Peindl KS, et al: Prevention of recurrent postpartum major depression with nortriptyline: a randomized clinical trial. J Clin Psychiatry 62:82–86, 2001

World Health Organization: International Statistical Classification of Diseases and Related Health Problems, 10th Revision. Geneva, World Health Organization, 1992

Chapter 4

Neurohormonal Aspects of Postpartum Depression and Psychosis

Deborah Sichel, M.D.

> The coexistence of the organic state raises an interesting question of pathologic physiology[:] one immediately asks if there exists a connection between the uterine condition and . . . the mind . . .
>
> *Louis Victor Marcé (1858)*

The emergence of a postpartum psychiatric illness carries ramifications for mother, baby, and family for altered family development, inadequate bonding between mother and infant, and the potential for subsequent poor attachment (Cooper and Murray 1995; Watson et al. 1984). Postpartum psychiatric illness constitutes a serious complication of birth, with the most tragic outcomes being infanticide and suicide. Yet, postpartum disorders often remain undiagnosed and untreated. One of the reasons may be that once a pregnancy has resulted in a live, healthy birth, health personnel have not been trained to appreciate how seriously ill women may become after delivery. In addition, providers may find it difficult to reconcile a previously well woman with the degree of psychiatric symptoms, so they ascribe problems to normal feelings of inadequacy and early motherhood. Furthermore, a large body of literature has focused on the woman's psychological state, childhood, and personality structure to account for symptoms. As a result, ill women have often been characterized as having a personality disorder because there was no other explanation within the scientific arena to account for the illness.

However, in the past few years, some data that have emerged indicate neurohormonal alterations associated with postpartum psychiatric disorders. Still in its infancy, the field is advancing, albeit slowly, as it incorporates these new findings. Women who suffer with these illnesses will be provided with a better understanding of the biological underpinnings of symptoms. Further, treatments and preventive strategies, both for postpartum psychosis and postpartum depressive illnesses, have emerged, indicating that a distinct neurobiology is associated with these disorders (Austin 1992; Cohen et al. 1995; Sichel et al. 1996; Stewart et al. 1991; Wisner and Wheeler 1994). Although no single neurochemical factor has yet emerged to completely account for this vulnerability, a number of different hormonal factors may contribute to the development of a postpartum illness.

A comprehensive discussion of the classification and nosology of postpartum disorder can be found in Chapter 3 ("Postpartum Disorders") of this volume. Studies of postpartum disorders suggest that some are first episodes of illness (Bell et al. 1994; Hunt and Silverstone 1995). Other studies indicate that up to 50% of women with prior histories of mood disorder are at substantial risk for postpartum episodes and relapse after subsequent pregnancies (Dean et al. 1989; Klompenhouwer and van Hulst 1991). Our own clinical experience suggests that prior subclinical mood disorder is common in many women postpartum. In an unpublished series, 24 of 26 postpartum psychotic women on a mother-baby unit demonstrated subclinical symptoms of mood disorder for many years prior to the florid episode of postpartum psychosis (Sichel and Driscoll 1999). Women either had minor depressive illness interspersed with short-lived major depressive episodes or demonstrated cyclothymic, hypomanic, or bipolar symptoms that were not detected on the usual scales for bipolar and major depressive illness (Akiskal et al. 2000). Further, the diagnosis of a long period of mood cycling or hypomanic features prior to a severe postpartum illness is important, because the rate of suicidality among women with these features is generally high (Rihmer and Pestality 1999).

Intensive questioning to elicit these features in a postpartum mother may be crucial, because it may suggest increased risk factors for suicide and possibly infanticide in this cohort of women. Since many of these women have never sought psychiatric help, they often deny that they have any psychiatric history, unaware that their previous mood swing symptoms are important. It behooves the clinician to identify previous history, using language the patient can understand. The use of psychiatric jargon like "Have you ever had any psychiatric symptoms?" or "Have you ever had depression before?" may well meet with an answer in the negative because women are not versed in its meaning. The fact that large numbers of women are prone to decompensation in the early postpartum period or even later in the postpartum year suggests there are particular neurochemical mechanisms that underlie the acute onset of illness within the proximity of childbirth. It is possible that onset of illness more than 3 months after delivery reflects psychosocial factors related to stress and genetic factors (McEwen 1995).

Jeanne Driscoll and I have also observed that many women whose episodes of depression and/or psychosis were adequately treated and in remission become ill again with the introduction of an oral contraceptive agent or any depot hormonal preparation such as Depo-Provera, a long-acting progesterone. Symptoms range from severe depression to hostility, agitation, rage attacks, rapid cycling, and frank psychosis. When the contraceptive agent is discontinued, they regain their former treatment response.

The premenstrual period has also been noted to be a time when symptoms recur (Endicott and Halbreich 1988; Pearlstein et al. 1990); the symptoms can last 7–14 days prior to the onset of menses. Occasionally, a patient becomes ill enough to warrant repeat hospitalization.

Steroid hormones constitute a group of compounds that have specific and designated actions on receptors in the body. For the purposes of this chapter, the steroids that are pertinent to the neurobiology of postpartum disorders are estrogen and progesterone, made in the ovary; cortisol (the stress hormone), made in the adrenal gland; and androgens and testosterone, made in the male testes and in the female ovaries.

The specific conditions of pregnancy and postpartum reflect complex endocrine states. My purpose in this chapter is to review the state of current knowledge in the neurohormonal arena, even though studies available still reflect a simplistic approach to a very complex psychobiological system and process.

General Factors and Mood Disorders in Women

As a group, women are more vulnerable to mood disorders across their lifetime, experiencing twice the incidence of depression that men do (Kornstein 1997; Weissman and Klerman 1977). This vulnerability is highest during the childbearing years, with the prevalence rate ranging from 7.5% to 10.4%. Now, with more sophisticated ways of measuring brain volume, involving positron emission tomography (PET) scanning techniques, we can look at the brain's functioning, albeit in a crude way. Some factors implicated in these higher rates probably involve differences in men and women at many levels, including different brain structure, organization, and functioning (Allen et al. 1991; George et al. 1996; Gur and Gur 1990; Harasty et al. 1997) and different responses to stress mediated by the stress feedback loop in the brain (Young et al. 1993). We have also been able to discern the multiple effects of estrogen, progesterone, and other hormones produced during pregnancy on the chemical systems in the brain (McEwen 1998a).

The known occurrence of specific mood changes at particular times of the reproductive life cycle (including the premenstrual period, pregnancy, and the postpartum period and during perimenopause and sometimes postmenopause); after surgical removal of the ovaries; and with use of both depot and oral contraceptives suggests that hormones are implicated at some level in these particular problems (Spinelli 2000). Despite these observations, to date, large epidemiological studies have not adequately characterized the groups of women for whom mood disorder is associated with a hormonal event. For instance, what renders women with various forms of bipolar disorder so particularly vulnerable to hormonal fluctuations (Blehar et al. 1998), and to what extent are women with major depressive disorder and anxiety disorders predisposed to hormonally related worsening of their disorders across their lifetime?

One outcome of undertreated and underrecognized postpartum illness is disruption of the mother-infant relationship (Cooper and Murray 1995), and suicide and infanticide are also potential outcomes. Even when the illness is recognized, inadequate treatment is an ongoing problem, because many clinicians do not treat the illness aggressively enough to achieve a state of wellness but rather define improvement of symptoms as a response. When inadequate treatment occurs, a flare-up of symptoms can lead to worsening of the illness and potential suicide or infanticide later in the postpartum year. This timing of the recurrence may lead an investigator to believe erroneously that the act is not related to the postpartum state.

The emergence of scientific data that indicate how the mental state of the mother is significantly affected by a particular neurochemical vulnerability to the event of childbirth will add scientific weight to the outcome of legal proceedings that occur subsequent to the act of infanticide (see Chapter 8: "Criminal Defenses in the Cases of Infanticide and Neonaticide"). Some of the problems encountered by defense attorneys during the trial of a woman who commits infanticide are due to the abysmal lack of biological data that point to particular neurochemical alterations as a consequence of childbirth. Although infanticide often occurs within the framework of a postpartum psychotic process in a mother who had been well, it can also occur within the throes of a nonpsychotic illness. Identifying and documenting the capacity of the events of childbirth that are associated with brain dysfunction triggered by neurohormonal changes is vitally important to the future understanding of psychosis and serious postpartum nonpsychotic illness, to the development of better treatments, and to prevention. Identification of susceptible groups of women in obstetric clinics and practices is crucial so that treatment can occur early and prevention can be achieved.

Depression and Regulation of Neurochemicals in the Brain

One of the first hypotheses about the etiology of depressive illness involved chemical messenger substances in the brain called the *monoamines* or *neurotransmitters* (Schildkraut et al. 1989). Those involved included serotonin, norepinephrine, and dopamine. These neurotransmitters carry signals from one neuron or brain cell to the next. This theory of depression suggested that negative mood states were caused by a deficiency of these chemical substances.

The monoamine theory was succeeded by the hypothesis that in depression, receptors, which regulate the activity of the chemical messengers, were damaged. These damaged receptors caused depletion of the neurotransmitters at the synapse or in the space between neurons. The most recent theory suggests that the primary dysregulation in depression is within the cell and is directed by genes. The receptor and neurotransmitter problems are secondary to, and a result of, the disorder of the signaling process. Therefore, the underlying cause of depression and manic-depressive illness is one or more defective genes, which are further altered by environment and social and psychological stress factors throughout life (Kendler et al. 1995). These illnesses can manifest at any age, from childhood to adulthood, with equal prevalence in boys and girls until adolescence, when hormonal shifts signal the onset of puberty. At this time, depression occurs in females at twice the rate it occurs in males.

Although it is more likely that altered gene signaling occurs between cells and, ultimately, within a particular pathway, the brain chemicals and their specific receptors are still involved in the process. The main thrust of treatment continues to be drug therapy, which targets specific neurotransmitters and their receptors. Treatment may in turn induce more normal signaling at a gene level.

Each messenger is made from a specific chemical precursor in the nerve cell. Dopamine and norepinephrine are made from tyrosine, and serotonin is made from tryptophan. Both estrogen and progesterone have profound effects on these chemical substrates in the brain (Pajer 1995) and serve as one possible mechanism of hormonal regulation on neurotransmitter activity.

Basic Brain Structure

Sex differences in brain physiology are reflected in the electrical activity of the brain and are related to the hormonal states of the reproductive life cycle (Becker et al. 1982; McEwen 1998a). The most primitive brain structure began as a shaft (brain stem) connected to the spinal cord. Around and out of this shaft developed a ring of structures, the limbic brain, also known as the reptilian brain. It is responsible for the sleep-wake cycle, appetite, thirst, aggressive impulses, sex drive, memory, body temperature, and the menstrual cycle. In depression, most of these functions are disturbed. For the purposes of this discussion, the important structures in the brain stem are the hypothalamus, hippocampus, and amygdala. Around the emotional brain developed the cortex, which served the functions of language, judgment, intelligence, reasoning, and complex thought processes, including the capacity for abstract thought.

Each chemical has its own particular circuit in the brain, arising from a storage area in the lower or more primitive areas of the brain and progressing through a number of structures in the emotional or limbic brain. From there, the chemicals progress to the cortex, the most recently evolved area of the brain.

Until recently, specific neurotransmitter chemicals were associated with particular psychiatric symptoms. For instance, traditionally, dopamine was associated with psychosis, and serotonin was associated with depression and obsessionality. However, it is now evident that the explanation is not so clear-cut. Although much research has focused on serotonin, it is clear that other chemicals also play a significant role in depression (Duman et al. 1997). A substantial role for serotonin in depression was elucidated when the brains of depressed suicide victims showed decreased levels of serotonin, a reduction in 5-HT receptor activity, and an increase in 5-HT receptor number compared with the brains of homicide victims (Mann et al. 1989).

These neurotransmitters are stored in vesicles in the nerve cells and then released into the synaptic cleft, or the space between nerve cells (see Figure 4–1). As these chemicals diffuse across to the next nerve cell, they

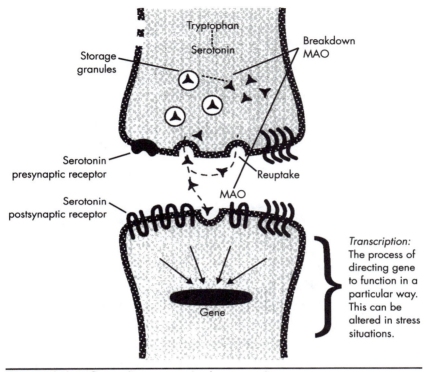

Figure 4–1. Cascading events in the synaptic space.

Note. MAO = monoamine oxidase.

Source. Reprinted from Sichel D. Driscoll JW: *Women's Moods: What Every Woman Must Know About Hormones, the Brain, and Emotional Health.* New York, HarperCollins, 1999, p. 50. Copyright 1999, Deborah Sichel and Jeanne Watson Driscoll. Reprinted with permission of HarperCollins Publishers, Inc.

stimulate their receptors on the postsynaptic nerve cell membrane. By this mechanism messages are communicated from one nerve cell to the next.

The entire system in the brain is imbued with a network of checks and balances, which serve to slow or speed up nerve cell firing. Receptors are one form of regulation. Some receptors have the ability to release the chemicals; some enhance absorption back into the cells, and others release enzymes, which break down the neurotransmitters. Two such important enzymes in the brain are monoamine oxidase (MAO) and catechol O-methyltransferase (COMT). Whereas chemical messengers such as dopamine, norepinephrine, and serotonin promote neural transmission and communication, receptors and enzymes inhibit neural transmission. Other neurotransmitters, such as γ-aminobutyric acid (GABA), also inhibit transmission. This continuous process of facilitation and inhibition contributes to the system of checks and balances within the brain.

Hormones themselves constitute yet one more method of regulation. For example, estrogen and progesterone may facilitate or inhibit the synthesis, degradation, and receptor activity of the above-mentioned brain chemicals. Estrogen decreases brain MAO and COMT, whereas progesterone increases these enzymes. Theoretically, it follows that estrogen is more likely to induce improved mood effects, whereas progesterone would tend to induce depressive symptoms.

Brain-Body Relationships in Depression

Three important circuits permit communication between the brain and the organs in the body: the hypothalamic-pituitary-thyroid (HPT) axis, the hypothalamic-pituitary-adrenal (HPA) axis, and, in women, the hypothalamic-pituitary-ovarian (HPO) axis. These axes are mechanisms of communication between the brain chemicals and hormones and explain how such communication can create mood and mental status changes.

The axes constitute another system of checks and balances. Each controls a biological cascade of events that effects communication between the brain and other body functions (Figure 4–2). Communication occurs both ways between each target organ and back to the pituitary and hypothalamus in the brain stem.

Hypothalamic-Pituitary-Thyroid (HPT) Axis

Thyroid disorders are also known to affect mood. Women are more vulnerable to thyroid disorders than are men. The relationship between the hypothalamus, pituitary, and thyroid is also involved in depression in women, in that women appear more vulnerable to hypothyroid and hyperthyroid states. Thyroid dysfunction has been reported in 30%–45% of women who demonstrate the rapid-cycling form of bipolar disorder (Whybrow 1995). Because bipolar disorder prior to pregnancy is a significant risk factor for postpartum psychosis, the state of the thyroid must be taken into account in assessment and treatment (see Chapter 3: "Postpartum Disorders").

One of the most consistent aspects of hormonal differences between men and women is the abnormally elevated rates of thyroid dysfunction in women with mood disorder and blunting of the thyrotropin-stimulating hormone (TSH) response to thyrotropin-releasing hormone (TRH) (Bauer et al. 1993). In general, thyroid disorder appears to be associated with mood and psychiatric symptoms more frequently in women (Whybrow 1995). Yet, the role of thyroid hormone in the acute induction of any of the postpartum illnesses remains unclear. Because of the elevated rates of thyroid illness in women across their lifetime, one would expect some association of thyroid illness with postpartum depression.

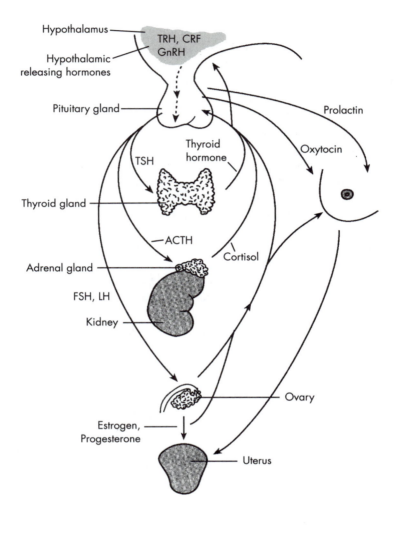

Figure 4–2.   Hormonal relationships in women.

Note.   ACTH = adrenocorticotropic hormone; CRF = corticotropin-releasing factor; FSH = follicle-stimulating hormone; GnRH = gonadotropin-releasing hormone; LH = luteinizing hormone; TRH = thyrotropin-releasing hormone; TSH = thyrotropin-stimulating hormone.
Source.   Reprinted from Sichel D. Driscoll JW: *Women's Moods: What Every Woman Must Know About Hormones, the Brain, and Emotional Health.* New York, HarperCollins, 1999, p. 98. Copyright 1999, Deborah Sichel and Jeanne Watson Driscoll. Reprinted with permission of HarperCollins Publishers, Inc.

In fact, Harris et al. (1996) did show an association between postpartum depression and transient thyroid dysfunction, but this does not mean that the thyroid problem caused the depression. In a further study, Harris (1999) showed that 3 of 100 postpartum women experienced depression related to the presence of positive antithyroid antibodies. However, the author concluded that the depression was not related to the presence of the thyroid antibodies. Another preliminary study, by Pedersen (1999), suggested that low thyroid hormone levels in late pregnancy may be related to postpartum mood or psychosis. Because different populations of women, such as those with a history of bipolar disorder or depression, are more likely to have different vulnerabilities to altered thyroid function, the cause is not easy to establish.

The most valuable and important finding about postpartum thyroid status is the contribution of altered thyroid function to mood. Since adequate response to antidepressants and mood-stabilizing medications is contingent on normal thyroid function, treatment of postpartum disorders underscores the need to evaluate thyroid function in the postpartum period. Both conditions must be independently and adequately treated.

Hypothalamic-Pituitary-Adrenal (HPA) Axis

One of the important endocrine links with the brain is the reciprocal connection between the hypothalamus, pituitary, and adrenal gland. This axis, also known as the *stress axis* in the body, is activated when the body is mobilized to meet any stress, physical or emotional.

This stress circuit ("fight or flight" response) is activated through the release of norepinephrine and serotonin from their stores in the primitive brain. Serotonin and norepinephrine stimulate the hypothalamus to release corticotropin-releasing hormone (CRH), which activates the pituitary gland to release adrenocorticotropic hormone (ACTH). ACTH signals the adrenal gland, sitting on top of the kidney, to release cortisol.

Cortisol is the body's main stress hormone and is often elevated in depression, suggesting disturbed hypothalamic-pituitary-adrenal regulation. In depression, some brain structures (hippocampus and amygdala) help to switch off this circuit, bringing the axis back to normal (McEwen 1998b). Hence, many patients with depression are found to have elevated levels of cortisol. With successful antidepressant treatment, the function of this axis normalizes, and cortisol levels return to normal.

Since we now understand that the HPA axis is involved in depression, it seems reasonable to examine how cortisol might contribute to postpartum depressive illness. In pregnancy, the plasma concentration of cortisol increases. A doubling of cortisol occurs in the first trimester, followed by a threefold increase by the third trimester, mainly due to an increase in transcortin, the protein that holds and binds cortisol.

One test that measures the ability of the brain to switch off cortisol involves giving the patient dexamethasone, a very potent steroid that ordinarily will reduce cortisol levels. In many patients with depression, it does not have this effect. We term this lack of effect *dexamethasone resistance*. Interestingly, the inability to reduce cortisol via this method is also a characteristic of pregnancy (Nolten and Ruechert 1981).

After delivery, cortisol levels remain elevated for 12–15 days, although most women continue to demonstrate this resistance to reduction of cortisol up to 6–8 weeks postpartum (Greenwood and Parker 1984). In women who are vulnerable to the onset of postpartum depression by virtue of previous episodes of depression, the sustained high cortisol levels may contribute to postpartum depressed mood, because functioning of this axis, instead of normalizing after pregnancy, may remain abnormal, contributing to postpartum symptoms of depression. At this time it is not clear how to identify women whose cortisol levels do not normalize and how increased cortisol is associated with postpartum depression.

Pedersen et al. (1993) showed a more prolonged recovery of the biological mechanisms of the HPA axis in women who are at risk for postpartum depression. However, Cizza et al. (1997) suggested that in postpartum depressed women, the reduction of cortisol is resisted for at least 12 weeks. This may be the result of increased or decreased CRH secretion, which may suggest a hypothalamic dysfunction (see Chapter 3: "Postpartum Disorders"). In contrast to these results, Harris et al. (1996) demonstrated an association between low evening cortisol levels in antepartum depressed women that continued until the fifteenth day postpartum, although the classic elevation of cortisol secretion twice a day continued.

More recent findings regarding the stress axis and depression after delivery may provide further information about postpartum depression or psychosis. Douglas (1999) found that a protein chemical called a *peptide* inhibits the effects of higher cortisol levels in the brain during pregnancy. This peptide restraining effect is lost after delivery, so women with a history of depressive illness may develop a severe postpartum mood episode because of the elevated levels of cortisol after delivery.

Hypothalamic-Pituitary-Ovarian (HPO) Axis

The HPO axis, which involves the hypothalamus, the pituitary, and the ovaries, is the body's messenger circuit between the brain and the reproductive system. To maintain the menstrual cycle, gonadotropin-releasing factor is released from the hypothalamus, which in turn stimulates release of luteinizing hormone from the pituitary. The final event in this chemical cascade is the rise in levels of gonadal steroids or sex hormones. If a pregnancy occurs, estrogen and progesterone levels gradually rise throughout the pregnancy until delivery, when the levels are the highest they will achieve during life. After delivery of the placenta, these levels drop precipitously. Estrogen usually reaches very low levels within 24 hours after birth. Progesterone takes about 3–5 days to reach negligible levels.

Estrogen and progesterone influence structures within the brain that are involved in depression (McEwen and Woolley 1994). Estrogen receptors are widely found in the brain—in the hypothalamus, pituitary, front part of the limbic brain, cortex, and brain stem. In particular, estrogen's impact on the brain parallels the effects that antidepressants induce in the receptors, the breakdown enzymes, and the system of checks and balances (Spinelli 2000). For instance, estrogen reduces the levels of MAO, which in turn increases levels of serotonin, norepinephrine, and acetylcholine (Pajer 1995). It increases dopamine levels and norepinephine receptor density in the hypothalamus and decreases cortex norepinephrine receptor density.

Estrogen exerts its influence by entering the cells and activating gene expression by impacting the DNA. The gene then produces other factors that directly influence serotonin, norepinephrine, and dopamine levels in women, thus affecting mood stability. Under the influence of estrogen, certain neurons of the hippocampus are stimulated to grow, actively forming connections with other neurons, whereas progesterone induces the opposite effect (McEwen and Woolley 1994).

Progesterone increases MAO and COMT levels, increases serotonin metabolism in the limbic brain, and decreases the risk for seizures. The overall effect is reduced amounts of chemical messengers and potential influence on the effects that estrogen has on genes. Overall, progesterone tends to induce depression or dysphoria. Some metabolites of progesterone (e.g., allopregnanolone) combine with the GABA complex to produce an anti-anxiety or calming effect, whereas another form, pregnanolone, combines to produce an effect in the opposite direction.

Recent studies have focused on how withdrawal of these hormones acts as a trigger to precipitate the emergence of a postpartum psychiatric illness through the events of the HPO axis. The endpoint is marked by the profound effects of estrogen and progesterone on the neurotransmitters and structures involved in depression when their production abruptly ceases at delivery. Acute withdrawal of the gonadal hormones appears to induce a range of negative mood effects in vulnerable women (Pajer 1995).

Although we still do not know the specific details of how these withdrawal effects catalyze and induce altered mood effects, a number of studies point to a role for hormone withdrawal in the etiology of postpartum illnesses. The hormone that appears to have the most profound postpartum effect, because of its antidepressant properties in the brain and its acute withdrawal after delivery, is estrogen (Wieck et al. 1991).

James Hamilton first explored the role of estrogen in postpartum psychosis in an uncontrolled treatment trial (Hamilton and Sichel 1992). Fifty women at risk for postpartum depression or psychotic recurrence were treated with a single, long-acting intramuscular estrogen (dose unspecified). Although at least a third to a half of these patients would have been expected to experience symptoms, none did. Hamilton also found that these women were surprisingly free of "baby blues"—a self-limiting mood disturbance occurring within 1–2 weeks after delivery (see Chapter 3). Although there was no long-term follow-up of these patients, the study suggested that the administration of estrogen immediately after delivery prevented the early onset of illness.

In a subsequent uncontrolled treatment trial, Sichel et al. (1996) administered oral estrogen in a single large dose (10 mg) at delivery, followed by oral estradiol in decreasing doses over 4 weeks. Subcutaneous heparin was given to prevent any chance of thrombosis with the high doses of estrogen. Relapse occurred in only one patient—which is fewer than the three to five one would have expected (see Chapter 3). None required psychotropic medications for the first year. In a group of women who were assessed to be at high risk for recurrent postpartum depression or psychosis, these results suggest that the estrogen may have acted as a prophylactic agent, stemming the acute withdrawal of estrogen and allowing them to remain well. Two of the patients subsequently developed nonpuerperal bipolar disorder, and one relapsed with major depressive disorder that was unassociated with birth.

Gregoire and colleagues (1996) described the use of estradiol skin patches 200 µg administered in a randomized, double-blind fashion to 61 women who were severely depressed. The treatment group, compared with the controls, showed improvement, as measured by the Edinburgh Postpartum Depression Scale (EPDS). The overall treatment effect at 3 months was 4.38 points. Major criticisms of this study were that it was uncontrolled and nonblinded and that some of the women were still taking antidepressant medication.

A few other studies have reported the efficacy of estrogen in treating and preventing postpartum illness. Ahokas and colleagues (2000) reported improvement in 10 women with postpartum psychosis, with recurrence in 1 patient who discontinued estrogen (see Chapter 3).

Although this research moves our knowledge forward, there is an important need for double-blind, randomized trials in the use of hormonal therapies. The fact that estrogen use postpartum often precludes breast-feeding and may lead to undernutrition in infants who are breast-fed (Ball and Morrison 1999) must be factored in when treatment or prophylaxis is considered.

Bloch and others recently conducted the first study that indicated direct involvement of the reproductive hormones in the development of postpartum depression (Bloch et al. 2000). Eight women with a history of postpartum depression and eight women without such a history had their menstrual cycles stopped with the use of leuprolide acetate, to which was added a large dosage of estradiol (4 mg/day, increasing to 10 mg/day) and progesterone (400 mg/day, increasing to 900 mg/day). Both estrogen and progesterone were then withdrawn under double-blind conditions. Women with postpartum depression showed increased symptoms in the add-back phase of hormones and a peak in the withdrawal phase. Women without such a history of postpartum depression demonstrated no such symptom pattern. The authors conceded that this study did not accurately reflect the milieu of the postpartum period but suggested that some women are particularly vulnerable to the effects that estrogen exerts in the brain. It is still unclear whether the persistent state of low estrogen for 2–3 weeks *after* delivery and/or the abrupt withdrawal of estrogen *at* delivery induced the depressive symptoms. However, these findings have important implications for future treatment and preventive strategies with estrogen.

In an earlier study, O'Hara and colleagues (1991) reported little difference in levels of free estriol, total estriol, progesterone, and prolactin in depressed and nondepressed subjects. Levels were drawn at weeks 34, 36, and 38 antepartum and on days 1 through 4 and 6 through 8 postpartum. Wisner's group (see Chapter 3) reexamined these data and reported that mean estradiol levels were lower in depressed subjects, compared with nondepressed subjects, at all times of assessment. Interpretation of such results is difficult, because we have no central nervous system measures that would correlate with the lower estrogen levels. Possible explanations are that there was inadequate suppression of the HPA axis in women who became depressed postpartum or that there is indeed a group of women who are very sensitive to persistence of lower-than-normal estrogen levels. These findings point to the need for multiple-system examination in future studies.

Another neurotransmitter system implicated in estrogen and mental status changes is the dopaminergic system. Women who have developed postpartum psychosis have sensitive dopamine receptors when challenged by apomorphine, which results in an increase in growth hormone. Since growth hormone is a measure of hypothalamic dopamine$_2$ receptors, and

15 women who demonstrated recurrence of psychosis showed elevations of growth hormone (Wieck et al. 1991), these findings suggest a role for abnormal receptor function induced by a withdrawal state of estrogen after delivery.

McIvor and colleagues (1996) reported similar findings in their study, in which 5 of 14 women who developed depression in the postpartum period demonstrated increased sensitivity of dopamine receptor function and activity. Both Wieck et al. and McIvor et al. concluded that dopamine activity predicted anxiety and depressive illness in the postpartum period.

Riley and Watt (1985) reported elevated levels of serum calcium in women with postpartum psychosis (see Chapter 3). This finding, although apparently robust, has not been replicated. It is possible that estrogen modulation of calcium occurs in some postpartum women, but it remains unclear how this pertains to the occurrence of psychosis.

The fact that postpartum psychosis usually occurs within the first 1–4 weeks after delivery suggests that the findings for a role of the gonadal hormones in inducing an acutely dysregulated state in the brain are important. In fact, Wisner and Wheeler (1994) described postpartum psychosis prominently associated with disorganization, confusion, delirium, bizarre behaviors, and unusual hallucinations (both paranoid and auditory) as somewhat different from psychosis occurring at other times, again implicating an acute, almost toxic brain reaction (see Chapter 3).

Dalton (1985), who administered intramuscular progesterone to 27 women with a previous postpartum depression at delivery and then daily for 7 days, postulated a role for progesterone withdrawal as a cause of postpartum depression. The author reported that 6 months after delivery, none of the women had developed postpartum depression, but these results are inconclusive because of a lack of double-blind conditions.

More recently, progesterone was given to postpartum women at 48 hours after delivery in a randomized, placebo-controlled trial (Lawrie et al. 1998). Increased depression ratings on the EPDS and the Montgomery-Åsberg Depression Rating Scale and decreased β-estradiol levels predicted depression in those women. The authors concluded that administration of progesterone within a short time of delivery is associated with an increased risk of developing depression and that, therefore, progesterone should not be given to postpartum women.

Conclusion

It is clear that numerous neurohormonal factors contribute to the emergence of affective disorder in pregnancy and in the postpartum period.

Moreover, a subgroup of women appear to be sensitive to the withdrawal effects of estrogen and, possibly, progesterone. Given the multiplicity of beneficial effects that estrogen has in the brain, significant changes are understandable when these women are subjected to acute hormonal change in the postpartum period. Contributions of the other hormones, cortisol and thyroid, are also important, although the exact roles that these hormones play are at this time not entirely as clear as the role of estrogen. Brain mood homeostatic mechanisms are so complex that an understanding of the contribution of all the parameters, particularly postpartum, is still in its infancy. However, the new results reviewed in this chapter establish a clear role for alterations in the brain related to the massive change in different hormone systems in the postpartum period.

Future studies must evaluate multiple systems to clarify the complex interrelationships that are involved. Such an approach will require cooperation between specialties of perinatal psychiatry and obstetrics and gynecology. Clearly, the etiology of postpartum mood and psychotic disorders lies in the biological and physiological elements associated with pregnancy and childbirth.

Psychiatrists, psychologists, and other health care providers must be cognizant of the neurohormonal underpinnings of severe puerperal psychiatric illness. In addition, it behooves the psychiatric community to educate our colleagues in the criminal justice system about these facts. Lawyers who represent women with mental illness in the postpartum period must also educate themselves about the new findings so that they can effectively and fairly represent their clients.

Moreover, expert witnesses are responsible for educating juries in a manner that provides a greater understanding of the physiological events involved in the etiology of acute postpartum illnesses. Women must be accorded this justice in light of the new neurochemical findings described in this chapter.

References

Akiskal HS, Bourgeois ML, Angst J, et al: Re-evaluating the prevalence of and diagnostic composition within the broad clinical spectrum of bipolar disorders. J Affect Disord 59 (suppl 1):S5–S30, 2000

Ahokas A, Aito M, Rimon R: Positive effect of estradiol in postpartum psychosis: a pilot study. J Clin Psychiatry 61:166–169, 2000

Allen LA, Richey MF, Chai YM, et al: Differences in the corpus callosum of the living human being. J Neurosci 11:933–942, 1991

Austin MVP: Puerperal affective psychosis: is there a case for lithium prophylaxis? Br J Psychiatry 161:692–694, 1992

Ball DE, Morrison P: Oestrogen transdermal patches for post partum depression in lactating mothers—a case report. Cent Afr J Med 45:68–70, 1999

Bauer MS, Halper LR, Schriger DL: Screening depressives of causative medical illness. The example of thyroid function testing, 1: literature review, meta analysis, hypothesis generation. Depression 1:210–219, 1993

Becker D, Creutzfeldt OD, Schkwibbe M, et al: Changes in physiological, EEG and psychological parameters in women during spontaneous menstrual cycle and following oral contraceptives. Psychoneuroendocrinology 7:75–90, 1982

Bell AJ, Land NM, Milne S: Long term outcome of postpartum psychiatric illness requiring admission. J Affect Disord 31:67–70, 1994

Blehar MC, DePaulo JR, Gershon ES, et al: Women with bipolar disorder: findings from the NIMH Genetics Initiative Sample. Psychopharmacol Bull 34: 239–243, 1998

Bloch M, Schmidt PJ, Danaceau M, et al: Effect of gonadal steroids in women with a history of postpartum depression. Am J Psychiatry 157:924–930, 2000

Cizza G, Gold PW, Chrousos GP: High-dose transdermal estrogen, corticotropin-releasing hormone, and postnatal depression (letter). J Clin Endocrinol Metab 82:704, 1997

Cohen LS, Sichel DA, Robertson LM, et al: Postpartum prophylaxis for women with bipolar disorder. Am J Psychiatry 152:1641–1645, 1995

Cooper PJ, Murray L: The course and recurrence of postnatal depression: evidence for the specificity of the diagnostic concept. Br J Psychiatry 166:191–196, 1995

Dalton K: Progesterone prophylaxis used successsfully in postnatal depression. Practitioner 229:507–508, 1985

Dean C, Williams RJ, Brockington IF: Is puerperal psychosis the same as bipolar manic depressive disorder? A family study. Psychol Med 19:637–647, 1989

Douglas AJ: Endogenous opioid regulation of oxytocin and ACTH secretion during pregnancy and parturition. Paper presented at the Maternal Brain Conference, Bristol, UK, 1999

Duman RS, Henniger GR, Nestler EJ: A molecular and cellular theory of depression. Arch Gen Psychiatry 54:597–606, 1997

Endicott J, Halbreich U: Clinical significance of premenstrual dysphoric changes. J Clin Psychiatry 49:486–489, 1988

George MA, Ketter TA, Parekh PI, et al: Gender differences in regional cerebral blood flow during transient self induced sadness or happiness. Biol Psychiatry 40:859–871, 1996

Greenwood J, Parker G: The dexamethasone suppression test in the puerperium. Aust N Z J Psychiatry 18:282–284, 1984

Gregoire AJP, Kumar R, Everitt B, et al: Transdermal estrogen for treatment of severe postnatal depression. Lancet 347:930–933, 1996

Gur RE, Gur RC: Gender differences in regional cerebral blood flow. Schizophr Bull 16:247–254, 1990

Hamilton JA, Sichel DA: Postpartum measures, in Postpartum Psychiatric Illness: A Picture Puzzle. Edited by Hamilton JA, Harberger PN. Philadelphia, University of Pennsylvania Press, 1992, pp 214–254

Harasty J, Double KL, Halliday GM, et al: Language associated cortical regions are proportionally larger in the female brain. Arch Neurol 54:171–176, 1997

Harris B: Postpartum depression and thyroid antibody status. Thyroid 7:699–703, 1999

Harris B, Lovett L, Smith J, et al: Cardiff Puerperal Mood and Hormone Study, III: postnatal depression at 5 to 6 weeks' postpartum and its hormonal controls across the peripartum period. Br J Psychiatry 168:739–744, 1996

Hunt N, Silverstone T: Does puerperal illness distinguish a subgroup of bipolar patients? J Affect Disord 34:101–107, 1995

Kendler KS, Kessler RC, Walters EE, et al: Stressful life events, genetic liability and onset of an episode of major depression in women. Am J Psychiatry 152:833–842, 1995

Kornstein SG: Gender differences in depression: implications for treatment. J Clin Psychiatry 58 (suppl 15):12–18, 1997

Lawrie TA, Hofmeyer GJ, DeJager M, et al: A double blind randomized placebo controlled trial of postnatal norethisterone enanthate—the effect on postnatal depression and serum hormones. Br J Obstet Gynecol 105:1082–1090, 1998

Mann JJ, Arango V, Marzuk PM, et al: Evidence for the 5-HT hypothesis of suicide: a review of post-mortem studies. Br J Psychiatry 155 (suppl 8):7–14, 1989

Marcé DLV: Traité de la folie des femmes enceintes, des nouvelles accouchées et des nourrices. Paris, JB Bailliere et Fils, 1858

McEwen BS: Stress experiences, brain and emotions: developmental, genetic and hormonal influences, in The Cognitive Neurosciences. Edited by Gazzaniga MS. Cambridge, MA, MIT Press, 1995, pp 1117–1135

McEwen BS: Multiple ovarian hormone effects on brain structure and functioning. Journal of Gender Specific Medicine 1:33–41, 1998a

McEwen BS: Protective and damaging effects of stress mediators. N Engl J Med 338:171-179, 1998b

McEwen BS, Woolley CS: Estradiol and progesterone in regulation of neuronal and synaptic connectivity in adult as well as developing brain. Exp Gerontol 29:431–436, 1994

McIvor RJ, Davies RA, Wieck A, et al: The growth hormone response to apomorphine challenge at 4 days' postpartum in women with a history of major depression. J Affect Disord 40:131–136, 1996

Nolten WE, Ruechert PA: Elevated free cortisol index in pregnancy: possible regulatory mechanisms. Am J Obstet Gynecol 139:492–498, 1981

O'Hara MW, Schlecte JA, Lewis DA, et al: Controlled prospective study of postpartum mood disorders: psychological environmental and hormonal variables. J Abnorm Psychol 100:63–73, 1991

Pajer K: New strategies in the treatment of depression in women. J Clin Psychiatry 56 (suppl 2):30–37, 1995

Pearlstein TB, Frank E, Rivera-Tovar A, et al: Prevalence of Axis I and Axis II disorders with late luteal phase dysphoric disorder. J Affect Disord 20:129–134, 1990

Pedersen C: Postpartum mood and anxiety disorders: a guide for the nonpsychiatric clinician, with an aside on thyroid associations with postpartum mood. Thyroid 9:691–697, 1999

Pedersen CA, Stern RA, Pate J, et al: Thyroid and adrenal measures during late pregnancy and the puerperium in women who have been major depressed or who become dysphoric postpartum. J Affect Disord 29:201–211, 1993

Rihmer Z, Pestality P: Bipolar II disorder and suicidal behavior. Psychiatr Clin North Am 22:667–673, 1999

Riley DM, Watt DC: Hypercalcemia in the etiology of puerperal psychosis. Biol Psychiatry 20:479–488, 1985

Schildkraut JJ, Green AL, Mooney JJ: Mood disorders: biochemical aspects, in Comprehensive Textbook of Psychiatry/V, 5th Edition, Vol 1. Edited by Kaplan HI, Sadock BJ. Baltimore, MD, Williams & Wilkins, 1989, pp 868–879

Sichel DA, Driscoll JL: Women's Moods: What Every Woman Must Know About Hormones, the Brain and Emotional Health. New York, William Morrow, 1999

Sichel DA, Cohen LS, Robertson LM, et al: Prophylactic estrogen in recurrent postpartum affective disorder. Biol Psychiatry 38:814–818, 1996

Spinelli M: Effects of steroids on mood/depression in menopuase: biology and pathobiology. Edited by Lobo RA, Kelsey J, Marcus R. New York, Academic Press, 2000, pp 563–582

Stewart DE, Klompenhouwer JL, Kendell RE, et al: Prophylactic lithium in puerperal psychosis: the experience of three centers. Br J Psychiatry 158:393–397, 1991

Watson JP, Elliot SA, Rugg AJ, et al: Psychiatric disorders in pregnancy and the first postnatal year. Br J Psychiatry 144:453–462, 1984

Weissman MM, Klerman GL: Sex differences in the epidemiology of depression. Arch Gen Psychiatry 34:98–111, 1977

Whybrow PC: Sex differences in thyroid axis function: relevance to affective disorder and its treatment. Depression 3:33–42, 1995

Wieck A, Kumar R, Hirst AD: Increased sensitivity of dopamine receptors and occurrence of affective psychosis after childbirth. BMJ 303:613-616, 1991

Wisner KL, Wheeler SB: Prevention of recurrent postpartum major depression. Hosp Community Psychiatry 45:1191–1196, 1994

Young EA, Katun J, Haskett RF: Dissociation between pituitary and adrenal suppression to dexamethasone in depression. Arch Gen Psychiatry 50:395–403, 1993

Chapter 5

Denial of Pregnancy

Laura J. Miller, M.D.

On the uncertainty of the signs of murder, in the case of bastard children . . . though no doubt there will be many exceptions to the general rule, that women who are pregnant without daring to avow their situation, are commonly objects of the greatest compassion; and generally are less criminal than the world imagine.

William Hunter, M.D., F.R.S.
Read to the members of the British Medical Society, July 14, 1783

"**A**nd then the little baby was born, when I didn't expect it; and the thought came into my mind that I might get rid of it and go home again. The thought came all of a sudden . . ." Thus Hetty Sorrel, a 17-year-old girl from the village of Hayslope in England in the year 1799, explains why she killed her newborn infant following a precipitous delivery after a pregnancy she'd never acknowledged. Hetty is a fictional character in George Eliot's novel *Adam Bede* (Eliot 1859). Yet her experiences of a forbidden relationship, a hidden pregnancy, the shock of unexpected birth, and the desperate solution of neonaticide have been all too real for many new mothers at many times, in many places.

Neonaticide, the killing of a baby by the mother on the day of birth, is a unique form of infanticide (see Chapter 6: "Neonaticide"). Neonaticide is often preceded, as it was in Hetty's case, by denial and/or concealment of the pregnancy. Understanding pregnancy denial is an important prelude to understanding and preventing neonaticide.

In this chapter, I describe various types of pregnancy denial. I examine possible reasons for such denial, including individual and sociocultural risk factors, and summarize its potential consequences. Finally, I delineate interventions that can help minimize the risks of neonaticide.

Types of Pregnancy Denial

Denial can be defined as "behavior that indicates a failure to accept either an obvious fact or its significance" (Chao 1973). Behavior is emphasized because a person may cognitively acknowledge a condition (e.g., a medical illness or a pregnancy) but disavow its implications (Strauss et al.1990). Denial can occur in the context of a psychiatric illness, such as schizophrenia, bipolar disorder, depression, anorexia nervosa, or posttraumatic stress disorder (PTSD). It can also occur without any other manifestations of a psychiatric illness; in such cases, it resembles adjustment disorder (Strauss et al. 1990).

As with other forms of denial, denial of pregnancy occurs along a spectrum of severity. Sometimes the existence of pregnancy is cognitively acknowledged but its emotional significance is denied. Sometimes the knowledge of pregnancy is briefly recognized but suppressed to the point of unawareness. Sometimes pregnancy denial becomes grossly delusional, persisting in the face of any and all proof. The presence and severity of denial can vary at different times during a pregnancy.

For descriptive purposes, three qualitatively distinct types of pregnancy denial can be identified: affective denial, pervasive denial, and psychotic denial.

Affective Denial

Affective denial is associated with feelings of detachment from the infant. This detachment contradicts the usual heightened emotional state of the pregnant woman that is associated with the process of early bonding. Women differ greatly from one another in their emotional reactions to pregnancy (Rofe et al. 1993). Many pregnant women develop a heightened cognitive and emotional sensitivity (Mothander 1992). Most women also begin a relationship with the fetus that is partly projection and partly reality-based. For example, a woman may develop the sense that her fetus "likes" certain foods, prefers certain positions, and has a certain level and pattern of activity (Zabielski 1994). Many women fantasize about what their child will be like, select a name, and talk to the fetus. Most women make behavioral changes, such as wearing maternity clothes, modifying physical activities, preparing space for their babies, negotiating maternity leaves, and planning for child care. These manifestations of emotional connection with the fetus can include transient feelings of indifference, detachment, or resentment. This type of ambivalence during pregnancy is normative and does not constitute clinically problematic denial.

Affective denial occurs when a woman acknowledges intellectually that she is pregnant but experiences very few or none of the accompanying emotional and behavioral changes. There is a blunting, rather than a heightening, of sensitivity. Women with this form of denial continue to think, feel, and behave as though they were not pregnant. They do not fantasize about, talk to, or interact with the fetus. They may not wear different clothes or alter their lifestyles in any way. They make no concrete or emotional preparations for the arrival of a baby.

In its less extreme guise, this type of denial is built into many cultural practices. In some cultures and religions, for example, babies are not thought to have souls until a fixed period of time after birth. Such customs, which evolved under conditions in which infant mortality was high, may cushion people from the emotional devastation of losing newborns (see Chapter 7: "Culture, Scarcity, and Maternal Thinking"). In cultures without such beliefs, affective denial of pregnancy is seen in just those situations in which emotional protection is most needed.

Women who have experienced a prior perinatal loss have a higher likelihood of emotionally distancing themselves during a subsequent pregnancy (Phipps 1985–1986). Women with substance addictions may also experience affective denial of their pregnancies (Spielvogel and Hohener 1995) that is posited to be due to an attempt to stave off guilt feelings about harming the fetus while continuing to use addictive substances.

Although affective denial can be adaptive in protecting against overwhelming feelings, it can have adverse consequences. It can compromise fetal and maternal health by decreasing prenatal care. It can also preclude a woman's emotional readiness for parenthood, which can be experienced as a more abrupt transition after an emotionally blunted pregnancy experience.

A, a 32-year-old woman, had previously given birth to a stillborn daughter but had never overtly grieved. When she began missing her menstrual period, she promptly went to a clinic for a pregnancy test, the result of which was positive. A acknowledged being pregnant but showed no emotion. When family members tried to discuss the pregnancy with her, A would make an excuse to leave the room. She missed several prenatal appointments before her mother realized this was happening and began to accompany her to the clinic. When her mother initiated prenatal visits, A would go along but would never ask questions. A remained expressionless when her obstetrician had her listen to the fetal heart tones. She would not make arrangements either to care for the baby or to have anyone else care for the baby. Throughout her pregnancy, A showed affect and expressed feelings about other topics; her emotional numbing was specific to pregnancy.

Pervasive Denial

A more extreme form of denial occurs when not only the emotional significance but the very existence of the pregnancy is kept from awareness. Often, the possibility of pregnancy, or even definite knowledge of pregnancy, has at some point been in conscious awareness. However, throughout long stretches of the pregnancy, sometimes up to or through the time of labor and delivery, awareness of pregnancy is suppressed (see Chapter 6). Even pregnancies that have been confirmed by ultrasound can subsequently remain outside of consciousness if the shock of pregnancy recognition was sufficiently traumatic to induce amnesia (Green and Manohar 1990).

During this type of denial, physical manifestations of pregnancy are either absent or misinterpreted. Available data suggest that women with profound pregnancy denial have fewer and less intense physical symptoms than do other women. There was little or no weight gain in the majority of women with pregnancy denial in one study (Brezinka et al. 1994). The woman's usual clothing may still fit, so that neither she nor others notice much change in her body habitus (Bascom 1977). When weight gain does occur, it may be attributed to other factors (Brozovsky and Falit 1971). Even the most reliable indicator of pregnancy, the cessation of monthly bleeding, may not occur throughout all or part of denied pregnancies (Bascom 1977; Finnegan et al. 1982). In a series of 27 women with pregnancy denial, most (18) reported vaginal bleeding during pregnancy, whether irregular spotting, continuous spotting, or regular, menstruation-like bleeding (Brezinka et al. 1994). When amenorrhea is noticed, it may be attributed to conditions other than pregnancy, such as stress, traveling, or menopause (Bonnet 1993; Brezinka et al. 1994; Milstein and Milstein 1983). Fetal movements may be attributed to intestinal gas (Jacobsen and Miller 1998).

Pregnancies denied are also pregnancies concealed. The phenomenon of collective deception and collusion in denial has been noted in nearly all cases of profound pregnancy denial. In a series of 27 cases of denied pregnancies, significant others vaguely suspected pregnancy in fewer than half and were totally unaware of the pregnancy in all the other cases; in no case was anyone fully cognizant of the pregnancy (Brezinka et al. 1994). Participation in denial by others can be so profound that a sexual partner may not have noticed pregnancy despite having had sexual inter-course just hours before labor (Bonnet 1993). Physicians sometimes col-lude in denial as well—for example, by attributing amenorrhea to stress without doing a workup (Milstein and Milstein 1983).

At the end of a denied pregnancy, labor can take a woman by surprise (Bonnet 1993). Labor pains may be misidentified as gastrointestinal symp-toms or the need to have a bowel movement (Arboleda-Florez 1976; Bonnet 1993; Finnegan et al. 1982; Jacobsen and Miller 1998). Some women visit emergency rooms with severe cramps and then deliver the baby (Brezinka et al. 1994); others have unassisted deliveries at home. Most women with pregnancy denial describe a feeling of dissociation dur-ing the birth experience (Finnegan et al. 1982; Wilkins 1985).

Pregnancy denial does not necessarily end with the birth of the baby. One woman, for example, heard her baby cry and thought someone else had delivered (Bascom 1977). In another case, placental remnants were found on examination of a woman who presented to an emergency room with vaginal bleeding, having no awareness that she had just delivered an infant (Bonnet 1993). Even women who intellectually accept that they have delivered a baby sometimes continue to distance themselves from emotional recognition of this reality (Bascom 1977; Finnegan et al. 1982).

> B, a 16-year-old girl, gave birth to a child amid the profound disapproval of her parents. Her mother helped her raise the child but felt particularly burdened by this because B's father was disabled by a heart condition. Her mother repeatedly told B that if she ever became pregnant again, it would be the death of her father, because he would surely have a heart attack.
>
> B had irregular menstrual cycles, so when she began to miss periods, she did not notice. Several months later, a friend of hers, noticing some weight gain, wondered aloud if B could be pregnant. B dismissed this fleeting thought. One day, she developed the sensation that she had to have a bowel movement. She sat down on the toilet. She later recalled being in a daze at that time and did not remember the next moments clearly. The next thing she knew, there was a dead baby in the toilet bowl.

Psychotic Denial

Women with psychotic disorders may deny pregnancy in a delusional way. In such cases, physical symptoms and signs of pregnancy generally occur but are misinterpreted, sometimes in bizarre fashion. One woman believed, for example, on sensing fetal movements, that her liver and kid-neys had become unmoored in her body and were rattling around loose. Some women have a delusional belief that these sensations are intestinal gas (Slayton and Soloff 1981).

Some women acknowledge that *something* is growing inside them but do not experience it as a fetus. It may feel to the woman like a blood clot (Miller 1990) or cancer (Cook and Howe 1984). Psychotic fantasies about what is inside her body may reflect psychological truths about the woman's emotional reaction to pregnancy. For example, the woman who believed her internal organs had come loose already had a 1-year-old baby. After treatment, she was able to explain that she'd been feeling overwhelmed at the prospect of having another baby so soon. She experienced herself as literally "coming apart," and she coped with this by maintaining delusional denial of pregnancy.

Psychotic denial may come and go during the course of a pregnancy. In addition, an internal contradiction can be sustained during psychosis, so that a woman can simultaneously maintain that she is pregnant and that she is not. Women who do not overtly acknowledge pregnancy may nevertheless allude to it; for example, a pregnant woman with three children denied being pregnant but spoke of a "fourth child." Like other symptoms, psychotic denial can be preceded or exacerbated by identifiable stressors, such as signing consent forms for adoption or learning of an abnormality on an ultrasound examination of the fetus (Miller 1990).

Unlike women with nonpsychotic denial, women with delusional denial do not usually conceal their pregnancies. Generally, others in their environment do not collude with the denial (Miller 1990). If a woman's psychotically denied pregnancy goes unrecognized, it is usually because the woman is so socially isolated that no one takes notice.

> C is a 35-year-old woman with schizophrenia who had lost custody of her first child. She lived with a boyfriend but had had sex with several other men. Her boyfriend had previously told her that if she became pregnant, she could no longer live with him. When C began to gain weight, her mother suspected pregnancy and took her to a clinic, where pregnancy was confirmed. C denied being pregnant, even after being shown an image of the fetus on ultrasound examination.
>
> C's mother tried to pressure her into having an abortion, even to the point of making up a story that C had threatened her with a knife so that C would be admitted to a hospital in order to have an abortion. However, C conveyed to hospital staff that if she were pregnant she would not want to abort the fetus. She carried the baby to term. After delivery, C acknowledged, "I guess I really was pregnant." She explained her previous denial by saying that she was torn between leading a boring, conventional life (e.g., taking medication, relinquishing her psychosis, being faithful to her boyfriend, and raising a child) and living the exciting but emotionally wrenching life of being psychotic, having many lovers, and having babies whose custody she lost. Unable to resolve this dilemma, she could not accept the existence of the pregnancy.

Reasons for Pregnancy Denial

Denial has diverse etiologies and contributory factors (Appelbaum 1998). The presence of denial does not necessarily imply a psychiatric disorder or a specific psychological conflict. A combination of physiological factors (e.g., irregular menses, few physical symptoms of pregnancy), external stress, and rationalization can cause pregnancy to be denied under circumstances of minimal to no psychopathology (Spielvogel and Hohener 1995). Nevertheless, certain cognitive and emotional processes appear to promote the likelihood of pregnancy denial in many cases.

Cognitive Models of Denial

People's responsiveness to painful or anxiety-provoking situations falls along a spectrum from highly reactive ("sensitizing") to less reactive ("repressing"). During pregnancy, women with a repressing cognitive style report less pain, anxiety, and depression than women with a sensitizing cognitive style (Rofe et al. 1993). This mental set exerts a more powerful effect on experienced level of emotional stress during pregnancy than does socioeconomic status or primiparity. Except among women with the most extreme repressing style, anxiety, depression, nightmares, and insomnia are frequent normative experiences during pregnancy, especially in the third trimester. Women who have a characteristically repressing cognitive style may be more apt to manage extreme pregnancy stressors with denial rather than some other way.

Having a repressing cognitive style, however, does not usually lead to pregnancy denial unless a conflict or stressor is also fueling the denial. Since pregnancy and motherhood call for major adjustments of lifestyle, relationships, career, and social role (Brezinka et al. 1994), it is not unusual for conflict and stress related to one or more of these changes to develop.

One cognitive model posits that when conflicts or stressors loom, people appraise the potential dangers they face. This process of appraisal can be conscious or preconscious. Potential dangers can include the threat of painful affects as well as physical or external threats. Once this appraisal is complete, the person chooses a response from his or her available repertoire of coping skills. Some strategies are problem-focused, in that they alter the relationship between the person and the environment in such a way as to reduce the threat or garner support. Denial is an emotion-focused, rather than a problem-focused, strategy; threatening information is actively excluded from conscious awareness. This strategy is more likely to be used when the external situation cannot be altered or when the person perceives it cannot be altered.

By reducing extreme anxiety, denial can be helpful. This is especially the case when it is the initial reaction to frightening news but is not sustained over time (Bluestein and Rutledge 1992). Initial denial can buffer the shock of the unexpected, giving a person time to collect herself and to mobilize other defenses. However, this strategy is risky, especially when sustained over time, because it decreases access to useful information and often prevents adaptive action (Forchuk and Westwell 1987).

A particular type of conflict that promotes use of denial is *cognitive dissonance* (Forchuk and Westwell 1987). This is a situation in which actions, behavior, or observed facts contradict a deeply held cognitive conviction. For this painful contradiction to be resolved, something must change—either the conviction or the fact. When the conviction is central to the person's sense of self, the fact may be denied in order for the conviction to be maintained. In the case of pregnancy denial, the conviction could be something like "Only bad girls get pregnant before marriage, and I'm not a bad girl." Rather than disavow that belief, the woman denies the fact of pregnancy. In the case of psychotic denial, there is often a need to reconcile antenatal feelings of attachment toward the fetus with the likelihood of being unable to parent the baby after birth. This dissonance between emotions and a reality-based appraisal of the likely outcome may result in delusional denial of pregnancy (Miller 1990).

Some evolutionary psychologists posit that the ability to conceal emotions has had adaptive value over time and therefore has been retained as a capability within the human psyche. The most effective way to conceal emotions from others is to deceive oneself; thus, a capacity for denial could be adaptive as well. However, it would be useful to store the denied information in case it is needed later. Thus, people may have evolved the capacity for dissociation in conjunction with denial (Pinker 1997).

Emotional Stressors Related to Pregnancy Denial

In most reported cases of pregnancy denial, two central areas of emotional stress emerge: conflicts related to sexuality (Bascom 1977; Spielvogel and Hohener 1995) and fears of interpersonal abandonment. Sometimes these two are closely intertwined. Pregnancy is a visible, public marker of having had a sexual relationship. Such acknowledgment of sexuality can be terrifying when past trauma has created profound confusion about sexuality or when cultural or familial attitudes forbid sexuality.

For many women, pregnancy raises fears of interpersonal abandonment and/or losses. In some cases, this is because there have been explicit threats of abandonment or experiences of loss linked to becoming pregnant. For example, some adolescents who denied their pregnancies had been told they would be kicked out of their homes if they became pregnant (Brozovsky and Falit 1971; Oberman 1996), or they had seen harsh familial treatment of an older relative who became pregnant (Arboleda-Florez 1976; Oberman 1996). In a study of teenagers, delayed pregnancy testing and associated pregnancy denial were linked to fear of parental response (Bluestein and Rutledge 1992).

Fear of being abandoned by a partner can also contribute to pregnancy denial. Sometimes the partner is jealous of the fetus or is jealous because the father of the fetus is a different man (Resnick 1970). Sometimes tensions arise because the pregnancy arose too early in a relationship (Brezinka et al. 1994). Sometimes denial occurs after a woman notes behavioral changes in her spouse early in pregnancy. For example, a woman who cognitively acknowledged but affectively denied her pregnancy related that as soon as she had become pregnant, her husband began to ignore her and spend long hours away from home. Her perception was that he now figured he no longer had to court her because she was "his" permanently because of the pregnancy. Anger toward the father of the fetus may contribute to pregnancy denial (Spielvogel and Hohener 1995), as a woman's means of distancing herself from a difficult relationship. Secure, committed relationships with the father of the fetus are rare among women with known cases of pervasive pregnancy denial (Oberman 1996). Communication difficulties with partners are a major reason why teenagers delay pregnancy testing (Bluestein and Rutledge 1992).

Past or anticipated loss of a child can lead to a woman's denying a subsequent pregnancy. In a study of psychotic pregnancy denial, there was a significant correlation between past or anticipated custody loss and current denial of pregnancy (Miller 1990). Sometimes the strong emotions from which a woman distances herself with denial show themselves in the content of delusions. For example, a woman who denied her pregnancy displayed bland affect when relating her history of miscarriage. However, she maintained the delusion that machines directed by the doctor who had treated her were tormenting her by grinding up the products of that miscarriage (Slayton and Soloff 1981).

A window into the emotions underlying pregnancy denial can be obtained by interviewing women who give birth in hospitals after denied pregnancies. In one such study (Bonnet 1993), many women recounted fantasies of violence toward their fetuses. These violent thoughts appeared in many cases to be related to the woman's efforts to get rid of traumatic associations.

D was a 23-year-old married woman who had recently immigrated to the United States from Ecuador. She was isolated from her family of origin and did not speak English, but she was happy with her marriage and found a satisfying job. When she became pregnant, she developed intense nausea and vomiting, which rendered her unable to continue working. Her husband then worked longer hours to compensate, so she felt very isolated. D showed no emotional or behavioral reactions to her pregnancy until the second trimester, when she began to feel fetal movements. At that point, she developed sudden angry thoughts toward the fetus, blaming the fetus for her nausea and vomiting and subsequent job loss. She made three apparent suicide attempts in rapid succession, one by nearly jumping out a window, one by overdose, and one by drinking cleaning fluid. Her husband rescued her each time. She later explained that she had no desire to kill herself but that these actions had been aimed at destroying the fetus. Her overt affect was bland during these events and while discussing them afterward.

Risk Factors for Pregnancy Denial

Individual Risk Factors

Youth

While women of any age can deny a pregnancy, this phenomenon is most commonly seen in pregnant adolescents. For example, the modal age of a sample of 47 women who had committed neonaticide, often after denying their pregnancies, was 17 (Oberman 1996). Denial in this age group can be put into perspective by understanding how commonly teenagers delay recognition of pregnancy. In a representative study, the mean delay in diagnosing pregnancy in a sample of 151 pregnant teens was 4.35 weeks (Bluestein and Rutledge 1992); 45% of the girls in the study sample had difficulty acknowledging that they were pregnant.

Teenagers who are pregnant often first seek medical attention for nonspecific, misleading complaints. Pregnancy is often missed on first visits to adolescent medical clinics (Causey et al. 1997). Studies of pregnant adolescents coming to emergency rooms (Causey et al. 1997; Givens et al. 1994) have found that less than 10% either requested a pregnancy test or mentioned the possibility of being pregnant. The rest had come for complaints such as gastrointestinal symptoms, vaginal discharge, or urinary symptoms. About 10% of these pregnant adolescents denied being sexually active. Some persisted in denying the possibility of pregnancy after being informed of positive pregnancy test results. One result of delayed acknowledgment of pregnancy is that less than 25% of pregnant teens in the United States receive prenatal care (Causey et al. 1997).

Passivity

A passive behavioral style has been noted in many women who deny pregnancy. The passivity begins with the sexual relationship that led to the pregnancy, in that women may be coerced into sex (Milstein and Milstein 1983; Resnick 1970). On suspecting or learning of pregnancy, some women who would otherwise have chosen to abort are prevented by their passivity from seeking abortion (Bonnet 1993).

Intellectual and Knowledge Deficits

For some women, impaired intellectual function contributes to lack of awareness of pregnancy (Brezinka et al. 1994; Oberman 1996). With other women, a striking lack of knowledge of the anatomy and physiology of reproduction, despite normal intellectual capacity, has been observed (Finnegan et al. 1982). However, pregnancy denial can also be seen in women with above-average IQ scores and good school performance.

Substance Addiction

Substance addiction can promote pregnancy denial, especially affective denial. When pregnancy is suspected, some women increase the use of addictive substances in an apparent effort to block out resultant feelings of guilt, self-loathing, and depression (Spielvogel and Hohener 1995). Many addicted pregnant women expect health professionals and family members to have a punitive attitude; when these women were surveyed, significantly more women with addiction doubted family support than did women with other high-risk conditions during pregnancy (Marcenko et al. 1994). This lack of support, perceived or actual, further serves to block pregnancy from awareness.

Affective denial of potential adverse consequences to offspring of substance use during pregnancy may persist after delivery. For example, new mothers who are heavy drinkers overestimate their infants' mental and physical development significantly more often than do new mothers who are abstainers and light drinkers, a finding not accounted for by education or socioeconomic status (Seagull et al. 1996).

Other Psychiatric Disorders

From available data, it appears that less than half of women with pervasive pregnancy denial have psychiatric disorders other than adjustment disorder (Brezinka et al. 1994). Specific psychiatric illnesses appear to affect pregnancy denial in different ways. Psychotic denial is most commonly found in the context of schizophrenia (Miller 1990). Symptoms of depression are associated not only with difficulty acknowledging pregnancy but also with dissatisfaction with family support while pregnant and with difficulty communicating with partners about pregnancy (Bluestein and Rutledge 1992). Eating disorders can promote misinterpretation of the appetite and weight changes that accompany pregnancy (Bonnet 1993; Kaplan and Grotowski 1996). Women with sexual abuse–related PTSD may experience a reemergence of traumatic memories connected to sexuality on suspecting pregnancy (Bonnet 1993; Spielvogel and Hohener 1995). The experience of being examined for pregnancy and being told of a pregnancy may be so traumatic for such women that they dissociate and do not register what the physician said (Bascom 1977).

Obstetric/Gynecological Factors

Women who have irregular menses prior to pregnancy may be more prone not to notice prolonged amenorrhea and are overrepresented in samples of women who deny pregnancy (Brezinka et al. 1994). Women who take oral contraceptive pills or intramuscular progestogens may have continued cyclic bleeding, which makes pregnancy more difficult to recognize (Brezinka et al. 1994; Kaplan and Grotowski 1996). Breech presentation can produce a less obviously pregnant body habitus, which renders denial and concealment easier (Brezinka et al. 1994).

Sociocultural Risk Factors

Women of all races, ethnicities, and social classes can deny pregnancies (Oberman 1996). However, certain familial and sociocultural contexts appear to foster pregnancy denial as well as resultant neonaticide. The common thread seems to be that something about the environment in which a woman becomes pregnant renders her pregnancy highly threatening to her well-being.

Rates of neonaticide have varied widely in different groups of people during different historical eras (Hrdy 1999; Oberman 1996). Examining these differences sheds light on sociocultural contexts that promote this most extreme correlate of pregnancy denial. Neonaticide rates have varied according to factors such as availability of birth control, abortion, environmental resources, and child care help. Circumstances in which a woman cannot choose *not* to be pregnant, might be abandoned or punished if pregnant, or has insufficient help or resources to raise a child promote neonaticide. Since it is more difficult for a mother to neglect, abandon, or kill an infant to whom she has become emotionally attached, many mothers faced with these desperate circumstances pave the way for rejecting their babies by failing to acknowledge pregnancy. Frank denial is part of a spectrum of maternal emotional distancing from offspring whose existence might pose great risks to their mothers.

A common thread in nearly all known cases of pervasive pregnancy denial is social isolation (Finnegan et al. 1982; Green and Manohar 1990; Oberman 1996). Even women surrounded by people may not feel emotionally connected to any of them. In many cases, the dread of being pregnant is associated with growing up in families, cultures, or religious contexts that stigmatize out-of-wedlock conceptions (Arboleda-Florez 1976; Finnegan et al. 1982; Green and Manohar 1990; Milstein and Milstein 1983; Resnick 1970; Spielvogel and Hohener 1995). The cultural prohibition may be so intense that prenuptial pregnancy becomes literally "unthinkable" (Bonnet 1993).

Consequences of Pregnancy Denial

Obstetric Complications

Any degree of pregnancy denial may delay the diagnosis of pregnancy and the initiation of prenatal care (Kinzl and Biebl 1991). In a study of pregnant adolescents, for example, difficulty acknowledging pregnancy was the only factor exerting a significant influence on delayed testing; race, education, financial barriers, and psychiatric symptoms did not (Bluestein and Rutledge 1992). By delaying prenatal care, pregnancy denial can contribute to higher incidences of preterm labor, perinatal mortality, and low-birth-weight infants (Joyce et al. 1983). One study, for example, found that mothers of very-low-birth-weight infants were 54% more likely than controls to have denied their pregnancies (Sable et al. 1997).

Some of the risks associated with pregnancy denial come from a woman's failing to protect herself and her fetus from toxins or potentially harmful conditions she might otherwise avoid. These include alcoholic beverages, cigarette smoke and tobacco products, radiation, teratogenic drugs, excessive job stress, or overly vigorous exercise (Brezinka et al. 1994; Kinzl and Biebl 1991). Other risks stem from a woman's failure to recognize warning signs of pregnancy complications (Brezinka et al. 1994; Kinzl and Biebl 1991). For example, unrecognized premature rupture of membranes can lead to infection. Uterine contractions, whether premature or from term labor, may be erroneously attributed to gastrointestinal discomfort; this can lead to precipitous or unassisted delivery.

Neonaticide

Neonaticide (see Chapter 6) is strongly associated with pregnancy denial (Saunders 1989; Spinelli 2001). Sometimes, confronted with a baby for whom she was not emotionally prepared, the mother actively kills her newborn (by, for example, battering or strangulation) (Bonnet 1993). In other cases, she does not actively attempt to kill the baby, but she does nothing to prevent the baby from dying. The most common way babies die after denied pregnancies is by being delivered into toilets and drowning (Green and Manohar 1990; Kellett 1992; Milstein and Milstein 1983; Mitchell and Davis 1984). In other cases, the baby may fall to the floor and sustain a skull fracture if the mother delivers from a crouching or standing position without assistance (Kellett 1992).

In some cases in which mothers have actively brought about their newborns' deaths, there were aggressive fantasies toward the fetuses prior to the birth. Some of these fantasies become enacted in the form of aggressive behavior directed toward the fetus—for example, a woman forced to confront a previously denied pregnancy may punch her abdomen (Kent et al. 1997). Sometimes such behavior can result in fetal injuries and/or placental abruption. In some cases in which women have later been able to discuss their fantasies, there is evidence to suggest that their behavior was prompted by identifying with an imagined aggressor. For example, some women did to their babies what they feared their own mothers would do to them (Bonnet 1993).

In many cases of neonaticide following denied pregnancies, the mothers appear to have killed their babies while in dissociative or near-dissociative states. Memory for the act is often hazy. Many women make little or no effort to conceal their acts.

Postpartum Psychiatric Problems

There is some evidence that women who deny pregnancies may be more vulnerable to postpartum psychiatric symptoms (Uddenberg and Nilsson 1975). In women with preexisting psychotic disorders, a complete absence of anxiety and depression during pregnancy predicts the development of postpartum psychosis (McNeil 1988). For some women, the sudden appearance of a baby after a denied pregnancy can lead to PTSD (Jacobsen and Miller 1998).

Parenting

For most women who acknowledge being pregnant, the psychological transition to motherhood begins during the pregnancy. Many pregnant women seek out and imitate maternal role models, fantasize about parenting, and "try on" different parenting behaviors and attitudes for fit with their self-definitions (Zabielski 1994). A woman who is aware of her fetus may develop the seeds of a reciprocal relationship. For example, she may note the activity patterns of the fetus and may begin to alter her daily rhythms accordingly. She may find that fetal movement is intensified when she lies down in one position and that the fetus calms when she lies in another position. In addition, many mothers take steps to learn concrete information and garner support. These steps may include attending classes, consulting relatives and friends, arranging child care, and having baby showers. As a result of these behaviors, by the ninth month of pregnancy, 85% of pregnant women in one survey felt that they were mothers already (Zabielski 1994).

None of this preparatory activity can occur during a denied pregnancy. Motherhood comes as a shock in the face of what may have already been stressful life circumstances (see Chapter 6). The nature and quality of parenting that ensues can be highly variable.

Despite the lack of preparation, a denied pregnancy can be followed by genuine joy and acceptance of the mothering role (Spielvogel and Hohener 1995). In a follow-up study of women who had denied their pregnancies, none of the offspring showed evidence of abuse or neglect, and only one was in substitute care (Brezinka et al. 1994). Even women who have committed neonaticide after denied pregnancies can successfully raise other children when circumstances change (Bartholemew 1989; Hrdy 1999; Jacobsen and Miller 1998; Wilkins 1985). Nevertheless, sometimes child welfare or health professionals may consider pregnancy denial, especially with a history of neonaticide, as automatically indicative of problem parenting. Hospital staff, for example, may try to convince mothers not to keep their babies after denied pregnancies or may seek judicial orders for foster placement of the infants (Brezinka et al. 1994).

Recurrence With Subsequent Pregnancies

For some women, pregnancy denial and resultant neonaticide recur in later pregnancies (Arboleda-Florez 1976; Bartholemew 1989). The risk of denying subsequent pregnancies may be greater if the reasons for denying the first pregnancy were never addressed (Joyce et al. 1983). The risk of recurrence of neonaticide seems higher in cases in which violence is a habitual part of the mother's life (Resnick 1970).

Interventions for Pregnancy Denial

Identification

The earlier pregnancy denial is identified, the more opportunity there is to prevent complications. Within prenatal clinics, affective denial can be best identified when staff are trained to understand the normal range of emotional reactions to pregnancy and to pay special attention to women at high risk for denial (e.g., women with prior pregnancy loss, women with substance addictions, teenagers with inadequate social support). Within emergency rooms and general medical clinics, it is important to remember to include pregnancy in the differential diagnosis of abdominal and pelvic symptoms. It is also helpful to obtain history from women, including teenagers, in the absence of family members (Malviya et al. 1996) and to obtain collateral history from significant others.

Medication

When pregnancy denial occurs in the context of a medication-responsive psychiatric condition, such as major depression, bipolar disorder, or schizophrenia, pharmacotherapy can alleviate the denial. The risks of the untreated symptoms, including denial, must be weighed against potential risks of medication during pregnancy (Miller 1998). In most cases, medication alone is not sufficient for treating denial, but it can help a woman feel ready to address the psychosocial problems that are contributing to the denial.

Psychotherapy

Even when a woman is not engaged in formal psychotherapy, a therapeutic stance on the part of health personnel working with her can help elucidate and work through the problems that led to the denial. The most important part of this therapeutic stance is conveying an open, nonjudgmental attitude. Reprimands or lectures may further alienate a woman whose emotional isolation may be fueling her denial (Joyce et al. 1983).

Since denial serves a protective function, a helpful therapeutic approach involves trying to understand the psychological purpose for the denial. Asking the woman directly before she is ready may increase anxiety and does not usually shed light, because she often does not know. Careful listening over time and use of collateral sources of information can provide clues. Once the underlying problems have become clear, it is necessary to find other ways of addressing those problems before the woman can relinquish the denial.

A therapeutic stance can also guide approaches to the mother-infant relationship after birth. For example, encouraging a woman to hold her baby may be frightening, and sometimes dangerous, if she maintains secret violent fantasies toward the infant. Helping her first to articulate the fantasies and then to link them to traumatic experiences in her own past may help her to feel ready to hold and care for the baby (Bonnet 1993).

> E, a 27-year-old woman in her eighth month of pregnancy, was brought to a prenatal clinic by her brother because she was losing weight. Her brother related that she was eating a lot—in fact, she was bingeing rapidly on large quantities of food—but that almost immediately after eating she would vomit. She did not try to conceal her bingeing and vomiting and did not appear to be inducing the vomiting. She had no body image disturbance. Her brother had brought her to the clinic 2 weeks earlier with the same complaint, and a nurse had lectured about nutrition and had admonished her to eat more slowly "for the sake of the baby." E had listened and nodded, appearing to understand. Since then, however, her brother noted that her bingeing had intensified and that the vomiting had worsened to the point of weight loss.
>
> This time, instead of lecturing, the nurse asked E open-ended questions about how things had been going for her and listened carefully. E disclosed that she believed there was no baby inside her. Rather, there was a devil inside her who was trying to steal all her nutrients, and she was eating rapidly in order to bypass the devil. E's brother revealed that E had a history of schizophrenia, which had been well controlled until she discontinued medication because of being pregnant.
>
> E agreed to resume antipsychotic medication. However, her delusion about a devil inside her persisted, as did her bingeing and vomiting, until a brief course of psychotherapy revealed that an unresolved emotional problem was fueling her delusion. Ever since she had become pregnant, E had felt jealous of the attention everyone was paying to the fetus instead of to her. When she became psychotic, this feeling expressed itself via a delusion that transformed the fetus into a devil and the emotional nutrients into physical ones. When this became clear, the therapist spoke to family members, who began paying more direct attention to E and talking about the baby less. E stopped maintaining her delusional belief and was able to eat normally.

Prenatal Care

Staff in prenatal clinics can help prevent and recognize pregnancy denial by paying close attention to the psychological impact on women when a pregnancy is first diagnosed (Green and Manohar 1990). If pregnancy is diagnosed early and the woman appears anxious, sad, or stunned by the news, she can be encouraged to discuss her reactions. Supportive follow-up visits, including outreach, may be appropriate. If the pregnancy is diagnosed very late, after a period of initial denial, it can be useful to ask in a nonjudgmental manner about awareness of bodily changes, life circumstances, and emotional reactions to the pregnancy.

Ultrasound examinations can have a profound emotional impact on women who are denying pregnancies. The manner in which the examination is conducted can make the difference between having a therapeutic impact or having a traumatic one. Sometimes viewing a fetus via ultrasound can facilitate maternal role formation (Zabielski 1994). Even psychotic denial can be reversed by a sensitively conducted ultrasound examination (Cook and Howe 1984), although in women who have strong emotional reasons to maintain their denial, ultrasound images can be easily misinterpreted (Miller 1990). For most women, the emotional impact of ultrasound examinations is more therapeutic when a high level of information is provided; this can decrease anxiety and increase adherence to prenatal health recommendations (Cox et al. 1987).

> F, a 34-year-old woman, became pregnant after having sex with a man who was not her husband. She had had two prior pregnancies, each resulting in miscarriage. She cognitively acknowledged the current pregnancy but had a striking absence of emotional response or behavioral preparation. Under pressure from her husband, she finally attended a prenatal visit and had an ultrasound examination. On seeing the image of her fetus, she cried profusely. She was then able to tell her midwife about her grief at the prior miscarriages as well as her fear that this was not her husband's child. She entered therapy and was able to emotionally accept the pregnancy.

Parenting Assessment and Rehabilitation

Some mothers clearly wish to parent their babies after denied pregnancies, and others clearly do not. Many have mixed feelings and could use help in sorting out their wishes and identifying available support. Information about options such as adoption, foster care, and standby guardianships can be helpful.

Since parenting capability cannot be predicted on the basis of pregnancy denial alone, a comprehensive parenting assessment is indicated for women who have denied their pregnancies but want to raise their babies. Optimal assessments rely on direct, systematic observation of parenting behavior, as well as multiple sources of data (Jacobsen et al. 1997). Parenting questionnaires with adequate reliability and validity can also be helpful (Budd and Holdsworth 1996). Identifying areas of parenting weakness can lead to parenting rehabilitation efforts such as parenting classes, parenting coaching, parent support groups, and therapeutic nurseries. When there is a risk of gross neglect or abuse, child welfare agencies can become involved to protect the baby and provide additional resources for the mother.

Social Support

For many women, inadequate social support is a central reason for having denied their pregnancies. Helping a woman realistically assess her available social supports can be of great help. If a woman perceives that significant others will be punitive and rejecting, it is important not to automatically assume that this perception is accurate or inaccurate, but to help the woman assess its basis in reality. If the woman's family and friends cannot be adequately supportive, linking the woman to community support structures can supplement her existing support. Many women who have given birth after a denied pregnancy need help with practical decisions, such as whom to notify and whether to place a birth announcement in the newspaper (Berns 1982).

Family Planning

Discussing family planning can feel intrusive if premature, in that some women who have denied pregnancies are not yet ready to acknowledge that they are sexually active (Berns 1982). This is especially the case for women who were passive in acquiescing to sex. Women with psychotic denial may be especially capable of maintaining the belief that they did not have sexual relations and did not give birth. Nevertheless, women who lose custody of babies because of psychotic illness often maintain a tremendous longing for motherhood and can be at high risk of subsequent unplanned pregnancies (Apfel and Handel 1993). In such cases, a combination of psychoeducation about sexuality and psychotherapy to help in grieving losses can help some women feel better able to make active choices about sexuality and family planning.

Among women with psychotic disorders, the most common reason given for not using birth control, even while sexually active and not desiring pregnancy, is that they did not expect to have sex (Miller and Finnerty 1998). Although this suggests that long-acting, reversible contraceptive methods would be useful options, women with schizophrenia spectrum disorders are significantly less likely to have ever heard of such options than non–mentally ill women of comparable educational and socioeconomic background (Miller and Finnerty 1998). Education about these and other options may help to prevent the type of emotionally overwhelming pregnancies that necessitate psychotic denial.

Medicolegal Issues

A pregnant woman is normally assumed to be competent to make informed decisions about recommended medical interventions on behalf of herself and her fetus. However, a woman's competency to make medical decisions may be compromised by denial of pregnancy (Muskin et al. 1998). If, for example, a woman consents to psychotropic medication or electroconvulsive therapy for herself but is not able to evaluate potential risks to her fetus because she denies having a fetus, her capacity to make a fully informed decision may be impaired (Miller 1994). Cases such as this nearly always involve psychotic denial, since in cases of nonpsychotic denial it would be unusual for others to be aware of the pregnancy to the extent of offering care. Since psychotic pregnancy denial often waxes and wanes and is not absolute, it is important to ascertain what the woman decides when she is acknowledging her pregnancy. Collateral historians may be able to provide information about what the woman would have wanted had she been fully competent. In cases in which a woman has profound psychotic denial and is unable to provide informed consent, some courts will appoint a guardian ad litem to represent the fetus.

Another major medicolegal issue that arises in the context of pregnancy denial is involuntary hospitalization. This problem usually arises when a woman is in her third trimester of a pregnancy that she is psychotically denying. Without intervention, she may fail to recognize labor and may deliver precipitously without assistance. This has led some clinicians to characterize third-trimester psychotic denial as an acute psychiatric emergency (Slayton and Soloff 1981) that justifies involuntary commitment to a hospital (Soloff et al. 1979). Although this may seem like an extreme measure for a woman who is not otherwise posing harm to herself or anyone else, the risks of not hospitalizing may be great, as illustrated in the following case:

> G is a 32-year-old woman who was brought to an emergency room by her boyfriend after she sustained lacerations from having jumped over a fence without fully clearing the barbed wire. Her wounds were treated, and she was found to be in a manic episode with psychotic features. She was in the 36th week of an intrauterine pregnancy, confirmed by physical examination and ultrasound, but she denied being pregnant. She initially agreed to be admitted to a psychiatric unit and agreed to take antipsychotic but not mood-stabilizing medication. After 4 days, she was much less psychotic but remained manic. She intermittently acknowledged her pregnancy. At this point, she demanded to leave the hospital. Her boyfriend and her family members backed her up, promising to take care of her and threatening to sue hospital staff if they did not discharge her. She had no suicidal or homicidal ideation and no longer had the sort of delusional

thinking and impulsivity that had prompted her to try to jump the fence. Accordingly, she was discharged against medical advice. She promptly discontinued her medication. About a week after discharge, she was found by a neighbor wandering the streets holding a baby, still fastened to her umbilical cord, which was dangling from her body. The neighbor brought G and the baby to a hospital, where the baby was admitted to the neonatal intensive care unit in poor condition, having sustained brain damage from presumed hypoxia.

Decisions about involuntary commitment of women because of psychotic denial of pregnancy must be made on a case-by-case basis, taking into account the nature of the patient's symptoms, the patient's insight into her illness, her history of adherence to prescribed medication and other mental health treatment, and her social support.

Public Policy and Health Care Delivery

A relatively recent type of law aims to alleviate the pressures that underlie pregnancy denial and neonaticide. The first such law, known as "Childbirth Under X," was passed in France in 1941 (Bonnet 1993). The law allows women to deliver babies anonymously in hospitals. A woman using this provision puts an identification card in a sealed envelope, for use only if she dies in labor. The costs of her labor and delivery are paid with government funds. Babies born under these circumstances become wards of the state at birth and are then adopted. Women using this service who agreed to be interviewed appeared to have feelings and life circumstances that were very similar to those of women who committed neonaticide. Because of the apparent success of this program, similar programs and laws have begun to appear elsewhere, including in the United States (see Chapter 13: "The Promise of Saved Lives").

Conclusion

The manner in which a society supports or condemns pregnant women has a strong influence on how a woman deals with a pregnancy she cannot adequately manage (Hrdy 1999). Cultures and subcultures in which it is relatively easy to obtain birth control, abortions, and adoptions have lower rates of neonaticide. Societies in which women are harshly punished or rejected for becoming pregnant, seeking abortion, or abandoning babies are more likely to give rise to pregnancy denial and resultant neonaticide. Health care systems that include easily available pregnancy testing and prenatal care, along with outreach to high-risk groups like teenagers, can also decrease the likelihood of pregnancy denial (Berns 1982).

Teachers and school counselors should be knowledgeable about identifying mood and personality changes in adolescents who appear gravid or who camouflage their physical appearance with oversized clothing.

Women with chronic mental illness who are likely victims of nonconsentual sexual activity and rape are at enormous risk for psychotic denial of pregnancy.

Denied pregnancies are associated with sequelae such as fetal abuse, neglect, unassisted labor and delivery, failure to resuscitate, or overt neonaticide. The fact that fetal and infant morbidity and mortality rates may be reduced implies a need for further education of health care providers and educators for early recognition of women at risk.

References

Apfel RJ, Handel MH: Madness and Loss of Motherhood: Sexuality, Reproduction, and Long-Term Mental Illness. Washington, DC, American Psychiatric Press, 1993

Appelbaum PS: Why denial of physical illness is not a "diagnosis." Int J Psychiatry Med 28:479–482, 1998

Arboleda-Florez J: Neonaticide. Can Psychiatric Assoc J 21:31–34, 1976

Bartholemew AA: Repeated infanticide. Aust N Z J Psychiatry 23:440–442, 1989

Bascom L: Women who refuse to believe: persistent denial of pregnancy. Am J Maternal Child Nursing, May–June 1977, pp 174–177

Berns J: Denial of pregnancy in single women. Health Soc Work 7:314–319, 1982

Bluestein D, Rutledge CM: Determinants of delayed pregnancy testing among adolescents. J Fam Pract 35:406–410, 1992

Bonnet C: Adoption at birth: prevention against abandonment or neonaticide. Child Abuse Negl 17:501–513, 1993

Brezinka C, Huter O, Biebl W, et al: Denial of pregnancy: obstetrical aspects. J Psychosom Obstet Gynecol 15:1–8, 1994

Brozovsky M, Falit H: Neonaticide: clinical and psychodynamic considerations. Journal of the American Academy of Child Psychiatry 10:673–683, 1971

Budd KS, Holdsworth M: Methodological issues in assessing minimal parenting competence. J Clin Child Psychol 25:2–14, 1996

Causey AL, Seago K, Wahl NG, et al: Pregnant adolescents in the emergency department: diagnosed and not diagnosed. Am J Emerg Med 15:125–130, 1997

Chao YY: Denial in a primigravida whose pregnancy terminated with hydatidiform mole. Maternal-Child Nursing Journal 1:243–250, 1973

Cook PE, Howe B: Unusual case of ultrasound in a paranoid patient (letter). Can Med Assoc J 131:539, 1984

Cox DN, Wittmann BK, Hess M, et al: The psychological impact of diagnostic ultrasound. Obstet Gynecol 70:673–676, 1987

Eliot G: Adam Bede (1859). New York, Signet, p 507

Finnegan P, McKinstry E, Robinson GE: Denial of pregnancy and childbirth. Can J Psychiatry 27:672–674, 1982

Forchuk C, Westwell J: Denial. Journal of Psychosocial Nursing 25:9–13, 1987

Givens TG, Jackson CL, Kulick RM: Recognition and management of pregnant adolescents in the pediatric emergency department. Pediatr Emerg Care 10: 253–255, 1994

Green CM, Manohar SV: Neonaticide and hysterical denial of pregnancy. Br J Psychiatry 156:121–123, 1990

Hrdy SB: Mother Nature: A History of Mothers, Infants, and Natural Selection. New York, Pantheon, 1999, p 292

Jacobsen T, Miller LJ: Mentally ill mothers who have killed: three cases addressing the issue of future parenting capability. Psychiatr Serv 49:650–657, 1998

Jacobsen T, Miller LJ, Kirkwood K: Assessing parenting competency in mental ill individuals: a comprehensive service. J Mental Health Admin 24:189–199, 1997

Joyce K, Diffenbacher G, Greene J, et al: Internal and external barriers to obtaining prenatal care. Social Work in Health Care 9:89–96, 1983

Kaplan R, Grotowski T: Denied pregnancy. Aust N Z J Psychiatry 30:861–863, 1996

Kellett RJ: Infanticide and child destruction—the historical, legal and pathological aspects. Forensic Sci Int 53:1–28, 1992

Kent L, Laidlaw JDD, Brockington IF: Fetal abuse. Child Abuse Negl 21:181–186, 1997

Kinzl J, Biebl W: Disavowal of pregnancy: an adjustment disorder. Am J Psychiatry 148:1620–1621, 1991

Malviya S, D'Errico C, Reynolds P, et al: Should pregnancy testing be routine in adolescent patients prior to surgery? Anesth Analg 83:854–858, 1996

Marcenko M, Spence M, Rohweder C: Psychosocial characteristics of pregnant women with and without a history of substance abuse. Health Soc Work 19:17–22, 1994

McNeil TF: A prospective study of postpartum psychoses in a high-risk group, 3: relationship to mental health characteristics during pregnancy. Acta Psychiatr Scand 77:604–610, 1988

Miller LJ: Psychotic denial of pregnancy: phenomenology and clinical management. Hosp Community Psychiatry 41:1233–1237, 1990

Miller LJ: Use of electroconvulsive therapy during pregnancy. Hosp Community Psychiatry 45:444–450, 1994

Miller LJ: Pharmacotherapy during the perinatal period. Directions in Psychiatry 18:49–63, 1998

Miller LJ, Finnerty M: Family planning knowledge, attitudes and practices in women with schizophrenic spectrum disorders. J Psychosom Obstet Gynecol 19:210–217, 1998

Milstein KK, Milstein PS: Psychophysiologic aspects of denial in pregnancy: case report. J Clin Psychiatry 44:189–190, 1983

Mitchell EK, Davis JH: Spontaneous births into toilets. J Forensic Sci 29:591–596, 1984

Mothander PR: Maternal adjustment during pregnancy and the infant's first year. Scand J Psychol 33:20–28, 1992

Muskin PR, Feldhammer T, Gelfand JL et al: Maladaptive denial of physical illness: a useful new "diagnosis." Int J Psychiatry Med 28:463–477, 1998

Oberman M: Mothers who kill: coming to terms with modern American infanticide. American Criminal Law Review 34:1–110, 1996

Phipps S: The subsequent pregnancy after stillbirth: anticipatory parenthood in the face of uncertainty. Int J Psychiatry Med 125:243–264, 1985–1986

Pinker S: How the Mind Works. New York, WW Norton, 1997, p 421

Resnick PJ: Murder of the newborn: a psychiatric review of neonaticide. Am J Psychiatry 126:1414–1420, 1970

Rofe Y, Blittner M, Lewin I: Emotional experiences during the three trimesters of pregnancy. J Clin Psychol 49:3–12, 1993

Sable MR, Spencer JC, Stockbauer JW, et al: Pregnancy wantedness and adverse pregnancy outcomes: differences by race and Medicaid status. Fam Plann Perspect 29:76–81, 1997

Saunders E: Neonaticides following "secret" pregnancies: seven case reports. Public Health Rep 104:368–372, 1989

Seagull FN, Mowery JL, Simpson PM, et al: Maternal assessment of infant development: associations with alcohol and drug use in pregnancy. Clin Pediatr (Phila) 35:621–628, 1996

Slayton RI, Soloff PH: Psychotic denial of third-trimester pregnancy. J Clin Psychiatry 42:471–473, 1981

Soloff P, Jewell S, Roth L: Civil commitment and rights of the unborn. Am J Psychiatry 136:114–115, 1979

Spielvogel AM, Hohener HC: Denial of pregnancy: a review and case reports. Birth 22:220–226, 1995

Spinelli M: A systematic investigation of 16 cases of neonaticide. Am J Psychiatry 158:811–813, 2001

Strauss DH, Spitzer RL, Muskin PR: Maladaptive denial of physical illness: a proposal for DSM-IV. Am J Psychiatry 147:1168–1172, 1990

Uddenberg N, Nilsson L: The longitudinal course of para-natal emotional disturbance. Acta Psychiatr Scand 52:160–169, 1975

Wilkins AJ: Attempted infanticide. Br J Psychiatry 146:206–208, 1985

Zabielski MT: Recognition of maternal identity in preterm and fullterm mothers. Maternal-Child Nursing Journal 22:2–36, 1994

Chapter *6*

Neonaticide

A Systematic Investigation of 17 Cases

Margaret G. Spinelli, M.D.

The meeting was called to order by Miss Susan B. Anthony. A large and influential meeting of ladies and gentlemen held in the Hall of the Cooper Institute . . . convened to take such steps . . . to obtain the liberation of the unhappy young woman, Hester Vaughan[,] at present under sentence of death for infanticide. . . . The Platform was principally occupied by ladies who have been conspicuous in the Women's Rights movement. Hester Vaughan . . . had been ill and partially unconscious for 3 days prior to her confinement and a child was born. Hours passed before she could cry for assistance, and when she did it was to be dragged to a prison and sentenced to be hanged. . . . Miss Anthony continued to plead for the liberation of Hester Vaughan . . .

Working Women's Association Meeting
to protest conviction of Hester Vaughan
News report in WORLD, Philadelphia, PA, December 1868

Neonaticide, or infant murder on the day of birth (Resnick 1970), is often preceded by denial of pregnancy. Although neonaticide has been the target of recent media attention, it has never been studied systematically. Well-documented clinical case reports of neonaticide describe a presentation of pregnancy denial (see Chapter 5: "Denial of Pregnancy"), dissociative symptoms, or psychosis (Bracken and Kasl 1976; Brezinka et al. 1994; Finnegan et al. 1982; Green and Manohar 1990). In this chapter, I describe the first systematic investigation of women charged with homicide after alleged neonaticide. Using contemporary diagnostic criteria and the biopsychosocial model of psychiatry, I identify risk factors and clinical presentations that may shed light on mechanisms for treatment, rehabilitation, and education.

In a court of law, expert witness testimony must be founded on scientific standards that are recognized in the psychiatric community (see Chapter 9: "Postpartum Psychiatric Disorders: Medical and Legal Dilemmas"). The defense of women who are alleged to have committed neonaticide is limited to early and outdated literature. In this chapter, I suggest that common variables exist in a subset of these women. Similarities in history, presentation, and circumstances of pregnancy and delivery suggest a pattern of shared psychopathology (Spinelli 2001). The aim of this chapter is to encourage further systematic exploration. Using a contemporary framework for psychiatric diagnosis and treatment, I introduce a preliminary paradigm for understanding denial of pregnancy and neonaticide (American Psychiatric Association 1994; Resnick 1970).

The Interviews

I performed forensic psychiatric interviews with 17 women who experienced denial of pregnancy followed by secret unassisted deliveries. Sixteen of the women allegedly committed neonaticide, and the remaining woman allegedly attempted neonaticide. There was a notable similarity in presentation, phenomenology, and family dynamics.

All of the women were interviewed in the United States. Psychiatric interviews were requested by defense attorneys (7 of the cases), public defenders (6), departments of probation (2), a colleague in psychiatry (1), and a presiding judge (1). The purpose of the interviews was to determine the mental status of the accused at the time of the alleged offense. The goal of the evaluations was to determine whether grounds for defense existed or to propose a plan of treatment and rehabilitation in the case of juveniles. All of the women gave their informed consent and were cognizant of the purpose of the interviews.

Eleven women were Caucasian, 5 were African American, and 1 was Asian in origin. The women ranged in age from 15 to 40 years (mean = 23 years, SD = 8 years). Twelve women were from middle-income families, and five were on public assistance. Three of the women had children from previous pregnancies.

In an effort to provide some quantitative measure of dissociative symptoms, the Dissociative Experiences Scale (DES; Carlson and Putnam 1993) was administered to each woman. The DES is a valid, reliable screening instrument that rates general dissociative experiences before and during pregnancy. A mean DES score of 15–20 suggests increased risk for dissociative disorder.

Clinical Findings

The psychiatric presentations of the women who were alleged to have committed neonaticide share similar characteristics (Table 6–1). Secret, unassisted deliveries were associated with dissociative psychosis (in 10 cases), dissociative hallucinations (14), and intermittent amnesia at delivery (14) (Steingard and Frankel 1985; Van der Hart et al. 1993). The women experienced delivery as watching themselves in a depersonalized state with little or no pain. Their characterological pictures were framed in a family dynamic of role confusion, emotional neglect, denial, and boundary violations, as illustrated in the following case:

Table 6–1. Neonaticide and denial of pregnancy

Denied pregnancy
Minimal or no physical changes of pregnancy
Depersonalization/"autoscopy"
Dissociative hallucinations
Labor: unassisted, minimal or no pain
Intermittent amnesia
Brief psychosis (+/–)
Childhood trauma (+/–)
Poor insight and abstract ability
"Good girl"—no history of sociopathy
Childlike, infantile

Family dynamic
  Social isolation and suspicion of others
  Boundary violations
  Emotional neglect
  Isolated, rigid or overtly chaotic
  Parental relationships: strained, estranged, or even bizarre
  Father: intrusive and prone to jealousy
  Mother: cold and hostile

Note.   +/– = may or may not be present.

W, a 16-year-old high school student, delivered a full-term infant into the toilet of her family bathroom. During her pregnancy, she was depressed and unable to function at school. Despite her chaotic home, she was an honor student who was active in theater and basketball. Both parents abused drugs and alcohol and separated before she was born. F, her older brother of 6 years, protected her from her mother's abuse and kept boys at a distance. W shared a bed with him until she was 16 years old, when she moved into her mother's bed coincident with her pregnancy. Although the probation department suspected that F had impregnated her, W denied incest or his paternity. W was too frightened of her mother to disclose her pregnancy.

W describes dissociative hallucinations during pregnancy and delivery as a running commentary of voices inside her head. W explains, "I felt the pregnancy was not real. At times, the voice is me arguing with me and at other times, it is me arguing with my mother. 'W you should tell her.' Another voice disagrees: 'No W. Don't tell her because you don't know what she's going to do. Just go to her. No, don't think about it.' Then a mother-like voice warned, 'Bitch, I hate you. I'll kill you.'" When labor began, W attributed food poisoning to her abdominal pains: "I tried to feel the baby's heart beat. I thought she was dead. I panicked and threw the baby out of the window. I forgot about it until the police arrived. On the next day, it was like it never happened. I felt like I was asleep or like I was in a coma. I know I did it, but it did not feel like me."

During interview, W's mother said, "I never liked her. I don't know why." W denied physical abuse by her mother despite reports by relatives and child protection services.

This case describes a picture of pregnancy denial in a young unmarried adolescent—a "good girl" in a chaotic and dysfunctional family who fail to notice her pregnancy. She denied abuse despite official reports to the contrary. An almost painless delivery takes place in her family bathroom. Classical dissociative hallucinations in commentary represent the self and the dissociative other.

Denial of Pregnancy

Although every woman in this clinical sample denied the fact of her pregnancy, a spectrum of disavowal was described (see Chapter 5), and several themes were outlined. Five denied knowledge of their gravid state until the delivery itself. Twelve described intermittent awareness of the intolerable reality, which was subsequently recompartmentalized. One woman had psychotic denial.

For some, pregnancy had been conscious for a brief period and then was denied throughout pregnancy and even delivery. Others became aware of their pregnancy late in gestation, convinced that the delivery was only a miscarriage. Physical symptoms of pregnancy were absent or misinterpreted. Family members, friends, and even live-in boyfriends did not realize the women were pregnant.

Depersonalization

Depersonalization accounts for the unusually low level of pain. Twelve women denied awareness of pain, and 5 described pain as minimal or "not bad." They went through labor quietly in the family home while others were in adjacent rooms.

> On the evening of her delivery, J went through labor in the bathroom, a place that she describes as a "black tunnel." She watched herself, powerless to direct her body below to perform what she wanted. Her observing self could not influence her participating self. "I could hear myself scream, but sound was not coming out of my mouth."

Although depersonalization is described as a dissociative symptom, this phenomenon is also described as *autoscopy* (see Neppe and Tucker 1989). Autoscopy involves illusions or hallucinations of self (symptoms) that are assigned to the atypical psychosis. The double is not an imposter but another self that is colorless and transparent but with a defined outline.

Dissociation

Kluft (1990) describes dissociation as the internal struggle and confusion over the nature of one's self-representation or identity.

> C disclosed her pregnancy to no one, including her fiancé. She states that "now I find it hard to remember how I felt. I didn't realize something was wrong. It is not you these things are happening to. You push everything away with no conscious effort. On the inside, you desperately hope that someone else will recognize something is wrong."

Dissociative Hallucinations

The internal confusion over identity is frequently characterized as an internal conversation with another identified object (Kluft 1990). Dissociative hallucinations are interactive dialogues between the observing self and participating self that are not concerned with problem solving (Steinberg et al. 1991). Fourteen (82%) of the women experienced dissociative hallucinations as a commentary of internalized voices distinct from psychotic hallucinations, which are heard outside of the head. One woman recalled, "It was like I was a third party. They had control over my decisions."

Labor and Delivery

With the onset of labor pains described as symptoms of the "flu" or "food poisoning," the women expect only a bowel movement. Fourteen experienced amnesia for various aspects of the birth, which they reexperienced as a "dream or coma." When they resumed conscious awareness, they insisted the baby was dead. When the women were confronted with the unbelievable reality of the infant (Bonnet 1993; Brozovsky and Falit 1971), the usual dissociative defense was insufficient in the face of such trauma. Because the reality was intolerable, a brief dissociative psychosis occurred. On reintegration, they could not account for the dead infant. Although some may have killed the infant during the dissociative psychotic state, neonates born under such hazardous conditions without prenatal care or resuscitation are already in a perilous circumstance.

> On the night of her delivery, V attributed her abdominal cramps to menstruation. While in the shower, she described vaginal pressure and bleeding and "felt something come out." She reported minimal discomfort: "When I saw the baby's head and body, I did not realize it came from me. It did not hurt, and I did not feel unusual. I could see it but not feel it. It was not happening."

Dissociative Psychosis

The inability to mount a successful dissociative response may result in psychosis (Hollender and Hirsch 1964). Fifteen women experienced brief amnesia, 10 of these women described associated psychotic symptoms at the sight of the infant (Brezinka et al. 1994; Green and Manohar 1990). Once called "hysterical psychosis," *dissociative psychosis* is associated with amnesia and is experienced as a waking dream that cannot be differentiated from normal perceptions (Van der Hart et al. 1993). The ego's inability to cope with the trauma of delivery apparently causes a break with the very reality denied (Steingard and Frankel 1985). Such individuals with immature ego development use primitive defenses and are therefore predisposed to experience brief psychotic episodes.

Dissociative Experiences Scale

The mean (22.5 ± 7.8) DES scores (Carlson and Putnam 1993) of this small clinical sample support an increased rate of dissociative psychopathology before and during pregnancy. Twelve of the women (71%) had DES scores greater than 15, which suggests existing dissociative disorders. The unusually high DES scores for 2 women suggest malingering.

One woman, hostile at interview, refused to endorse psychopathology and had a score below the mean cut-off (6). Three other women had DES scores of 12, 14, and 14.33.

Family Dynamics

In each case the family's denial of the pregnancy supported existing psychopathology complicated by role confusion, boundary violations, and emotional neglect (Courtois 1988). Social isolation and suspicion of others were themes reported during patient and family interviews. Family dynamics were portrayed as explicitly chaotic or rigid and religious, seemingly intact to others. Interestingly, this picture is similar to that of abusive families, as described by Dietz et al. (1999) and Courtois (1988).

Parental relationships were strained, estranged, or even bizarre. Fathers were intrusive and prone to jealousy or abuse. Mothers presented as cold, hostile, and withdrawn or as absent due to physical illness, substance abuse, or psychopathology.

> Although sexual abuse is denied, S and her parents describe an intense relationship between S and her father. Her mother prefers to have them away as much as possible. S and her father feel "hated" by the mother and believe "she is nuts." S's father spends all his time at home, except mealtimes, in the barn, where S joins him for company. Paradoxically, the mother reports her and her husband's marital relationship as "good."

The inappropriate actions of S's father were illustrated during the interview when he moved a chair across the room and sat down with his knees touching the interviewer's chair. He had to be asked to return his chair to the former position.

Daughters were parentified substitutes for their mothers and yet presented as childlike and even infantile. College and other opportunities for growth and independence were discouraged. Most of the women were isolated except for having a superficial or chance relationship with the baby's father, who usually remained unidentified. Neediness and poor self-esteem made these women vulnerable to abusive relationships. Fourteen of the women were "good girls" with no history of sociopathy, problems with the law, violence, or irresponsible behavior. To the contrary, they were honor students, champion swimmers, and volunteers. Two older women had previous legal problems and/or a history of alcohol abuse.

Childhood Trauma

Nine of the 17 women (53%) reported a history of overt childhood sexual trauma; in 7 of the cases, the trauma was corroborated by independent sources. Nine of the 17 women (53%) reported physical abuse, while 11 (65%) experienced either sexual or physical trauma. Emotional abuse (Courtois 1988) was prominent in all homes. Many of these women, protective of abusive parents, idealized these relationships as "perfect," "good," or "close."

> Although B denied sexual abuse, her father was terminated for showing pornographic films to his adolescent employees.

Corpse

Many women demonstrated bizarre behaviors with their infant's corpse. Some made no effort to hide the corpse from authorities, whereas others placed them in dumpsters. Often, the woman kept the dead infant close to her. Some returned to bed with their dead infant, where they remained until discovered.

> Airport police arrested J for murder when she carried her dead baby in a knapsack, planning to bring her home to France.

> Fifteen-year-old B wrapped her baby in a towel and returned to bed. When her cousin asked what was on the bed, she replied, "It's a dolly."

> Although M denied psychotic symptoms, she transported her baby's corpse to a shared office file cabinet. After 2 weeks, the foul odor prompted the staff to pry open the locked file, where they found the putrefied and maggot-ridden corpse. During her interview at the sixth postpartum month, M was indifferent to the peculiar nature of her actions.

Cognition

In general, the women presented as much younger than their ages and possessed almost no ability to problem solve. They lacked abstract ability and insight into their dilemma. Judgment was poor. They had nonsensical or paradoxical attitudes toward pregnancy. Although school records were usually unavailable, most young women had limited intelligence, a lack of general knowledge, poor cognitive skills, and few resources for coping. Three had available school records with reported formal IQ; each had a Full Scale IQ of 84, which placed them in the 14th percentile, representing the low-average range of intellectual ability.

The Biopsychosocial Model

Dissociation/Trauma Paradigm and Denial of Pregnancy

Denial is an attempt to avoid an intolerable reality. Psychotic denial is a primitive defense commonly found in psychotic patients and, less frequently, in healthy adults under unusually severe stress (Slayton and Soloff 1981). Denial frequently occurs during major illness such as myocardial infarction. Denial of pregnancy (see Chapter 5) has been described in cross-cultural contexts, in incest victims (Silverblatt and Goodwin 1983), in psychotic women (Miller 1990), and in women with dissociative disorders (Van der Hart et al. 1991).

For a fact to be denied, prior knowledge of the fact must exist. When the women admitted even brief knowledge of their pregnancy, their denial was interpreted as a manipulation. Denial resulted when intolerable emotions were aroused by their conscious awareness of pregnancy and culminated in disavowal (Van der Hart et al. 1991). Pregnancy is intrinsically frightening for women with dissociative disorder. Janet (1907) suggested that patients rarely have a precise notion of what is wrong with them and consequently ignore their own dissociative symptoms. Janet emphasized *retraction of the field of consciousness* that limits their ability to focus on one idea at a time or to plan for options. They resort to the attitude of *la belle indifférence d'une hysterique*.

The findings in this small sample suggest that dissociative disorder precipitates pregnancy denial. Although these data argue for a common presentation, there is likely heterogeneity in the psychopathology of women who commit neonaticide.

Findings in this sample are similar to those of case reports of pregnancy denial, which describe similar phenomenology in a subset of neonaticidal women (Brezinka et al. 1994; Green and Manohar 1990; Spinelli 2001). However, cases published in isolation that use various interview techniques preclude reliable and replicable data collection. The presentation of pregnancy denial requires systematic investigation.

Brezinka et al. (1994) observed 27 women in an obstetrical environment who professed disavowal of pregnancy until term or the onset of contractions en route to the hospital. Although neonaticide was not the outcome for these women, pregnancy was denied until birth. Many of the women claimed to have no symptoms of pregnancy, whereas others attributed symptoms to other causes.

Brozovsky and Falit (1971) described "evanescent awareness" by adolescents from strict families who colluded in denial. The authors argued that when birth makes denial impossible, the adolescents respond with acute disorganization and psychosis, at which time they murder the infant.

Finnegan et al. (1982) described three cases of denied pregnancy with a "brief psychotic break at delivery." Most striking was the case of a 39-year-old woman who presented in labor and was told by the obstetrician that she was pregnant. She replied, "That's ridiculous," and then immediately delivered an infant who succumbed after 1 minute. Emergency resuscitation efforts by staff went unnoticed by the patient. She was discharged from the hospital after 3 days, denying pregnancy and delivery.

Bonnet (1993) described "unthinkable pregnancies" with similar findings in psychodynamic evaluations of 22 adoptive mothers—women who experienced denial of pregnancy only to interpret signs of labor as "food poisoning" or illness. Four women were accused of neonaticide. Consistent with this case series, the family dynamic described was one of neglect in violent or incestuous homes as well as failure to recognize the pregnancy. Sexual abuse was experienced by 20% of Bonnet's sample, compared with 53% of the sample described in this chapter.

Although vulnerable to ego disruption, these women maintain reality testing that breaks down under overwhelming circumstances (Hirsch and Hollender 1969). This sudden psychotic disintegration (Martin 1971) is associated with amnesia.

Because underlying reality testing is maintained, rapid reintegration follows (Bonnet 1993; Martin 1971) when reality is tolerable (i.e., the infant is dead). Psychosis and amnesia resolve, leaving the woman confused over the sight of the dead infant, who has succumbed without benefit of resuscitation or has been murdered by the mother.

Biological Model

The hypothalamic-pituitary-ovarian (HPO) axis influences biological substrates in the central nervous system (CNS) and end organs such as the ovaries (Wisner and Stowe 1997). On the one hand, the gonadal hormones regulate chemical events in the brain; on the other hand, CNS changes influence hormone fluctuations.

The concept of pregnancy denial is often met with disbelief because it is associated with the absence of physical signs and symptoms such as enlarged abdomen and breasts and amenorrhea. That "psychic stimuli may produce observable endocrine change " has been suggested by Gerchow (1957; quoted in Harder 1967) and others. Starkman and colleagues (1985) described a similar but reverse psychophysiological phenomenon in hysterical pregnancy or pseudocyesis.

Pseudocyesis is manifested when the desire for pregnancy induces the onset of pregnancy symptoms such as amenorrhea, lactation, colostrum secretion, increased abdominal girth, and the subjective experience of fetal movements (Cohen 1982). Moreover, an enlarged uterus and softened congested cervix have been detected on pelvic examination (Brown and Barglow 1971). These findings suggest underlying psychophysiological mechanisms, which may be common to both states, whereby pregnancy denial and hysterical pregnancy have similar neurohormonal underpinnings but opposite somatic manifestations.

Cohen (1982) hypothesized that CNS changes influence the HPO axis in pseudocyesis to inhibit follicle-stimulating hormone and luteinizing hormone, which suppress ovulation. At the same time, prolactin supports the persistent lutenization of the corpus luteum. This theory is supported when depletion of brain biogenic amines induces lactation and amenorrhea in humans and reserpine induces pseudocyesis in animals. The potential for similar but opposite neurohormonal processes may endorse denial of pregnancy as a "mirror image " of pseudocyesis.

Whether the denial and associated CNS changes are powerful enough to influence the biological manifestations of pregnancy is unclear. However, the fact that the HPO axis regulates estrogen and progesterone, both of which are implicated in the physical changes of pregnancy, and oxytocin "bonding hormone," which reverses rat infanticidal activity (Insel 1992), supports a psychobiological theory of pregnancy denial.

A Psychodynamic Paradigm

Freud (1893–1995/1955) suggested that hysterical psychosis is a failure of repression in response to a current stress caused by eruption of material that is wholly or partially out of awareness. In a transient hysterical psychosis (Hollender and Hirsch 1964), conflict is severe, environmental escape routes are barred, and there is an inability to manipulate or influence the factors contributing to the conflict situation (labor and delivery). The hysterical character has a limited repertory of responses available for coping. As anxiety mounts, an altered ego state, along with hallucinations or delusions, is experienced as a manifestation of ego disruption. This breakdown of ego boundaries impairs the ability to evaluate reality or to distinguish what is outside from what is inside.

Brozovsky and Falit (1971) suggested that neonaticide develops out of disorganized ego states when denial is so tenaciously clung to even when it is no longer tenable (upon the birth of the child). In Kleinian terms, mother is the "bad object." The girl identifies with the aggressor mother, while the infant represents the patient herself. She kills the infant—

what she has always feared would be done to her.

Bonnet (1993) provided a psychodynamic formulation for 27 cases of denial of pregnancy. She suggested that the women discovered the fetus when the mechanism of denial had become less efficient and decompensation resulted. Bonnet hypothesized that the presence of the fetus triggered the reemergence of traumatic childhood memories connected to sexuality and revealing sexual pleasure. The boundaries between the fetus and the psychic experience became fluid. Rather than confront the traumatic unthinkable past, they eliminated the fetus. They could not make the connection with their traumatic childhood and put it into words.

Conclusion

The preliminary data presented in this chapter suggest a method of systematic evaluation based on contemporary diagnostic criteria. Recognition that a diagnostic dilemma exists is the first step in the resolution of the diagnostic differential between dissociative pathology and sociopathy. Classification of symptoms with a common presentation and course suggests a need for phenomenological studies. Once psychopathology is identified, strategies for treatment and prevention can be devised. Such programs could mobilize support systems and facilitate family intervention, prenatal care, family planning, adoption alternatives, and parenting classes (Miller 1990).

Risk management is a concern for the professional who treats or testifies in these cases. Questions posed by the court may involve other living children or future pregnancies. Guidelines do not exist. In this case series, one woman had previously killed a neonate after a prior denied pregnancy. One woman is safely and successfully raising another child. Questions about treatment, rehabilitation, and parenting potential cannot be answered by systematically collected data. Decisions are based on clinical judgment and individual case evaluations.

Although this clinical inquiry is limited by the small sample size, it is the only sample of alleged neonaticides systematically evaluated and reported. The DES is a valid and reliable objective test that can be used to determine the risk for dissociative disorder. On the other hand, malingering is a primary concern in this population, for whom secondary gain plays a pivotal role. Use of the Structured Clinical Interview for Dissociative Disorders (SCID-D; Steinberg et al. 1991) should be considered in future studies. Objective personality, neurocognitive testing, and tests of personality, intelligence, and malingering should be performed.

In the absence of treatment, these women leave prison in their child-bearing years with the same psychopathology that brought them into the system. This investigation is intended to provide a preliminary framework for designing research strategies for development of clinical trials. Neonaticide remains a subject of both psychiatric and judicial debate. Further systematic and scientific inquiry is warranted.

References

American Psychiatric Association: Diagnostic and Statistical Manual of Mental Disorders, 4th Edition. Washington, DC, American Psychiatric Association, 1994

Bonnet C: Adoption at birth: prevention against neonaticide. Child Abuse Negl 17:501–513, 1993

Bracken MB, Kasl SV: Psychosocial correlates of delayed decisions to abort. Health Education Monographs 4(1):6–44, 1976

Brezinka C, Huter O, Biebl W, et al: Denial of pregnancy: obstetrical aspects. J Psychosom Obstet Gynecol 15:1–8, 1994

Brown E, Barglow P: Pseudocyesis: a paradigm for psychophysiological interactions. Arch Gen Psychiatry 24:221–229, 1971

Brozovsky M, Falit H: Neonaticide: clinical and psychodynamic considerations. Journal of the American Academy of Child Psychiatry 10:673–683, 1971

Carlson EB, Putnam FW: An update on the dissociative experiences scale. Dissociation 6:16–27, 1993

Cohen LM: A current perspective of pseudocyesis. Am J Psychiatry 139:1140–1144, 1982

Courtois CA: Healing the Incest Wound. New York, WW Norton, 1988

Dietz PM, Spitz AM, Anda RF, et al: Unintended pregnancy among adult women exposed to abuse or household dysfunction during thieir childhood. JAMA 282:1359–1384, 1999

Finnegan P, McKinstry E, Robinson GE: Denial of pregnancy and childbirth. Can J Psychiatry 27:672–674, 1982

Freud S: Studies on hysteria (1893–1895), in Standard Edition of the Complete Psychological Works of Sigmund Freud, Vol 2. Translated and edited by Strachey J. London, Hogarth Press, 1955, pp 203–240

Gerchow J: Die arzlich-forensische Beurteilung vor Kindesmonder-inner. Halle, 1957

Green CM, Manohar SV: Neonaticide and hysterical denial of pregnancy. Br J Psychiatry 156:121–123, 1990

Harder T: The psychopathology of infanticide. Acta Psychiatr Scand 45:196–245, 1967

Hirsch SJ, Hollender MH: Hysterical psychosis: clarification of the concept. Am J Psychiatry 125:909–915, 1969

Hollender MH, Hirsch SJ: Hysterical psychosis. Am J Psychiatry 120:1066–1074, 1964

Insel TR: Oxytocin—a neuropeptide for affiliation: evidence from behavioral, receptor autoradiographic, and comparative studies. Psychoneuroendocrinology 17:3–35, 1992

Janet P: The Major Symptoms of Hysteria: Fifteen Lectures Given to the Medical School at Harvard University. London, Macmillan, 1907

Kluft RP (ed): Incest-Related Syndromes of Adult Psychopathology. Washington, DC, American Psychiatric Press, 1990

Martin PA: Dynamic consideration of the hysterical psychosis. Am J Psychiatry 128: 745–748, 1971

Miller LJ: Psychotic denial of pregnancy: phenomenology and clinical management. Hosp Community Psychiatry 41:1233–1237, 1990

Neppe VM, Tucker GJ: Atypical, unusual or cultural psychosis, in Comprehensive Textbook of Psychiatry/V, 5th Edition, Vol 1. Edited by Kaplan HI, Sadock BJ. Baltimore, MD, Williams & Wilkins, 1989, pp 842–852

Resnick PJ: Murder of a newborn: a psychiatric review of neonaticide. Am J Psychiatry 126:1414–1420, 1970

Silverblatt H, Goodwin J: Denial of pregnancy. Bulletin of Birth Psychology 4: 13–25, 1983

Slayton RI, Soloff PH: Psychotic denial of third-trimester pregnancy. J Clin Psychiatry 42:471–473, 1981

Spinelli M: A systematic investigation of 16 cases of neonaticide. Am J Psychiatry 158:811–813, 2001

Starkman MN, Marshall JC, LaFerla J, et al: Pseudocyesis: psychologic and neuroendocrine interrelationships. Psychosom Med 47:46–56, 1985

Steinberg M, Rounsaville B, Cicchetti D: Detection of dissociative disorders in psychiatric patients by a screening instrument and a structured diagnostic interview. Am J Psychiatry 148:1050–1054, 1991

Steingard S, Frankel FH: Dissociation and psychotic symptoms. Am J Psychiatry 142: 953–955, 1985

Van der Hart O, Faure H, Van Gerven M, et al: Unawareness and denial of pregnancy in patients with MPD. Dissociation 4:65–73, 1991

Van der Hart O, Witztum E, Friedman B: From hysterical psychosis to reactive dissociative psychosis. J Trauma Stress 6:43–64, 1993

Wisner K, Stowe Z: Psychobiology of postpartum mood disorders. Semin Reprod Endocrinol 15:77–89, 1997

Chapter *7*

Culture, Scarcity, and
Maternal Thinking

Nancy Scheper-Hughes, Ph.D.

Maternal behavior begins in love, a love which for most women is as intense, confusing, ambivalent, and poignantly sweet as any they will ever experience.

Sara Ruddick (1980, p. 344)

So perhaps there is a middle ground between the two rather extreme approaches to mother love—the sentimentalized maternal "poetics" and mindlessly automatic "maternal bonding" theorists on the one hand, and the "absence of love" theorists on the other. Somewhere between these extremes lies the reality of maternal thinking and practice grounded in specific historical and cultural contexts, bounded by different economic and demographic constraints.

Nancy Scheper-Hughes (1992, p. 356)

Maternal practices always begin as a response to "the historical reality of a biological child in a particular social world."

Sara Ruddick (1980, p. 348)

This chapter is an abridged version of Chapter 8 of the author's book *Death Without Weeping: Mother Love and Child Death in Northeast Brazil* (Berkeley, University of California Press, 1992). Abridged and reprinted with permission from The Regents of the University of California and University of California Press. Copyright 1992, The Regents of the University of California.

T his chapter is about culture, scarcity, and maternal thinking. It explores maternal beliefs, sentiments, and practices as they bear on child survival on the hillside shantytown of Alto do Cruzeiro (Hill of the Crucifix). The argument builds on an earlier and controversial article I wrote on this topic (Scheper-Hughes 1985), which I have since restudied, rethought, and mulled over with the women of the Alto on three return field trips since 1987.

I trust I can do greater justice to the topic than when I began. If, however, I cannot establish here some basis for empathy, for a shared understanding of sentiments and practices that seem so very different from our own and therefore so profoundly disturbing, then I have failed. One difficulty for the reader is that over the years I have come to participate in the worldview expressed by these women. Their sentiments and practices now seem to me all quite commonsensical and predictable. I must struggle to recapture a sense of the initial "strangeness" so as to identify, at least initially, with the reader's possible reluctance to accept a set of practices driven by an alternative womanly morality, one that will seem quite foreign to many. It is a dilemma common to all ethnographic writing: how do we represent the "other" to the "other"? But here the stakes are very high indeed.

The ethnographer, like the artist, is engaged in a special kind of quest through which a specific interpretation of the human condition, an entire sensibility, is forged. In the act of writing about culture, what emerges is always highly subjective, partial, and fragmentary but also deeply felt. So-called participant observation has a way of drawing the ethnographer into witnessing a kind of human life that she or he might really prefer to avoid. Once there, the ethnographer may not know how to go about getting out except through writing, which in turn draws others into the process as well, making them party to the act of witnessing.

Because of the difficult subject of this research, I am forced to create a pact with the reader. These are not "ordinary" lives that I am describing. Rather, they often are short, violent, and hungry lives. Reading this report entails a descent into a Brazilian heart of darkness, in a town called Bom de Jesus. As this chapter begins to touch on and evoke, as Peter Homans (1987) noted, some of our worst fears and unconscious dreads about "human nature," the reader may feel righteous indignation. Conversely, what is an appropriate and respectful distance to take toward the subjects of my inquiry, one that is neither so close as to violate their own sense of decorum, nor so distancing as to render them the mere objects of anthropology's discriminating, and sometimes incriminating, "gaze"? I begin, as always, with stories, because storytelling, intrinsic to the art of ethnography, offers the possibility of a personal, yet respectfully distanced, rendering of events.

Mother Love and Child Death

The subject of my study is love and death on the Alto do Cruzeiro, specifically mother love and child death. What effects do deprivation, loss, and abandonment have on the ability to love, nurture, trust, and have and keep faith in the broadest terms? I treat the individual and the personal as well as the collective and cultural dimensions of maternal practices in an environment that is hostile to the survival and well-being of mothers and infants. I argue that a high expectancy of child death is a powerful shaper of maternal thinking and practice, as is evident, in particular, in the delay of attachment to infants, who are sometimes thought of as temporary household "visitors." This detachment can be mortal at times, contributing to the severe neglect of certain infants and a failure to mourn the death of very young babies. I am not arguing that mother love, as we understand it, is deficient or absent in this threatened community, but rather that its life history, its course, is different, shaped by overwhelming economic and cultural constraints. In its attempts to show how emotion is shaped by political and economic context as well as by culture, this discussion can be understood as a political economy of the emotions.

What I discovered while working as a medic in the Alto do Cruzeiro during the 1960s was that while it was possible, and hardly difficult, to rescue infants and toddlers from premature death, from diarrhea and dehydration, by using a simple sugar, salt, and water solution, it was more difficult to enlist the mothers themselves in the rescue of children they perceived as ill-fated for life or as better off dead. It was more difficult still to coax some desperate young mothers to take back into the bosom of the family a baby they had already come to think of more as a little winged angel, a fragile bird, or a household guest or visitor than as a permanent family member. And so Alto babies, "successfully" rescued and treated in the hospital rehydration clinic or in the crèche and returned home, were sometimes dead before I had the chance to make a follow-up house call. Eventually I learned to inquire warily before intervening: "Dona Maria, do you think we should try to save this child?" or, even more boldly, "Dona Auxiliadora, is this a child worth keeping?" And if the answer was no, as it sometimes was, I learned to keep my distance.

Later, I learned that the high expectation of death and the commensurate ability to face death with stoicism and equanimity produced patterns of nurturing that differentiated those infants thought of as "thrivers" and "keepers" from those thought of as born "already wanting to die." (Bhattacharyya 1983; Scrimshaw 1978). The survivors and keepers were nurtured, while the stigmatized or "doomed" infants were allowed to die *a mingua,* of neglect. Nonetheless, the mortally neglected infants and babies I am referring to here are often (although not always) prettily kept washed and combed, and their emaciated little bodies are dusted with sweet-smelling talcum powders. When they die, candles are often propped up in tiny waxen hands to light their way to the afterlife. At least some of these little "angels" have been freely "offered up" to Jesus and His Mother, although "returned" to whence they came is closer to the popular idiom.

Ambiguities of Mother Love: Lordes and Zezinho

In 1966 I was called on to help Lordes, my young neighbor, deliver a child. The baby was a fair and robust little tyke with a lusty cry. But while Lordes showed great interest in the newborn, she ignored Zezinho, an older child who spent his days miserably curled up in a fetal position and lying beneath his mother's hammock. Zezinho's days seemed numbered. I finally decided to intervene. When I took Zezinho away from Lordes and brought him to the relative safety of the crèche, Lordes did not protest. The crèche mothers laughed at my efforts to rescue a *crianca condenada* (condemned child). Zezinho himself resisted the rescue. The crèche mothers said, "If a baby wants to die, it will die." There was no sense in frustrating him so.

The boy finally relented; he began to eat with minimal interest. Indeed, it did seem that Zezinho had no *gosto*, no "taste" for life. Gradually, Zezinho developed an odd and ambivalent attachment to me. Once he became accustomed to it, Zezinho liked being held, and he would wrap his spindly arms tightly around my neck. As the time approached to return Zezinho to his mother, my first doubts began to surface. Could it be true, as the crèche mothers hinted, that Zezinho would always live in the shadows, "looking" for death, a death I had tricked once but would be unable to forestall forever?

When I returned to Bom de Jesus and the Alto in 1982 to be among the women who formed my original research sample, Lordes was no longer living in her lean-to but was still in desperate straits. Zezinho was now a young man of 17. Much was made of my reunion with Lordes and Zezinho. Zezinho laughed the hardest of all at these "survivor tales" and at his own near-miss encounter with death at the hands of an "indifferent" mother who often forgot to feed and bathe him. Zezinho and his mother obviously enjoyed a close and affectionate relationship, and while we spoke, Zezinho draped his arm protectively around his little mother's shoulders.

Love is always ambivalent and dangerous. Why should we think that it is any less between a mother and her children? And yet, it has been the fate of mothers throughout history to appear in strange and distorted forms. Mothers are often portrayed as larger than life, as all-powerful, and sometimes as all-destructive. Or mothers are represented as powerless, helplessly dependent, and angelic. Historians, anthropologists, philosophers, and the public at large are influenced by old cultural myths and stereotypes about childhood innocence and maternal affection as well as by their opposites. The "terrible" power attributed to mothers is based on the perception that the infant cannot survive for very long without considerable nurturing, love, and care, and historically that has been the responsibility of mothers.

Whenever we try to pierce the meanings of lives very different from our own, we face two interpretive risks. We may be tempted to attribute our own ways of thinking and feeling to "other" mothers. Any suggestion of radically different existential premises (such as those, for example, that guide selective neglect in Northeast Brazil) is rejected out of hand as impossible and unthinkable. To describe some poor women as aiding and abetting the deaths of certain of their infants can only be seen as "victim blaming." But the alternative is to cast women as passive "victims" of their fate, as powerless, without will or agency. Part of the difficulty lies in the confusion between causality and blame. There must be a way to look dispassionately at the problem of child survival and conclude that a child died from mortal neglect, even at the mother's own hands, without also blaming the mother— that is, without holding her personally and morally accountable.

Attributing "sameness" across vast social, economic, and cultural divides is a serious error for the anthropologist, who must begin, although cautiously, from a respectful assumption of difference. Here we want to direct our gaze to the ways of seeing, thinking, and feeling that characterize these women's experience of being-in-the-world and, as faithful Catholics, their being-beyond-this-world.

Seen in the context of a particular social world and historical reality, the story of Lordes and Zezinho conveys the ambiguities of mothering on the Alto do Cruzeiro, where mortal selective neglect and intense maternal attachment coexist. These same "neglectful" mothers can exclaim, as Lordes did, that they live only for their grown children, some of whom survived only in spite of them. In so doing, these women are neither hypocritical nor self-delusional.

Holding On and Letting Go

Sara Ruddick (1980) has suggested that although some economic and social conditions, such as extreme poverty or social isolation, can erode maternal affection, they do not kill maternal love. Her understanding of mother love carried resonances of Winnicott (1986) as she referred to the metaphysical attitude of "holding"—holding on, holding up, holding close, holding dear (Ruddick 1980).

But here I want to reflect on another set of meanings and practices of mothering. Among the women of the Alto, to let go also implies a metaphysical stance of calm and reasonable resignation to events that cannot easily be changed or overcome. I asked Doralice, an older woman of the Alto who often intervened in poor households to rescue young and vulnerable mothers and their threatened infants, "What does it mean, really, to say that infants are like birds?" She replied,

> It means that . . . well, there is another expression you should know first. It is that all of us, our lives, are like burning candles. At any moment we can suddenly "go out without warning" ["*a qualquer momento apaga*"]. But for the infant this is even more so. The grown-up, the adult, is very attached to life. One doesn't want to leave it with ease or without a struggle. But infants are not so connected, and their light can be extinguished very easily. As far as they are concerned, *tanto faz*, alive or dead, it makes no real difference to them. There is not that strong *vontade* to live that marks the big person. And so we say that "infants are like little birds," here one moment, flying off the next. That is how we like to think about their deaths, too. We like to imagine our dead infants as little winged angels flying off to heaven to gather noisily around the thrones of Jesus and Mary, bringing pleasure to them and hope for us on earth.

Perhaps we should say "hoped for" by Doralice, because she added this disclaimer: "Well, this is what we say, this is what we tell each other. But to tell you the truth, I don't know if these stories of the afterlife are true or not. We want to believe the best for our children. How else could we stand all the suffering?"

And so, a good part of learning how to mother on the Alto includes knowing when to *let go* of a child who shows that he or she wants to die. The other art is knowing just when it is safe to let oneself go enough to love a child, to trust him or her to be willing to enter the *luta* that is this life on earth.

A Criança Condenada

What does it actually mean to let go of a baby? What is the logic that informs this traditional practice? Alto mothers spoke, at first covertly, of a folk syndrome, a cluster of signs and symptoms in the newborn and young baby that are greatly feared and from which mothers (and fathers) recoil. Inevitably, premature death is in the cards for these babies, and parents hope that it will be a rapid and not particularly "ugly" death. They certainly do not want to see their little ones suffer. These hopeless cases are referred to by the general and euphemistic terms child sickness *(doença de criança)* and child attack *(ataque de menino)*. Mothers avoid repeating the specific and highly stigmatizing names or descriptions of the conditions subsumed under "child sickness" and "child attack." These include *gasto* (wasted, spent, passive), *batendo* (convulsed), *olhos fundos* (sunken eyes), *doença de cão* (frothing, raving madness), *pasmo* (witless), *roxo* (red), *pálido* (white), *susto* (soul shocked), *corpo mole* (body soft, uncoordinated), and *corpo duro* (body rigid, convulsed).

The infant afflicted with one or more of these "dangerous" and "ugly" symptoms is generally understood as doomed, "as good as dead," or even as "better off dead." Consequently, little is done to keep him or her alive. The sequelae of a folk diagnosis of child sickness may be understood as a *folk* tradition of passive euthanasia, not uncommon to the people of the Alto. The vast majority of all deaths occur in the first 12 months of life; the condemned child syndrome is in reality the condemned infant syndrome.

Difference and Danger: Stigma, Rejection, and Death in Other Cultures

I approach the topic of stigma as it is related to child attack and child death with some trepidation, for I do not wish to add to the burden of lives already pushed close to the margins of endurance. But fear and rejection of certain "condemned" babies result in infant and child death on the Alto do Cruzeiro. Stigma involves all those exclusionary, dichotomous contradictions that allow us to draw safe boundaries around the acceptable and the desirable in order to contain our own fears about sickness, death and decay, madness, and violence. These tactics of separation allow us to say that this person is *"gente,"* one of us, and that person is "other," barely human, if at all.

Cultural responses to defective newborns are varied. The African Nuer studied by E. E. Evans-Pritchard (1956) referred to the physically deformed infant as a "crocodile" child and to twins (another kind of birth anomaly) as birds. Few Nuer twins or crocodile infants survived, and when they died, Nuer said of them that they "swam" or "flew" away. Birds return (or are returned) to air, and amphibious infants return (or are returned) to water, the medium in which each really belongs.

Elsewhere, physically different and stigmatized infants may be rejected as "witch babies" or as "fairy children." Among the rural Irish of West Kerry, old people still speak of "changelings," sickly or wasted little creatures that the fairies would leave in a cot or a cradle in the place where the healthy human infant should have been (Eberly 1988; Scheper-Hughes 2000). Irish changelings, like Nuer bird-twins, were often "helped" to return to the spirit world from whence they came, in some cases by burning them in the family hearth.

Carolyn Sargent (1987) studied birth practices among the West African Bariba of the People's Republic of Benin, where until very recently a traditional form of infanticide was practiced to rid the community of dangerous witches held responsible for all manner of human misfortune. Witches were believed to present themselves at birth in the form of various physical anomalies, among them breech presentation, congenital deformity, and facial or dental abnormalities. Such infants were traditionally exposed, poisoned, or starved. When the Bariba came to live in ethnically diverse urban communities and to give birth in modern hospitals, the killing of stigmatized witch infants was, of course, prohibited. Instead, such marked infants now live, carrying their stigmas with them and suffering an inordinate amount of consequent physical abuse and neglect. Witch babies grow up into witch children and, later, into community scapegoats, blamed for all manner of unfortunate events.

Dorothy and Dennis Mull, a husband-wife, anthropologist-physician team, worked in the mid-1980s among the Tarahumara Indians of the Sierra Madre mountains in Mexico. The Mulls discovered a common Tarahumara belief that gazing at an unattractive deformity can cause *susto*, magical fright, and soul loss. The presence of physical abnormalities put the whole community at risk of serious illness, so that allowing a damaged neonate to die was understood as a kind of public health measure (Mull and Mull 1987).

In the Brazilian Amazon, infanticide was normatively practiced by some Amerindian peoples in the interests of social hygiene. Today, the Brazilian church and state intervene, as they do in most parts of the world. Nevertheless, Thomas Gregor reported that infanticide is still practiced today, although covertly, by the Mehinaku Indians in the case of twins, illegitimate births, or infants with birth defects. At birth each infant is carefully examined: "We look at its face, at its eyes, its nose, and at its genitals, its rectum, its ears, its toes and fingers. If there is anything wrong, then the baby is forbidden. It is disgusting to us. And so it is buried" (Gregor 1988).

Sacrifice and the Generative Scapegoat

Indeed, this is the very same advice that Dona Maria the midwife gives to Alto mothers in cases of suspected child sickness or child attack in a newborn. Dona Maria bases it on her own sad experience: "It is harsh to say this, but sometimes, I warn the new mother right away, 'This one we won't need to wash, no.'"

The afflicted infant or small baby is isolated. She or he will often remain hidden away in the folds of a too-large hammock. Although slowly starving to death, such babies rarely demand to be fed or held. Many such babies die alone and unattended, their faces set into a final, startled grimace—an ultimate *susto*—that they will take with them into their tiny graves. A mother's single responsibility is to thrust a candle into the dying infant's hands to help light the path on the journey to the afterlife. After the hurried burial of such a baby, the older children, who form the funeral procession, come home and change their clothes to remove all traces of the stigmatized illness.

I do not wish to suggest, however, that poor Brazilians are more prone to stigmatizing the sick or the different than we are. Social life in rural Northeast Brazil tends, if anything, to be more, rather than less, tolerant of human difference than elsewhere. The sickly and the disabled who survive childhood are, with few exceptions, well integrated into public and community life. Meanwhile, madness circulates freely in the marketplace and in the downtown plazas of Bom de Jesus in the form of known and tolerated village fools, clowns, and madmen and madwomen. There is little to exclude them from active participation in town life. What motivates the social exclusion and induced death of a *criança condenada* is not hate but sacrifice.

In a way, we can consider the offered-up angel-babies of Bom de Jesus as prototypic generative scapegoats, sacrificed in the face of terrible domestic conflicts about scarcity and survival. The Christian notion of the sacrificial lamb provides a means of deriving meaning from the otherwise "senseless" assertions women made to the effect that their babies "had" to die.

In such societies, where a 30%–40% mortality is expected in the first year of life, the normative practice of infanticide—or weeding out, as it were—the "worst bets" for survival enhances the life chances of healthier siblings. From the safe distance of the affluent first world, it is difficult to refrain from "child saving" efforts when our own cultural values promote the idea of the intrinsic right to life of each individual person born, no matter how malformed, how unattractive, or how frail. There is no intent here to discredit these humanitarian values, but rather to suggest that they are not universally shared and that they are context- and culture-specific. We might want to question the relatively greater stress (and value) placed on the rescue of newborns and very young children over the rescue of older children, adolescents, and adults in our society—values that I was unconsciously translating into practice in the Brazilian shantytown context.

Child Maltreatment

Korbin (1981) reported on cross-cultural patterns of child maltreatment and found that child battering was rare or absent in sub-Saharan Africa, in the South Pacific, among Native Americans in the North and South Pacific, and among Native Americans in North and South America. Conversely, Korbin noted in her introduction that intentional cruelty and sadism toward toddlers and older children seem to be phenomena of more technologically advanced industrial societies. The doomed neonate in traditional societies practicing infanticide is pitied, not hated. Some indigenous societies fail to recognize the sickly, deformed, or wasted infant as a fully human creature. In contrast, child abusers in industrial societies perpetrate malicious child battering as a hostile attack on the defective child.

I would not want the reader to confuse the Brazilian shantytown practice of "letting go" a weak or sickly child born of an ethos of survivalist triage with malicious child abuse in the United States that is sometimes directed against an ungainly, unattractive, slow, or disabled child. Rather than their behaviors being forced by economic exigency, the abusing parents in more affluent societies may simply feel themselves shamed or otherwise reduced by the presence of less than excellent or beautiful or "below average" children and may lash out in perverse anger at the "offending" child. It is also true, of course, that some parents are simply violent and abusive.

Conclusion

Anthropological thinking defies boundaries. Insights come to us by way of cross-cultural juxtaposition, making the strange seem familiar and the familiar seem strange. Cultural responses to birth defects are shaped by reproductive and parenting goals that are themselves influenced by bioevolutionary, demographic, political, economic, and ecological constraints. The ethnoeugenic infanticide practiced in some traditional societies in response to the birth of infants viewed as anomalous, different, and dangerous has all but disappeared in the contemporary urban context, and the vigilance of child protective service workers and clinicians has done much to eradicate mortal forms of selective neglect directed against abnormal children. Yet, the physical and psychological abuse of some of these stigmatized children remains a feature of societal life in the United States (Gil 1970).

But what of mothering in an environment like the Alto where the risks to child health and safety are legion—so many, in fact, that mothers must necessarily concede to a certain "humility," even "passivity," toward a world that is in so many respects beyond their control? Among the mothers of the Alto, maternal thinking and practice are often guided by another, quite opposite metaphysical stance—one that can be called, in light of the women's own choice of metaphors, "letting go." If holding has the double connotations of loving, maternal care (to have and to hold), on the one hand, and of retentive, restraining holding on or holding back, on the other, letting go also has a double meaning. In its most negative sense, letting go can be thought of as letting loose destructive maternal power, as in child battering and other forms of physical abuse. But malicious child abuse is extremely rare on the Alto do Cruzeiro, where babies and young children are often idealized as "innocents" who should not be physically disciplined or restrained. But letting go in the form of abandonment is not uncommon on the Alto, and an occasional neonate is found from time to time in a backyard rubbish heap.

But, ultimately, I remained frustrated. The folk category of child sickness was impossibly loose, fluid, elastic, and nonspecific. It was ambiguous. How could a mother be certain that she was dealing with a case of nontreatable *gasto* as opposed to an ordinary case of pediatric diarrhea?

It might be suggested, somewhat provocatively, that the current "epidemic" of child abuse (from which physically different and "unattractive" children suffer more than their share) may actually represent, in part, a paradoxical effect of the suppression of the former, traditional patterns of selective neglect directed against babies seen as ill-fated for survival. I have elsewhere explored the meanings and consequences of the transition from "traditional tolerant" to contemporary "child abuse tolerant" societies (Scheper-Hughes 1987). The differences between allowing certain neonates to die for economic, ecological, or "ethnoeugenic" reasons in a traditional society and the hostile battering of a stigmatized child in a modern industrialized society need to be emphasized. The two patterns are not only distinct but nearly mutually exclusive. They represent the difference between cultural norm and cultural pathology, between human exigency and malicious intent.

References

Bhattacharyya AK: Child abuse in India and the nutritionally battered child, in International Perspectives on Family Violence. Edited by Gelles R, Cornell C. Lanham, MD, Lexington Books, 1983, pp 107–118.

Eberly SS: Fairies and the folklore of disability: changelings, hybrids, and the solitary fairy. Folklore 99:59–77, 1988

Evans-Pritchard EE: Nuer Religion. Oxford, UK, Oxford University Press, 1956

Gil DG: Violence Against Children: Physical Child Abuse in the United States. Cambridge, MA, Harvard University Press, 1970

Gregor T: Infants are not precious to us: the psychological impact of infanticide among the Mehinaku Indians. 1988 Stirling Prize paper at the annual meeting of the American Anthropological Association, Phoenix, AZ, November 16–20, 1988

Homans P: Comments on Nancy Scheper-Hughes's "Mother Love and Child Death." Chicago Symposium on Culture and Human Development, Chicago, IL, November 6, 1987

Korbin JE: Child Abuse and Neglect: Cross-Cultural Perspectives. Berkeley, University of California Press, 1981

Mull DS, Mull JD: Infanticide among the Tarahumara of the Mexican Sierra Madre, in Child Survival. Edited by Nancy Scheper-Hughes. Dordrecht, the Netherlands, D Reidel, 1987, pp 113–132

Ruddick S: Maternal thinking. Feminist Studies 6:342–367, 1980

Sargent CF: Born to die: the fate of extraordinary children in Bariba culture. Ethnology 23:79–96, 1987

Scheper-Hughes N: Culture, scarcity, and maternal thinking: maternal detachment and infant survival in a Brazilian shantytown. Ethos 13(4):291–317, 1985

Scheper-Hughes N: The cultural politics of child survival, in Child Survival. Edited by Nancy Scheper-Hughes. Dordrecht, the Netherlands, D Reidel, 1987, pp 1–29

Scheper-Hughes N: Death Without Weeping: The Violence of Everyday Life in Brazil. Berkeley, University of California Press, 1992

Scheper-Hughes N: Saints, Scholars and Schizophrenics: Mental Illness in Rural Ireland, New Expanded Edition. Berkeley, University of California Press, 2000

Scrimshaw S: Infant mortality and behaviour in the regulation of family size. Population and Development Review 4:383–403, 1978

Winnicott DW: Home Is Where We Start From: Essays by a Psychoanalyst. New York, WW Norton, 1986

Part III

Contemporary Legislation

Chapter 8

Criminal Defense in Cases of Infanticide and Neonaticide

Judith Macfarlane, J.D.

In those unhappy cases of the death of . . . children, as is every action indeed that is either criminal or suspicious, reason and justice demand an enquiry into all the circumstances; and particularly to find out from what views and motives the act proceeded. For, as nothing can be so criminal but that circumstances might be added by the imagination to make it worse; so nothing can be conceived so wicked and offensive to the feelings of a good mind, as not to be somewhat softened or extenuated by circumstances and motives. In making up a just estimate of any human action, much will depend on the state of the agent's mind at the time; and therefore the laws of all countries make ample allowance for insanity. The insane are not held to be responsible for their actions.

William Hunter, M.D., F.R.S.
Read to the members of the British Medical Society, July 14, 1783

The killing of an infant by its own mother is an act that at once captivates and repels popular attention. Flying in the face of "mother love," infanticide both shocks common notions of decency and calls out for punishment at law. Yet, many infanticides are committed not by women

---

The views expressed in this chapter are those of the author and not necessarily those of The Council of The City of New York Office of the General Counsel.

intent on callously ridding themselves of their children but rather by women who are experiencing a psychosis precipitated by gross postpartum mental illness. That a woman suffered some form of mental illness at the time of the killing calls into question her criminal culpability.

Postpartum mental illness has been the subject of study for centuries. Modern debates center primarily on whether postpartum mental illnesses can properly be considered as clinical entities, separate from other mental disorders that may be experienced at any time by either men or nonpregnant women (e.g., schizophrenia, affective psychosis). Whatever answer results from this unfolding debate, the fact remains that observable, clinical symptoms of mental illness appear in some women during the puerperium. The degree of that mental illness runs the gamut from psychosis arriving on the heels of delivery to postpartum depression that may or may not be associated with psychotic symptoms (see Chapter 3: "Postpartum Disorders").

In some cases, the postpartum mental illness a woman suffers is so severe that it leads her to cause the death (either by affirmative act or by omission) of her newborn or infant, turning her not only into a subject of psychiatric interest but into a criminal defendant as well. In the United States, a woman accused of killing her newborn or infant is typically charged with some gradation of homicide. All homicide statutes contain a criminal intent requirement *(mens rea)* that the prosecution must prove beyond a reasonable doubt in order to obtain a conviction. For example, a murder statute applied to a woman who kills her newborn or infant may require that the prosecution show that she *intentionally* killed her infant or newborn. Depending on the facts of her case, her defense attorney may raise a number of defenses, such as involuntary act, diminished capacity, or insanity, in fighting the prosecution's intentionality claim. These defenses are used to show that at the time of the killing, the woman did not possess the level of intent to kill specified by the statute under which she is prosecuted or that she was unable to refrain from the impulse to kill because her mental faculties were undermined by mental illness, namely a postpartum mental disorder.

In reviewing the facts of any given case of infanticide or neonaticide, a defense attorney must take extreme care to ascertain whether his or her client was suffering from any mental illness at the time of the killing so that he or she may consider asserting a suitable defense to the crime. Clearly, the final determination of whether the defendant actually suffered from one of these disorders can be made and attested to only by a psychiatrist. However, the defense attorney is likely to be one of the first individuals to come into contact with a woman accused of killing her infant or newborn and will be sufficiently informed of the facts surrounding the case to suspect mental illness as a potentially exculpating factor.

Therefore, it is critical that the practitioner seeking to defend his or her client in such a case be familiar with the psychiatric attributes frequently apparent in cases of neonaticide and infanticide.

The aim of this chapter is to consider those mental illnesses consistently appearing in cases of neonaticide and infanticide within a framework of criminal law defenses in an effort to offer guidance to the defense attorney exploring available defenses. In this chapter, I pay particular attention to those features that are most critical to establishing a defense of diminished capacity, involuntary act, or insanity in a criminal trial. These disorders will then be applied to the above-mentioned criminal law defenses to illustrate how they may work to undermine the prosecution's claim that a woman intentionally killed her newborn or infant. A successful defense would result in acquittal, conviction for a lesser offence, or a verdict of not guilty by reason of insanity or guilty but mentally ill.

Since homicide statutes in American jurisdictions are distinguished only by degree, neonaticide and infanticide are not recognized as kinds of homicide but rather are terms used informally to designate the victim (see Chapter 1: "A Brief History of Infanticide and the Law" and Chapter 6: "Neonaticide"). In this chapter, I maintain a distinction between infanticide and neonaticide, not only to highlight the unique clinical qualities inherent in the two cases but also to identify the victim. The terms *postpartum depression* and *postpartum psychosis* are used to describe aggregate symptoms often present in women who commit infanticide.

Clinical Considerations in Neonaticide and Infanticide

Certain patterns have emerged from documented cases of neonaticide. Typically, mothers who commit neonaticide are teenagers or young women (Green and Manohar 1990). While neonaticides are most often committed by women between the ages of 16 and 38, close to 90% of the killings are committed by women under 25 years of age (Brockington 1996; Kaye et al. 1990). Another significant factor is the marital status of the mother: less than 20% are married (Kaye et al. 1990). These women usually have had no prior contact with the criminal justice system (Brockington 1996; Kaye et al. 1990). Studies indicate that women who commit neonaticide do not suffer from any preexisting mental illness such as schizophrenia or depression and typically are not suicidal (d'Orbán 1979; Green and Manohar 1990; Kaye et al. 1990; Saunders 1989). Even more striking than demographic similarities among women who commit neonaticide are the behavioral and psychological features apparent in this group. These features have been so consistent as to lead one group of investigators to view them as falling within a discrete "clinical entity" (Brozovsky and Falit 1971).

Certainly, the most significant similarity in cases of neonaticide is the denial of pregnancy "through psychotic or hysterical mechanisms" (Brockington 1996; Spinelli 2001). This denial occurs throughout the pregnancy and, in some cases, even continues after childbirth. Although in the case of a normal, albeit unsought, pregnancy the recognition of the pregnancy is often delayed, some women accused of neonaticide continue to disavow their pregnancy even through the childbirth itself (Brockington 1996; Finnegan et al. 1982; Jacobsen 1999).

Like neonaticide, infanticide horrifies our most basic sensibilities. However, it is clear that the postpartum mental illness suffered by some women leads them to kill their infants during a period of psychosis. At the outset, it is important to note that postpartum mental illness consistently evades tidy classification. Perhaps the most prominent reason for this resistance is the plasticity of the illness and the waxing and waning of its presentation: psychotic symptoms such as delusions and hallucinations may abruptly surface, followed by periods of deep depression, only to be replaced with psychoses.

The delusions in postpartum psychotic depression are usually related to pregnancy and childbirth are often accompanied by suspicion and themes of possession (Attia et al. 1999; Brockington 1996; Hamilton et al. 1992). These delusions, coupled with homicidal ideation (Wisner et al. 1994), present great danger to the newborn or infant. Examples of delusions in these cases include the woman's belief that she is being controlled by outside forces, that her thoughts are not her own and are inserted into her mind by other people or beings, that the infant is the devil incarnate, that the baby has not yet been born and is still within the womb, and that the child is going to be kidnapped.

Hallucinations are also extremely common in these cases (Attia et al. 1999; Brockington 1996; Hamilton et al. 1992; Sneddon 1992). These hallucinations are dangerous because they frequently involve themes regarding the death or murder of the infant (see Chapter 3). Hallucinations may be auditory, visual, tactile, or olfactory (Attia et al. 1999). Command hallucinations, typically auditory, may direct the woman to kill herself or her infant. Visual hallucinations can take the form of, for example, a smoke- or fire-filled room and can lead the woman to believe that her baby will die if not rescued, causing her to throw her baby in water in an attempt to save him or her. As is the case with delusional thinking, hallucinations can act as the precipitating event leading to the death of an infant when a mother acts on the basis of those hallucinations.

Perhaps the most remarkable aspect of postpartum psychotic depression is its lability. Symptoms are those of an organic psychosis associated with confusion, delirium, and marked mood changes characteristic of depression or panic (Attia et al. 1999; Hamilton 1992).

Neonaticide and Infanticide as Criminal Acts

Punishment for neonaticide and infanticide is almost as old as the crimes themselves. At first widely accepted (if not encouraged) on eugenic grounds (Kumar and Marks 1992) and pressures of "overcrowding and overpopulation" (Kaye et al. 1990), infanticide slowly became the subject of legal censure. Arguably more a mechanism for regulating the sexual behavior of women than for curtailing high rates of infant deaths at the hands of their mothers, neonaticide and infanticide prosecutions yielded varied punishments, from diets of bread and water for 1 year (Kumar and Marks 1992) to penance terms of 15 years, public whippings (Brockington 1996), or execution.

In countries such as England and Canada, women accused of neonaticide or infanticide are prosecuted under statutes that specifically address those crimes. Prosecution of women under these statutes has resulted in lenient sentencing, with probation and psychiatric treatment as common outcomes (Oberman 1996). Indeed, no woman found guilty of infanticide has been incarcerated in England for over 50 years (Barton 1998). Similar statutes making infanticide a lesser crime than murder have been enacted around the world: Austria, Colombia, Finland, Greece, India, Italy, Korea, New Zealand, New South Wales, the Philippines, Tasmania, Turkey, and Western Australia all have statutes whose effect is to recognize infanticide as a less culpable form of homicide (Oberman 1996).

In the United States, early laws regarding infanticide focused primarily on determining punishment, usually quite harsh, for infanticidal mothers. The gradual evolution from harsh punishment in cases of infanticide to more lenient treatment of these women, similar to those reforms in England and across the world, has not yet occurred in American jurisdictions. The failure of American law to evolve toward a more lenient treatment of infanticidal women reflects a larger problem than simple ambivalence toward how these women are treated by the criminal justice system, although that is certainly a factor. As a nation comprising numerous autonomous states, no single sweeping "reducing" statute comparable to the amended and expanded British Infanticide Act of 1938 can be established, since each state has the power to adopt criminal laws within its jurisdiction as it sees fit. Hence, unlike their British counterparts, American mothers accused of killing their infants have never enjoyed a single law uniformly applied throughout the United States that automatically reduces the degree of homicide in cases of infanticide or neonaticide from murder to manslaughter. To date, no American state has a statute similar to the British Infanticide Act. Thus, in cases in which a woman has been suspected of killing her infant or newborn, criminal charges have ranged from first-degree murder, a felony, to the unlawful disposal of a corpse, a misdemeanor (Oberman 1996).

Since no de jure acknowledgment of the special nature of these killings and their relationship to postpartum mental illness exists in the United States, American women have had to expose that reality themselves on a case-by-case basis. That is, in order to submit evidence that would tend to negate the prosecution's claim that she acted with an intent to kill, an American woman accused of killing her newborn or infant while suffering from a postpartum mental illness must raise a defense such as insanity or diminished capacity. In the following subsection, I discuss the treatment of neonaticide and infanticide in American courts by way of several case studies.

Neonaticide in the Courts

Despite its relatively common occurrence, neonaticide has generated little case law. One explanation for this dearth may be that the bodies of dead newborns are rarely discovered because of the secret nature of their disposal. Another explanation may be that a neonaticide is difficult to attribute to any one person when the pregnancy was not, for whatever reason, disclosed or apparent to others. Indeed, one researcher was able to give the identity of the mother of a dead and discarded newborn in fewer than half of 62 cases (Brockington 1996). Many neonaticides remain unpublicized because the cases disappear through the pretrial plea-bargaining process or because of poor media coverage (Oberman 1996, p. 26). Even when cases are decided and appealed, the court may have failed to issue a written opinion. Finally, the "scarcity of appeals in these cases may reflect . . . that the outcomes are relatively lenient" (Oberman 1996). Given the stakes involved in a retrial, a woman convicted of neonaticide who is sentenced to community service, probation, or counseling has no real incentive to appeal. The following is a summary of two reported cases of neonaticide.

> Having complained of intense menstrual cramps, a 15-year-old, Ms. Doss, gave birth alone in the bathroom of her home (her mother was at the store buying menstrual provisions for her daughter). When Doss's mother

returned home, she heard small cries coming from the kitchen. She discovered a newborn baby wrapped in plastic and placed on top of a trash can. Doss's mother promptly brought her daughter and the newborn to the hospital. At the hospital, the newborn died of multiple stab wounds inflicted to its chest.

At her trial, Doss claimed that she had been unaware of her pregnancy until she began her eighth month because she had continued to menstruate until that point. Her mother also denied knowledge of the pregnancy. The trial court concluded that the wounds had not occurred as a result of her attempts to detach the umbilical cord from the newborn and that Doss had intentionally stabbed the newborn. Doss was convicted of first-degree murder and sentenced to 30 years in prison.

On appeal to the Appellate Court of Illinois (People v. Doss 1987), Doss challenged her conviction on several grounds. First, she contended that the prosecution had supplied insufficient evidence to support a conviction of first-degree murder and that she should instead have been convicted of involuntary manslaughter, which carried a far less lengthy sentence. The court rejected her argument, stating that the Illinois first-degree murder statute required a mental state that showed that "in performing the acts that cause[d] death, [the] accused kn[ew] that such acts create[d] a strong probability of death or great bodily harm" (People v. Doss 1987). The court construed the statute to mean that the prosecution needed to show not that Doss had specifically intended to kill the newborn, but rather that the action was "voluntarily and willfully done" and would naturally lead to the newborn's death (People v. Doss 1987). The court concluded that the stab wounds were not the result of an attempt to detach the umbilical cord, but instead had been intentionally dealt by Doss and constituted sufficient evidence to support that the acts leading to the newborn's death had been "voluntarily and willfully done."

Doss also argued that her conviction should be reduced from first-degree to second-degree murder on a justification theory. Doss asserted that the "shock and fear of family disgrace" (People v. Doss 1987) created by the delivery and birth of the newborn led her to unreasonably believe that the killing of the newborn was justified. The court held that a reduction of Doss's conviction of first-degree murder to second-degree murder under a justification theory could occur only if she was "able to prove that either she was acting under a sudden and intense passion resulting from serious provocation, or she believed the circumstances, if they existed, justified the killing" (People v. Doss 1987). However, the court dismissed her argument that she was acting under the heat of passion once confronted by the reality of the birth, holding that "a young child cannot cause the serious provocation required of second-degree murder" (People v. Doss 1987). Doss's conviction was upheld.

Bernadette Reilly gave birth unattended to a baby girl. She spent the remainder of the day of the delivery in her bed, weak from continuous bleeding. Her landlady persuaded her to go to a hospital later that evening. On examination, hospital staff realized that she had just given birth hours before. Reilly denied having given birth to the hospital staff and the police. A subsequent search of her room unearthed her dead newborn wrapped in a garbage bag, along with a pair of scissors and a book on childbirth. During subsequent questioning, Reilly admitted to giving birth to the child but that the baby did not move or cry after being born. Reilly said that she shook the baby to try to revive it, but it never awoke. An autopsy revealed that the newborn died from injuries inflicted by a blunt object. Reilly was charged with criminal homicide and child endangerment.

At her trial, Reilly asserted the insanity defense and presented two psychiatrists who each "testified that Reilly suffered a brief reactive psychosis at or immediately following the birth, causing her to break from reality" (Commonwealth of Pennsylvania v. Reilly 1988). Both psychiatrists concluded that Reilly was insane at the time of the newborn's death. The prosecution did not present any evidence rebutting Reilly's insanity defense. Nonetheless, her defense was rejected by the trial court, and she was found guilty of third-degree murder and child endangerment. She was sentenced to 3–10 years in prison. The Supreme Court of Pennsylvania affirmed her conviction.

Infanticide in the Courts

The earliest reported case in which a postpartum mental disorder was used as the basis of an insanity defense is the 1951 case of *State v. Skeoch*:

Dorothy Skeoch was accused of suffocating her 6-day-old baby when he was found dead with a diaper tied around his neck. Skeoch was charged with murder. Initially, Skeoch maintained that a robber had broken into her house, whereupon she fainted and awoke to find some of her possessions stolen and her baby with a diaper tightly tied around his neck. However, when further questioned by the police, Skeoch confessed to killing the infant. At her trial, Skeoch's husband and mother-in-law testified that she appeared to be "insane" immediately after the birth of the infant and on the day of his death. Moreover, a neurologist and psychiatrist testified that she was suffering from "postpartum psychosis with infanticide, a mental disorder that frequently occurs with the delivery of a child." (State v. Skeoch 1951)

Notwithstanding this testimony, Skeoch was convicted of murder and sentenced to 14 years in prison. On appeal, her conviction was reversed by the Supreme Court of Illinois on the grounds that the prosecution failed to rebut Skeoch's claim of insanity. The court held that even though there is a governing presumption of sanity in all cases, once Skeoch admitted evidence sufficient to raise a reasonable doubt as to her sanity at the time of the crime, the presumption of sanity no longer applied, and the State was required to show that she was sane beyond a reasonable doubt as a necessary element of the crime (State v. Skeoch 1951).

The following summarizes a widely publicized California case tried in 1987:

> Sheryl Massip threw her 6-week-old infant in front of a moving car. When the driver of the car swerved and avoided the baby, Massip drove over the infant herself. She threw the corpse in a garbage can. At first, Massip told the police that her infant had been kidnapped, but later she confessed to having run over her infant.
>
> At trial, it was revealed that Massip had been suffering from extreme mental illness in the 6 weeks after the birth of her child. Her infant cried frequently, causing Massip to be confused and to have feelings of worthlessness and inadequacy because she could neither determine the cause of his crying nor make his crying stop. After experiencing a "seizure," Massip spent a weekend at her mother's house, where she experienced visual and auditory hallucinations. She continued to have these hallucinations upon her return home. On the day of the killing, she took her son on a walk. While walking, "she heard voices telling her the baby was in pain and to put him out of his misery; she felt as if she were in a tunnel and everything was moving slowly. She was watching her own actions from outside herself" (People v. Massip 1990). Massip then threw the infant in the path of an oncoming car. When the car avoided the baby, Massip "picked him up and walked with him, but did not remember what he looked like. At this time she saw him as a doll or an object, not a person" (People v. Massip 1990). She brought the baby to her own car and ran him over.

Massip was charged with second-degree murder. She entered two pleas, not guilty and not guilty by reason of insanity. After 6½ days of deliberation, the jury found her guilty of second-degree murder, finding that she was sane at the time of the offense (Barton 1998). Massip moved for a new trial, and the trial court reduced her conviction from second-degree murder to voluntary manslaughter. The court additionally "set aside the [previous] finding of sanity, entering a new finding of not guilty by reason of insanity" (People v. Massip 1990). This judgment was affirmed, and Massip was required to attend an outpatient treatment program.

Criminal Law Defenses

Because our criminal law requires that a culpable state of mind be proven to justify a conviction, defenses such as insanity, diminished capacity, and the involuntary act are available to a defendant to counter the prosecution's proof of criminal intent and either negate the *mens rea* (guilty mind) element of the crime charged, show that the defendant did not know what she or he was doing at the time of the act, or simply show that the defendant was unable to control her or his behavior. Evidence to this effect ultimately compels the trier of fact (the judge or jury hearing the case) to decide that the defendant's true state of mind at the time of the offense was not criminally blameworthy and therefore does not meet the mental element required for a conviction (Table 8–1).

Table 8–1. Criminal law defenses

Defense	Requirements
Insanity	
M'Naghten Cognitive focus	At the time of the crime, the defendant suffered a mental disease, disability, or defect that caused her to: Not know right from wrong; **OR** Fail to appreciate the nature and quality of her actions.
Model Penal Code Cognitive / volitional focus	At the time of the crime, the defendant suffered from a mental disease, disability, or defect that caused her to: Lack substantial capacity to appreciate the criminality of her conduct; **OR** Fail to conform her conduct to the requirements of the law.
Involuntary act	At the time of the crime, the defendant suffered from a mental disease, defect, or disability that caused conduct that was not a product of her deliberate effort.
Diminished capacity	At the time of the crime, the defendant suffered from a mental disease, defect, or disability. Since she suffered from such as disease, defect, or disability at the time she committed the act, she was incapable of forming the intent (e.g., specific intent to kill, malice aforethought, premeditation) required by the statute under which she is prosecuted.

The literature on postpartum mental illness makes a convincing case that women who kill their newborns and infants suffer from distinct and recognized mental disorders at the very time of the killing. These disorders bear directly on the mother's ability to form the *mens rea* required for a conviction under any given homicide statute. Successful use of the involuntary act, diminished capacity, or insanity defenses works to undermine the proof of *mens rea* mounted by the prosecution and thus reduces the offense under which the defendant can be convicted, serves as a mitigating factor at the time of sentencing, or even leads to acquittal. These defenses are *affirmative defenses*, which place the burden on the defendant to raise the defense and, depending on the jurisdiction, to prove it by some considerable degree (usually by a preponderance of the evidence) (Robinson 1984).

Involuntary Act

The involuntary act defense, or automatism, is presented when a criminal act occurred at the precise moment when, because of a physical or mental disability, the person accused of the criminal act was unable to control her or his actions. A typical example of a crime committed involuntarily is the person who kills while sleepwalking. A defendant who asserts the involuntary act defense is essentially claiming that the action causing the criminal act was performed without a connection between her muscles and her mind (Robinson 1984). Although the specific formulation of the defense differs between jurisdictions, it can be summarized as such: "An actor is excused for his conduct constituting an offense if, as a result of (1) any mental or physical disability, (2) the conduct is not a product of the actor's effort or determination" (Robinson 1984, p. 260). The involuntary act defense is recognized in almost every American jurisdiction (Robinson 1984).

It is critical that the defense establish proof of a disability, as it makes the punishable conduct "blameless" because it was in no way intended by the actor. However, since the number of physical and mental disabilities that may bring about an involuntary act is virtually limitless, an exhaustive list of qualifying disabilities does not exist (Robinson 1984). This lack of specificity

> might be justified on the ground that the lack of control in many involuntary act cases is so complete and dramatic that no other requirement is needed to assure blameworthiness. It is irrelevant whether the muscular movement comes from a grand mal seizure or from a reflex action. Such total lack of volition is an obvious and convincing ground for exculpation. (Robinson 1994, pp. 897–898)

Hence, the disability's severity is scrutinized to determine whether the lapse in control rises to a level that makes the defendant blameless. Instances of unconsciousness (People v. Newton 1970) and dissociative states (People v. Lisnow 1978) have been accepted by courts as severe enough to satisfy the disability requirement imposed by the involuntary act defense (Robinson 1984).

Diminished Capacity

The diminished capacity defense involves the defendant's use of a mental disease or defect to negate the *mens rea* element of the crime charged (Robinson 1984). Diminished capacity is a failure-of-proof defense, meaning that the mental disease or defect claimed by the defendant made it impossible for her or him to formulate or possess the mental state required for a conviction under the statute with which she or he is charged (Robinson 1984). Consider, for example, a woman who is charged with first-degree murder for the death of her 6-week-old infant in a state that defines first-degree murder as premeditated. It may be shown that during the 6 weeks leading up to the infant's death and during the infant's death itself, the woman was experiencing severe hallucinations and psychoses, making it impossible for her to plan and premeditate her infant's murder. When a defense of diminished capacity is successful, the final result is the mitigation or elimination of criminal culpability, since the prosecution cannot show that the defendant possessed the requisite criminal intent beyond a reasonable doubt (Barton 1998). Thus, diminished capacity is employed by a defendant to show that, because of a mental disease or defect, she did not have capacity to form the intent specified by criminal statute under which she is charged, thereby negating the *mens rea* element of the crime.

In most cases, however, the diminished capacity defense offers but a partial victory, since most homicide statutes engulf lesser-included offenses that contain "lesser culpability requirements" (Robinson 1982, p. 475). Therefore, the failure of proof of the greater offense often leads to a conviction based on the lesser offense (e.g., murder to voluntary manslaughter). In the rare instance when "there is no lesser included offense, or if the mental illness also negates an element of any lesser included offense, the mental illness will prevent conviction altogether" (Robinson 1982, p. 476).

Insanity

Although controversial, the insanity defense, in one form or another, is recognized by all American jurisdictions. In honoring insanity as an excuse to criminal conduct, our "society has recognized . . . that none of the three asserted purposes of the criminal law—rehabilitation, deterrence and retribution—are satisfied when the truly irresponsible, those who lack substantial capacity to control their actions, are punished" (United States v. Freeman 1966). Thus, despite frequent and vehement attacks, such as the one mounted in the wake of the Hinckley verdict of not guilty by reason of insanity after Hinckley's shooting of President Ronald Reagan, the insanity defense has been preserved and is generally seen as essential in a system that punishes only when moral responsibility is present.

The two main formulations of the insanity defense used by American jurisdictions are the *M'Naghten* test (M'Naghten's Case 1843) and the Model Penal Code/American Law Institute (MPC) test (Model Penal Code 1985).

M'Naghten

The *M'Naghten* test, or the "right and wrong test," was derived from the landmark English case of the same name decided in 1843. Under *M'Naghten*, to raise a successful insanity defense, the defendant must clearly prove that "at the time of the committing of the act, the party accused was laboring under such a defect of reason, from disease of the mind, as not to know the nature and quality of the act he was doing; or, if he did know it, that he did not know he was doing what was wrong" (M'Naghten's Case 1843). The focus of the *M'Naghten* test involves nothing other than the cognitive capacity of the defendant to appreciate her actions. A defendant is judged insane only if she can prove that, because of a mental disability, she either did not know right from wrong at the time she committed the ultimately criminal act or did not understand the nature and quality of the act.

Despite criticisms that the test is too rigid, many states continue to use the *M'Naghten* rule as their test for insanity. Some few jurisdictions, such as Tennessee, have broadened *M'Naghten* by adding the "irresistible impulse test," which "relieve[s] [one] of criminal responsibility when his mental condition is such as to deprive him of his will power to resist the impulse to commit the crime" (Graham v. State 1977).

Model Penal Code

The MPC provides that "[a] person is not responsible for criminal conduct if at the time of such conduct as a result of mental disease or defect he lacks substantial capacity either to appreciate the criminality [wrongfulness] of his conduct or to conform his conduct to the requirements of law" (Model Penal Code 1985). The MPC approach has been adopted by about half of the states and the majority of the federal circuit courts of appeal (Robinson 1984). The approach to insanity in the MPC enjoys widespread appeal because it "views the mind as a unified entity and recognizes that mental disease or defect may impair its functioning in numerous ways" (United States v. Freeman 1966), as opposed to the compartmentalizing vision of *M'Naghten*. Thus, one prong of the MPC test focuses on *cognitive* aspects of behavior, while the other focuses on *volitional* aspects of behavior.

Therefore, evidence that a mental disorder suffered at the very moment of the crime caused the defendant to lack the substantial capacity to appreciate the wrongfulness of her or his conduct satisfies the cognitive aspect of the MPC test. Alternatively, proof that a mental disease or defect left the defendant unable to conform her or his conduct to the requirements of the law, notwithstanding any recognition on the defendant's part that what she or he was doing was wrong, satisfies the volitional prong of the MPC test. The satisfaction of *either* the cognitive or the volitional prong is grounds for an insanity verdict in a MPC jurisdiction.

Involuntary act, diminished capacity, and insanity are defenses that can be used by a woman accused of causing the death of her infant or newborn while she was suffering from a postpartum mental disorder. Both the *M'Naghten* and the MPC tests require that the defendant have a medically recognized mental disorder at the time of the offense to support the assertion that her conduct was not criminally culpable and therefore blameless (Robinson 1984). This disability requirement "lends the necessary credibility to this objectively unconfirmable claim of abnormality" (Robinson 1984, p. 287). The recognition of the disability by both the medical profession and the public at large (namely, a jury) serves a dual purpose: On the one hand, the disability requirement provides the basis for excusing the defendant of criminal liability for her actions in her particular case; on the other hand, the disability requirement serves as a limited exception to the general proscription against criminal behavior, thereby preserving that very prohibition of conduct in persons of sound mind (Robinson 1984).

Using DSM to Satisfy the Disability Requirements in Criminal Defenses

In this section, I discuss postpartum mental disorders apparent in cases of infanticide and neonaticide—disorders that may serve to satisfy the disability requirement in the involuntary act, diminished capacity, or insanity defenses. This discussion is not intended to be exhaustive and is limited to aspects of the disorders that are germane to asserting one of the above-discussed defenses.

The involuntary act, diminished capacity, and insanity defenses require that a mental disability be proved. Although professional recognition of the disability is not, by itself, dispositive of whether a defendant is ultimately judged to be mentally unsound at the time of the crime for legal purposes, courts require that the mental disability claimed by the defendant be one that is recognized by the psychiatric community. For example, in Stephanie Wernick's case (described later in this section), the court refused to hear evidence of "neonaticide syndrome" because it had not yet been generally accepted in the field of psychiatry (Barton 1998).

DSM-IV and the Postpartum-Onset Specifier

The *Diagnostic and Statistical Manual of Mental Disorders*, 4th Edition (DSM-IV) is a classification of mental illness developed for use by clinicians in diagnosing mental disorders in their patients. Compiled by the American Psychiatric Association, DSM-IV "reflects a consensus about the classification and diagnosis of mental disorders" (American Psychiatric Association 1994). (A text revision of DSM-IV, referred to as DSM-IV-TR, was published in 2000 [American Psychiatric Association 2000].) Although DSM-IV cautions that "clinical diagnosis of a DSM-IV mental disorder is not sufficient to establish the existence for legal purposes of a 'mental disorder,' 'mental disability,' 'mental disease,' or 'mental defect'" (American Psychiatric Association 1994, p. xxiii), the mental disorders listed in DSM-IV are routinely used and relied on by lawyers, expert witnesses, and judges in making that determination.

Notwithstanding considerable evidence that postpartum mental illnesses are marked by symptoms peculiar only to them (Kumar and Marks 1992), and that we may observe the common usage of terms such as "postpartum depression" and "postpartum psychosis" by practitioners around the country (Hamilton et al. 1992), these conditions have not yet been fully recognized by the American Psychiatric Association as discrete mental illnesses capable of providing a differential diagnosis. Instead, they are officially regarded as mental disorders with postpartum onset. Similarly, although the literature on neonaticide has identified an aggregation of psychiatric symptoms that defines these cases, neonaticide syndrome has not yet been recognized in the DSM system.

The association between childbirth and maternal mental illness has, however, been formalized by the American Psychiatric Association in DSM-IV. The American Psychiatric Association formalized that association—an association wholly lacking in previous editions of the manual—by including a postpartum-onset specifier for a number of mood and psychotic disorders catalogued in DSM-IV. Currently, episodes of several disorders are considered to have a postpartum onset if they occur within 4 weeks of childbirth (American Psychiatric Association 1994). In its discussion of the postpartum-onset specifier, DSM-IV points out that postpartum mental illness is more commonly labile than nonpostpartum cases. However, although DSM-IV includes only a postpartum-onset specifier for these cases, it discusses aspects of postpartum mental illness in other than temporal terms. For example, DSM-IV also points to the frequent presence of delusions (e.g., believing that the infant is the devil), suicidal ideation, and obsessional thoughts regarding violence to the child in these cases (American Psychiatric Association 1994). The postpartum-onset specifier is the most recent consensus in the debate over the presence of unique phenomenology of severe postpartum psychiatric illness (Miller et al. 1999).

Since postpartum psychosis and neonaticide syndrome do not exist as officially recognized disorders, they cannot be used, standing alone, to satisfy the disability requirement in any of the criminal law defenses discussed earlier. However, the neonaticide literature indicates that the disorders appearing in cases of neonaticide share features with a number of disorders, including depersonalization disorder, dissociative identity disorder not otherwise specified, and brief psychotic disorder. Similarly, infanticide frequently is committed by women with major depressive disorder, bipolar mood disorder, or major depressive disorder with psychotic features that include the above-mentioned postpartum-onset specifier. These disorders are listed in DSM-IV as recognized mental disorders and, as such, can be used to satisfy the disability requirement in the criminal law defenses. Since they are recognized as distinct disorders in the psychiatric community, they are powerful tools in establishing the mental disability, disease, or defect necessary to plead a defense such as insanity or to prove involuntariness or diminished capacity. The relationship between these mental disorders and criminal law defenses is described below.

Application of Disabilities Featured in DSM-IV to Criminal Defenses

The neonaticide literature is replete with showings of cognitive impairment, delusions, automatism, disorientation, hallucinations, grossly disorganized behavior, and catatonia. These behaviors are symptomatic of depersonalization and brief psychotic disorder and can serve as the mental disease or defect that negates the *mens rea* required for first-degree murder (e.g., the defendant, in a catatonic state, could not have the capacity to form the intent required for first-degree murder).

Depersonalization disorder can be asserted as the disability required to plead the involuntary act defense. Depersonalization disorder is the experience of persistent or recurrent episodes of depersonalization, changed self-perception, dreamlike states, and an inability to control behavior. These symptoms—being an automaton, feeling like an outside observer of mental and physical efforts, and experiencing the sensation of lacking control of one's actions—fit squarely within the involuntary act defense. Thus, when a review of the facts of a neonaticide reveals that at the time of the killing the woman suffered depersonalization disorder, the involuntary act defense should be raised. It should be argued that the dissociative state (depersonalization disorder) is a mental disability that makes the killing of the neonate not the result of the woman's effort or determination. As such, the woman's conduct is excused because it was not within her control. Since the involuntary act defense provides a complete defense to a crime (People v. Newton 1970), a woman who raises a successful involuntary act defense should be acquitted and excused of all criminal liability.

Depersonalization disorder can also be used to fulfill the disability requirement in an insanity defense in a jurisdiction that follows the MPC approach to insanity. Since depersonalization disorder may cause a woman to be unable to control her actions and behavior, a woman can assert that, as a result of mental disease or defect (depersonalization disorder), she lacked the substantial capacity to conform her conduct to the requirements of law. If this is proven to the satisfaction of the jury, the woman may be found insane under the MPC.

When a defendant asserts the defense of diminished capacity, she need only show evidence that, because of a mental disease or defect, she was unable to form the requisite intent to commit the crime charged. For example, since neonaticides are often brought on first-degree murder charges, a diminished capacity defense would work to introduce evidence of a mental disease or defect, which would show that the defendant did not have the capacity to form the intent statutorily required for a first-degree murder conviction.

Major depressive disorder with or without psychotic features, bipolar disorder, or *schizophrenia* may include symptoms such as delusions, hallucinations, and disorganized speech or behavior. In an infanticide case, a defendant can use one of these disorders to establish the disability requirement in her defense of diminished capacity or insanity under *M'Naghten* or the MPC. For example, a woman suffering from hallucinations and delusions may be assessed as having had a psychotic disorder at the time of the killing of the infant. If so, she may use that disorder to satisfy the disability requirement in a claim of diminished capacity or insanity.

In a *M'Naghten* jurisdiction, if the woman can show that, because of a defect of reason or disease of the mind, she did not know right from wrong at the time of the crime or that she did not understand the nature and quality of her act, she will be judged legally insane. In an MPC jurisdiction, evidence of a psychotic disorder is useful to satisfy either the volitional or the cognitive aspect of the MPC test. The cognitive impairment demonstrated in the literature on postpartum psychosis (e.g., hallucinations, delusions or disorganized behavior) is clearly relevant as to whether the defendant had the substantial capacity to appreciate the criminality of her conduct. Similarly, the volitional aspect of the MPC test can also be satisfied by a defense based on a psychotic disorder, because a woman with such a disorder can be expected to act on the basis of delusions, an impairment of one's ability to conform one's conduct to the law.

A psychotic disorder can be used as the foundation of the diminished capacity and insanity defenses in a case of infanticide or neonaticide. When the diminished capacity defense is employed, the defendant need only show evidence that, because of a mental disease or defect, she was unable to form the requisite intent to commit the crime charged. For example, since neonaticides and infanticides are often brought on first-degree murder charges (Oberman 1996), a diminished capacity defense using a psychotic disorder as the requisite disability would work to show that the defendant did not have the capacity to form the intent statutorily required for a first-degree murder conviction, such as premeditation.

As described earlier, an insanity defense in a *M'Naghten* jurisdiction focuses on the cognitive capacity of the defendant. Generally, if the defendant can show that, because of a defect of reason or disease of the mind, she did not know right from wrong at the time of the crime or that she did not understand the nature and quality of her act, she will be judged legally insane. Evidence of a psychotic disorder is probative of the issue of the defendant's state of mind at the time of the infanticide. DSM-IV includes delusions and hallucinations and disorganized behavior as criteria for a diagnosis of brief psychotic disorder of postpartum onset. Critically, and especially with regard to the requirements of the *M'Naghten* test, DSM-IV suggests that supervision of the individual may be necessary to protect the individual "from the consequences of poor judgment, *cognitive impairment*, or acting on the basis of *delusions*" (American Psychiatric Association 1994, p. 302; emphasis added). DSM-IV does not provide a detailed list of the stressors that commonly lead to such a disorder, but it does note that "[t]he precipitating event(s) [of the psychotic break] may be any major stress" and adds that the diagnosis should note whether the psychotic break occurred within 4 weeks postpartum (American Psychiatric Association 1994, p. 302).

The MPC test has both a cognitive aspect and a volitional aspect, the satisfaction of *either* being grounds for an insanity verdict. The cognitive aspect rids the defendant of criminal responsibility when it can be shown that the defendant suffered from a mental disease or defect that caused her or him to lack the substantial capacity to appreciate the wrongfulness of her conduct. The volitional aspect rids the defendant of criminal responsibility when it can be shown that, because of a mental disease or defect, the defendant was unable to conform her or his conduct to the requirements of the law.

Evidence of a psychotic disorder, such as brief psychotic disorder, is useful to satisfy the cognitive aspect of the MPC test. The cognitive impairment demonstrated in the literature and acknowledged by DSM-IV (e.g., hallucinations, delusions) is relevant to whether the defendant had the substantial capacity to appreciate the criminality of her conduct. Similarly, the volitional aspect of the MPC test can be satisfied by a defense also based on the presence of a psychotic disorder. Case studies suggest that although many of the homicides are actively and positively inflicted by the mother, in many cases the mother fails to rescue her baby from a toilet or is unable to move subsequent to the delivery and thus leaves the child to die. Similarly, depersonalization disorder may be a good defense under the MPC's volitional approach, since this dissociative state leaves the mother with the sensation that she is unable to control her own movements (e.g., sensory anesthesia, sensation of lacking control over one's own actions).

Emergence of a "Neonaticide Syndrome"?

Case Illustration

A New York State court was the first to discuss, in the case summarized below, the aggregate symptoms commonly present in cases of neonaticide (e.g., denial, dissociation) as a potential neonaticide syndrome.

> Stephanie Wernick, a student living in a college dormitory, awoke several times one night because she was bleeding heavily (Wernick Brief 1996). Throughout the night, Wernick went to the bathroom to tend to the bleeding, which she attributed to heavy menstruation. Two dorm residents heard quiet cries coming from the bathroom and went to investigate. They found Wernick in a bathroom stall, standing in a pool of blood. When they asked whether Wernick was sick, she replied that she was fine and asked them to get her a tampon. She stayed in the stall for an extended period, during which time her friends checked on her. Later, her roommate found her in the shower. Wernick later asked her to dispose of

an untied bag that she said was filled with her soiled clothes. Unbeknown to the roommate, the bag contained the body of a newborn boy. When Wernick finished her shower, she went to her room, leaving the bathroom without cleaning the blood from the floor. She went to bed and, since she had not yet delivered the placenta, continued to bleed through the night.

Later that night, a college custodian found the bag containing the newborn. He called the police. Given the dramatic events of the night, the bag was easily traced back to Wernick. The first police officer on the scene (who was also an emergency medical technician) described Wernick as appearing "in shock, pale green [in] appearance[,] agitated, shivering while wrapped up in a blanket in a room described as very hot, lying in bed with blood on the sheets" (Appellate Brief on Behalf of Defendant-Appellant Stephanie Wernick 1996). Despite the urging of her friends, Wernick refused to go to the hospital, stating that she had to take a final exam in the morning. Eventually, she consented to be taken to the hospital by ambulance. While in the ambulance, Wernick began to speak about the delivery and told the ambulance technician "that she delivered a baby in the toilet, wrapped the baby in a pink towel, cleaned herself up with toilet paper, took a shower[,] and when she came out of the shower, the baby was gone." (Appellate Brief on Behalf of Defendant-Appellant Stephanie Wernick 1996)

Wernick was charged with first- and second-degree manslaughter. At her trial, the prosecution offered evidence that Wernick had asphyxiated the newborn by "stuffing toilet paper down his throat" (People v. Wernick 1995). Her attorney asserted the insanity defense, "claiming that she lacked substantial capacity to know and appreciate the nature and consequences of her conduct or that such conduct was wrong" (People v. Wernick 1995). To establish her defense, several expert witnesses testified about Wernick's mental state at the time of the crime and testified that "upon giving birth, [she] suffered from a brief reactive psychosis because she could no longer deny the reality of her pregnancy" and that "during this psychotic state, [she] was able to perform purposeful acts, such as stuffing toilet paper in the infant's mouth, but that she was unable to appreciate the nature and consequences of her conduct" (People v. Wernick 1995). The experts' testimony "tended to establish that (1) she completely denied the existence of her pregnancy, (2) such denial occurs in almost all cases in which women kill their newborn infants immediately after birth, and (3) in a large number of those cases the women believed that they were not pregnant" (People v. Wernick 1996).

Foreseeing an attempt by the defense to assert a neonaticide syndrome as proof of Wernick's insanity, the prosecution had moved for an evidentiary proceeding so that the court could determine whether this so-called syndrome had gained sufficient acceptance from the psychiatric community to be admissible in court. The defense opposed the hearing, stating that it had no intention of eliciting testimony from its experts regarding neonaticide syndrome. No evidentiary hearing was held, and the court therefore ruled that evidence tending to support the existence of a neonaticide syndrome or relying on the existence of such a syndrome could not be elicited during the trial. To allow such testimony, the court reasoned, would allow a neonaticide syndrome to be used as evidence without it first having to pass the rigors of an evidentiary hearing aimed at gauging the syndrome's acceptance in the scientific community. The court relied on an earlier New York case, stating

> [I]n an insanity defense case, the existence of a mental disease or syndrome or the validity of a theory of human behavior must be generally accepted in the field of psychiatry or psychology before experts may discuss such matters in their testimony at trial. If general acceptance has been attained, a psychiatric expert then "must be permitted" to state a diagnosis and to give a reasonable explanation for a finding that the defendant does or does not suffer from the mental disease, or that that person is or is not affected by the syndrome, or that a theory of human behavior does or does not explain the defendant's conduct. (People v. Weinstein 1992)

Since no evidentiary hearing was held on neonaticide syndrome, the court permitted the defense experts to testify only to their observations of Wernick and to their opinions of her conduct at the time of the killing and to the basis of their opinion (e.g., literature on the subject). The trial court made separate evidentiary rulings on the expert testimony, sustaining the prosecution's objections each time the expert's testimony seemed to refer to neonaticide syndrome. After one such objection, the trial judge explained:

> I am not preventing the witness from testifying as to the basis of his opinions. I am just preventing him, as I said, from setting up a specific profile that he has gleaned from the literature, as to why young mothers, or mothers kill their babies. . . . Certainly, the Doctor can testify as to this specific defendant, and what led him to his conclusions, based upon his own experiences, his reading of the literature, his studies of her, without quoting this common theme from the literature. (People v. Wernick 1995)

At the conclusion of the trial, Wernick was convicted.

Wernick raised several issues on appeal. First, she maintained that the trial court had wrongfully excluded portions of expert testimony relating to her mental state at the time of the crime. The New York Appellate Division affirmed the trial court's ruling on the admission of the expert testimony, stating that testimony was excluded where it tended to show that she suffered from neonaticide syndrome. Since no formal evidentiary hearing determining the general acceptance of neonaticide syndrome within the psychiatric community was held, the defense experts could not present evidence supporting the existence of such a syndrome or that Wernick had suffered from it at the time of the crime.

Wernick also argued that the trial court's refusal to admit the experts' testimony on neonaticide syndrome violated New York Criminal Procedure Law, which provides that psychiatrists or psychologists must be allowed to clarify and explain their diagnoses and opinions. The appellate court dismissed this contention, holding that the trial court's rulings did not prevent the defense's expert witnesses from referring to their experiences as practitioners or their reading of relevant literature when explaining their diagnosis, but rather prevented the defense's expert witnesses from "plugging" Wernick's symptoms into a larger, untested, and theretofore unaccepted profile of neonaticide syndrome.

The appellate court's decision was appealed to the New York Court of Appeals, the state's highest court. Wernick argued she had been denied her due-process rights when the trial court had refused to allow her expert witnesses from referring to the basis of their testimony (scientific literature on neonaticide). Wernick argued that her expert witnesses had not attempted to testify that she suffered from neonaticide syndrome or that such a syndrome even exists. Rather, they intended to testify that she had suffered a brief reactive psychosis and attempted to explain that diagnosis by referring to relevant literature. Wernick further argued that her expert witnesses had "merely attempted to show that clinical studies have established patterns of conduct of young women, reflecting certain similar characteristics, who have suffered from a genuine pathological denial of their pregnancies and subsequently killed their newborns immediately after birth" (People v. Wernick 1996).

The court rejected this argument, characterizing it as a "refined strategy" to allow the jury to hear evidence of neonaticide syndrome without the syndrome's having to be tested for its general acceptance in the scientific community. Turning to a section of the New York Criminal Procedure Law, which provides that psychiatrists or psychologists must be allowed to clarify and explain their diagnoses and opinions, the court concluded that precedents controlling that rule endorsed the policy that "evidence offered by a psychiatric expert be of a kind established as generally accepted in the profession as reliable" and that New York Criminal Procedure Law does not do away with the need for a evidentiary hearing in "instances when a party seeks to present novel scientific or psychiatric or medical evidence" (People v. Wernick 1996). The Court of Appeals affirmed Wernick's conviction.

The Need for Syndrome Evidence: Syndromes Generally and Rape Trauma Syndrome

DSM-IV defines a syndrome as a "grouping of signs and symptoms, based on their frequent co-occurrence, that may suggest a common underlying pathogenesis, course, familial pattern, or treatment selection" (American Psychiatric Association 1994, p. 771). In the courtroom, syndrome evidence is used when it is both relevant to an issue of fact that is in dispute and helpful to the finder of fact in reaching a verdict (People v. Taylor 1990). Critics of syndrome evidence claim that it addresses issues that juries are competent to understand without the help of complicated expert testimony. Proponents argue that the main strength of syndrome evidence is that it counters misconceptions about human behavior that, if unexplained, could eventually lead to erroneous decisions about the conduct. In other words, syndrome evidence serves to contextualize behavior for the purposes of legal judgment. A look at the commonly accepted rape trauma syndrome (RTS) is illustrative of the point.

RTS is a process of reorganization that occurs as a result of rape. The reaction to this life-threatening situation causes a syndrome of psychological, physical, and behavioral reactions (Burgess and Holmstrom 1974). Among other things, RTS is used in the courts to explain why a rape victim may remain silent after the rape and not expeditiously report it to the authorities. RTS has gained acceptance in courtrooms around the country.

A New York Court of Appeals case held that RTS is admissible in New York courts to explain why a rape victim might not appear distraught after being raped (People v. Taylor 1990). The court recognized that popular misconceptions about the effects of rape on a rape victim make jurors less likely to believe accusations made by a victim who did not immediately report the rape to the authorities. Underlying this misconception is the idea that rape is so offensive to bodily integrity that a person who does not promptly report a rape is fabricating her or his accusations, when in fact "prompt complaint is contrary to most . . . victims' experiences" (Torrey 1991). Any given pool of jurors could hold such misconceptions about how a person who has been raped "should act," however contrary to reality those conceptions may be. Absent an explanation of such conduct, it is likely that jurors would use those misconceptions to inform their decision to believe or disbelieve the testimony of a person who is claiming that she or he was raped.

While acknowledging RTS as a "therapeutic concept" (People v. Taylor 1990), the court maintained that, as an aggregate of symptoms and behaviors accepted within the scientific community, RTS could be helpful to a jury in deciding an issue of disputed fact. The court supported its position by noting that "patterns of response among rape victims are not within the ordinary understanding of the lay juror" (People v. Taylor 1990) and can therefore be explained by an expert witness. The court in this case limited the use of RTS to explain why a complainant might not have seemed distraught after the assault and expressly banned the use of RTS as proof that a rape actually occurred. Other courts have held that RTS is admissible to explain a delay in the reporting of the rape by the victim (People v. Hampton 1987).

RTS is not included in DSM-IV as a disorder. However, rape is recognized as a traumatic stressor that may lead the victim to suffer from post-traumatic stress disorder (PTSD), a disorder featured in DSM-IV. The fact that RTS is considered to fall within the umbrella of PTSD lends RTS the requisite credibility (general acceptance within the relevant scientific community) necessary for expert testimony to be admissible.

RTS is an example of the use of syndrome evidence to aid the finder of fact in deciding a contested issue. Syndromes help juries to explain behavior by fitting that behavior within a larger perspective of similarly situated people. The aim of such evidence is to provide the jury with information that may well be outside their common experience or knowledge. Despite the general perception and criticism of syndrome evidence as explaining issues the jury already understands and has been traditionally allowed to determine on its own, a layperson's knowledge cannot be assumed. Syndrome evidence

> differ[s] from the traditional use of expert testimony because [it does] not seek to educate the jury about a field with which the ordinary person is unfamiliar, such as a scientific process or specialized field of knowledge. Instead, [this] type . . . of psychological testimony address[es] an area once thought to be the one exclusive area of juror expertise—judgments about people's mental states, and how those mental states are reflected in a person's behavior. In some sense this testimony is subversive, because it questions society's existing morals by countering conventional myths and misconceptions of human nature. (Murphy 1992, pp. 281–282)

Syndrome evidence serves as a powerful means of combating myths by allowing experts to testify to "knowledge [that] would enable the jurors to disregard their prior conclusions as being common myths rather than common knowledge" (Murphy 1992, p. 298). Although such knowledge is perhaps "subversive," it is nonetheless necessary in order to fully contextualize a woman's behavior in the face of fundamentally extraordinary circumstances, such as a sexual assault or even a denied pregnancy. As long as a court is able to determine that syndrome evidence passes standards of reliability and admissibility, that the evidence is relevant to determining the fact at hand, and that it is narrowly admitted so as not to usurp the function of the jury, syndrome evidence serves as probative evidence that aids the finder of fact in coming to an informed conclusion on a disputed issue.

Novel Scientific Evidence and Admissibility

Before novel scientific evidence, including syndrome evidence, can be admitted as evidence at trial, it must undergo a hearing outside the presence of the jury so that its reliability can be assessed. There are two court-established tests for this purpose: the older is the *Frye* test, used in many state jurisdictions; the more recent is the *Daubert* test, which was enunciated by the U.S. Supreme Court and is controlling in the federal court system (Table 8–2).

Table 8–2.   Tests of admissibility

Admissibility standard	Admissibility factors
Frye test	Is the evidence generally accepted? Identify the field under which the proffered testimony falls; **AND** Determine whether the underlying theory offered in the expert's testimony is generally accepted by the appropriate scientific community. Note that the methods from which the theory is derived and implemented must be generally accepted in such community.
Daubert test[a]	Judge as gatekeeper: Is the evidence reliable and relevant? In order to be admissible, evidence must be: Reliable and relevant; and Assist the trier of fact to understand or determine a fact in issue. Some factors to consider: Has the theory or technique been tested? Has the theory or technique undergone the rigors of peer review and/or publication? Does the theory or technique have a known or potential rate of error? Has the theory or technique gained general acceptance from the appropriate community?

[a]The *Daubert* test applies to scientific, technical, and specialized knowledge.

Frye v. United States articulated the "general acceptance" standard, which served as the governing test for the admissibility of scientific evidence in the federal court system until its abrogation by the Supreme Court in 1993. *Frye* articulated the principle of "general acceptance" as the litmus test of reliability:

> Just when a scientific principle or discovery crosses the line between the experimental and demonstrable stages is difficult to define. Somewhere in this twilight zone the evidential force of the principle must be recognized, and while courts will go a long way in admitting expert testimony deduced from a well-recognized scientific principle or discovery, the thing from which the deduction is made must be sufficiently established to have gained general acceptance in the particular field in which it belongs. (Frye v. United States 1923, p. 1014)

The holding in *Frye* provided federal courts with a standard to use in deciding whether or not novel or controversial scientific evidence would be admissible. The *Frye* standard involves two parts: "First, there must be a theory that is generally accepted in the appropriate scientific community. . . . Second, there must be methods, implementing the theory, which are generally accepted in the appropriate scientific field" (Ebert 1993, p. 224). Therefore, in determining the reliability of novel scientific evidence, the court must first identify the field under which the proffered testimony falls. The court must next determine whether the underlying theory offered in the expert's testimony is generally accepted by the appropriate scientific community.

The "general acceptance" standard articulated in *Frye* was adopted by most state courts. Although only a district court decision, *Frye* has proven to be a tenacious holding: even though the U.S. Supreme Court held in *Daubert v. Merrell Dow Pharmaceuticals, Inc.* (1993) that *Frye* had been superseded by the adoption of the Federal Rules of Evidence, many state courts continue to employ the *Frye* test in determining the admissibility of scientific evidence in their respective jurisdictions.

Prior to its 1993 decision in *Daubert v. Merrell Dow Pharmaceuticals, Inc.*, the U.S. Supreme Court had never ruled on the place of scientific conclusions in the law. Instead, the Court had historically "relied upon the conclusions of scientific research without any consideration of the validity of the methods that produced those conclusions" (Laurens and Walker 1996, p. 841). *Daubert* came to the U.S. Supreme Court from a California tort action claiming that the plaintiffs had suffered birth defects because of Bendectin exposure. The trial court refused to allow the plaintiffs to admit expert testimony, based on live animal studies, pharmacological studies, and "re-analysis of previously published epidemiological (human statistical) studies" (Daubert v. Merrell Dow Pharmaceuticals, Inc. 1993), to contradict the defendant's claim that there was no link between the use of Bendectin and human birth defects. The U.S. District Court for the Southern District of California refused to hear the plaintiff's evidence because it did not meet the requirements delineated by the *Frye* test: the petitioner's evidence on Bendectin was not "sufficiently established to have general acceptance in the field to which it belong[ed]" (Daubert v. Merrell Dow Pharmaceuticals, Inc. 1993).

On review of the lower court's ruling in *Daubert*, the U.S. Supreme Court held that *Frye* had been superseded by the adoption of the Federal Rules of Evidence, which codifies the rules of evidence to be used in all federal courts. The Court specifically pointed to the language in the Federal Rules regarding the admissibility of relevant evidence, expert testimony, and the bases for the expert opinions in holding that *Frye*'s "general acceptance" standard had not been incorporated into the Federal Rules. With respect to expert testimony, at the time the *Daubert* decision was rendered, Federal Rule 702 stated, "If scientific, technical, or other specialized knowledge will assist the trier of fact to understand the evidence or to determine a fact in issue, a witness qualified as an expert by knowledge, skill, experience, training, or education, may testify thereto in the form of an opinion or otherwise" (Federal Rules of Evidence 1998). The Court reasoned that *Frye*'s "rigid 'general acceptance' requirement would be at odds with the 'liberal thrust' of the Federal Rules and their 'general approach of relaxing the traditional barriers to opinion testimony.'" (Daubert v. Merrell Dow Pharmaceuticals, Inc. 1993).

However, although the U.S. Supreme Court refused to incorporate *Frye*'s "general acceptance" standard into the Federal Rules of Evidence, it did not allow for the unfettered introduction of evidence. In clarifying the Federal Rules of Evidence standard, the Court listed two requirements that must be met by a party seeking to introduce novel scientific evidence. First, the relevance and reliability of the evidence continue to be threshold requirements. Second, a trial judge "must determine at the outset . . . whether the expert is proposing to testify to (1) scientific knowledge that (2) will assist the trier of fact (judge or jury) to understand or determine a fact in issue" (Daubert v. Merrell Dow Pharmaceuticals, Inc. 1993).

The Court provided a number of factors that courts could use in the determination of "whether the reasoning or methodology underlying the testimony is scientifically valid and of whether that reasoning or methodology properly can be applied to the facts at issue" (Daubert v. Merrell Dow Pharmaceuticals, Inc. 1993). One of the factors to be considered is whether the evidence can be tested. The Court stated, "Scientific methodology today is based on generating hypotheses and testing them to see if they can be falsified; indeed, this methodology is what distinguishes science from other fields of human inquiry" (Daubert v. Merrell Dow Pharmaceuticals, Inc. 1993). Another factor is whether the theory or techniques being identified have been subjected to the rigors of peer review and publication. Still, the Court recognized that, although publication and peer review may be considered in determining the admissibility of the evidence, the lack of either is "a relevant, though not dispositive, consideration in assessing the scientific validity of a particular technique or methodology on which an opinion is premised" (Daubert v. Merrell Dow Pharmaceuticals, Inc. 1993). A third factor is the "known or potential rate of error . . . and the existence and maintenance of standards controlling the technique's operation" (Daubert v. Merrell Dow Pharmaceuticals, Inc. 1993). Lastly, the Court noted that recourse to the "general acceptance" standard might be used to determine the validity of scientific evidence, although, like peer review and publication, it is not dispositive. In a later case, the U.S. Supreme Court noted that the factors articulated in *Daubert* for use in determining whether novel evidence is reliable were intended to be helpful but not definitive (Kuhmo Tire Company, Ltd. v. Carmichael 1999).

It is important to note that in 2000, Federal Rule 702 was amended to read as follows:

> If scientific, technical, or other specialized knowledge will assist the trier of fact to understand the evidence or to determine a fact in issue, a witness qualified as an expert by knowledge, skill, experience, training, or education, may testify thereto in the form of an opinion or otherwise, if (1) the testimony is based upon sufficient facts or data, (2) the testimony is the product of reliable principles and methods, and (3) the witness has applied the principles and methods reliably to the facts of the case. (Federal Rules of Evidence 2001)

The Advisory Committee notes accompanying Rule 702 explain that the rule was amended in response to the standards set forth in *Daubert* and subsequent decisions and point out that the 2000 amendment "affirms the trial court's role as gatekeeper and provides some general standards that the trial court must use to assess the reliability and helpfulness of proffered expert testimony." The amended Rule 702 is capacious enough to "require consideration of any or all of the specific *Daubert* factors where appropriate." Hence, under the amended Rule 702, the principles articulated in *Daubert* and subsequent cases persist as indicators to be used in assessing whether testimony proffered by an expert witness is reliable enough to go to the jury (Table 8–2).

"Neonaticide Syndrome": *Frye* and *Daubert*

The recognition of a neonaticide syndrome would serve to contextualize recognized mental disorders (e.g., depersonalization disorder, brief psychotic disorder) within a larger framework of characteristics typical in cases of neonaticide, such as denial of pregnancy. However, as the *Wernick* case makes clear, neonaticide syndrome will not be admissible in court until it has undergone a *Frye* or *Daubert* hearing (depending on the jurisdiction) to test its credibility as evidence. Since neonaticide syndrome has not yet undergone either of these tests in a court of law, its success at this point is purely speculative. However, the factors that would most likely be considered in a *Frye* or *Daubert* determination of the acceptance of neonaticide syndrome as evidence may be identified.

In a *Frye* jurisdiction, neonaticide syndrome would be checked against the "general acceptance" standard. It is difficult to say whether the literature on neonaticide reveals sufficient agreement in the psychiatric community that a neonaticide syndrome in fact exists. A review of the available literature demonstrates that neonaticides are considered to be a distinct "clinical entity" (Brozovsky and Falit 1971), with numerous characteristics repeatedly surfacing in the case studies on women who kill their newborns. In addition, besides the characteristics themselves, there are recognized mental disorders alluded to in the literature on neonaticide—for example, brief psychotic disorder and depersonalization disorder. It is beyond dispute that these two disorders are generally accepted within the scientific community according to the *Frye* standard: they are contained in DSM-IV, the authoritative book on mental disorders compiled by the American Psychiatric Association. The relevant articles on neonaticide appear in the major professional journals and are open to peer review. Of course, these considerations would also be supported by the testimony of psychiatrists who could affirmatively state whether neonaticide syndrome is in fact a legitimate syndrome with clinical dimensions.

In a *Daubert* jurisdiction, the inquiry would focus more broadly on whether neonaticide syndrome is reliable and relevant. Since neonaticide syndrome would be used as evidence to support the existence of a mental disease or defect for the purposes of mounting a defense to a charge of homicide, it would certainly be considered relevant. The second and more difficult issue is the reliability of neonaticide syndrome. The factors considered under a *Daubert* approach include the "testability" of the evidence, the rate of error and existence of standards by which the method is controlled, whether the theory has been subjected to peer review and publication, and the general acceptance of the theory within the relevant scientific community.

If neonaticide syndrome were to be considered as falling underneath the umbrella of either brief psychotic disorder or depersonalization disorder (much like RTS is understood as falling underneath the umbrella of PTSD), the inquiry on methodology would center primarily on whether DSM-IV reflects the use of an accepted methodology, namely, the formulation of hypotheses and their subsequent testing for falsification. Surely, DSM-IV meets those standards. Furthermore, as noted in the discussion on *Frye* earlier in this chapter, articles on neonaticide are published in the profession's leading journals and are thus exposed to peer review, a factor that the U.S. Supreme Court in the case of *Daubert* considered probative. Finally, the testimony of psychiatrists in the field conclusively affirming or disaffirming neonaticide syndrome would be crucial, given that there is no direct mention of a neonaticide syndrome in the literature.

Conclusion

It is clear from the research on the subject that a number of mental disorders, however they may be defined, often occur during the puerperium and can be so strong as to lead a new mother to kill her newborn or infant. However, while in theory it is easy enough to "plug" these disorders into governing affirmative defense statutes in order to achieve the necessary mental disability requirement, the end result of exculpation in one form or another is not as automatic or clear-cut as it would seem. Because of the shortcomings of the law and psychiatry, these cases of infanticide and neonaticide often end in the conviction and prolonged incarceration of a woman who, when all is said and done, was mentally ill at the time she caused the death of her child. Witness the case of Bernadette Reilly, whose insanity defense was rejected notwithstanding compelling evidence that she suffered brief reactive psychosis, a disorder recognized in the DSM classification. Reilly was found guilty of third-degree murder and was sentenced to 3–10 years in prison (Commonwealth of Pennsylvania v. Reilly 1988).

The obstacles, sometimes even failings, of the law and psychiatry with respect to the just treatment of women accused of murdering their newborns and infants are manifold. First, the United States does not—indeed, cannot—have an infanticide statute similar to that of England or Canada that provides *de jure* acknowledgment of postpartum mental illness and would apply universally to all infanticides prosecuted under state law. Such a statute would have to be established on a state-by-state basis through each state's own (often protracted) legislative process (Katkin 1992).

Because no statute in the United States regards infanticide as a crime qualitatively different from murder, a woman accused of killing her newborn or infant must invoke that difference by asserting a defense that is based on (and contingent on) proof that she suffered from a mental disorder at the time of the offense. The success of this undertaking is hampered by inadequacies in the law. For example, the *M'Naghten* formulation of insanity focuses solely on the cognitive aspect of the human personality, even though "we are told by eminent medical scholars that . . . [there are] those who can distinguish between good and evil but who cannot control their behavior" (United States v. Freeman 1966). Approximately half of the states follow the *M'Naghten* test. Such outmoded conceptions of the personality and of mental illness as maintained by the *M'Naghten* formulation of insanity severely limit the extent to which a defendant can show that a mental disability made her unable to conform her conduct to the law.

Furthermore, the "rigidity with which the legal system views mental illness" (Attia et al. 1999, p. 110) poses a major obstacle to successful defenses based on mental disorders. This rigidity is even more amplified when consensus regarding the existence of a mental disorder has not yet been reached by the psychiatric community. Thus, only when there has been agreement within the psychiatric profession as to the existence of a mental disorder may an expert testify that a defendant had the disorder at the time the crime was committed. The consensus that would permit a woman accused of killing her newborn or infant to assert an insanity defense based on a postpartum mental illness, such as postpartum psychotic depression, has not yet been sufficiently achieved. A woman is left to support her defenses with a recognized disorder, such as schizophreniform disorder, even though that disorder lends an incomplete and imperfect description of the actual mental state she possessed at the time of the homicide. It is absolutely imperative, therefore, that the psychiatric profession formalize the aggregate symptoms apparent in the various puerperal mental illnesses so that a woman accused of killing her child in the puerperium may adequately defend herself by way of using a recognized postpartum mental disorder as the basis of her defense.

Apart from the more theoretical problems posed by issues such as the definition of mental disorders or criminal defense formulations, equally obstructive practical considerations weigh against a woman attempting to defend herself against homicide charges in the death of her infant or newborn. For instance, the timing of a postoffense psychiatric evaluation is paramount to assessing the woman's mental state at the time of the act or omission that caused the death of her newborn or infant (Hickman and LeVine 1992). However, sometimes these examinations are made only after significant delays. The loss of memory associated with these cases makes such "waiting periods" problematic. Furthermore, investigative tactics used by police detectives eager to "crack a case" may result in the insertion of rationalizations and false or incomplete recollections into the memory of the woman (Hickman and LeVine 1992)—insertions that are ultimately detrimental to her case. Lastly, and rather ironically, the most pervasive characteristic of postpartum mental disorders, their changeability, renders it extremely difficult to convince a jury that a woman was insane at the time that she caused the death of her infant when at trial she appears to be totally "normal" (Hickman and LeVine 1992).

It is patently unjust that a woman who suffered from a mental disorder at the time she caused the death of her infant be convicted for murder and sentenced to a long term in prison. However, the penal treatment of infanticide and neonaticide apparently induced by postpartum mental disorder will gain uniformity and fairness only when the psychiatric community comes to an agreement on the nature and extent of those disorders. Postpartum disorders wait to be recognized by the American Psychiatric Association as codeable mental disorders. Until then, American women are placed in the unenviable position of asserting imperfect grounds of mental disability as the basis for their defense and hoping for the best.

References

American Psychiatric Association: Diagnostic and Statistical Manual of Mental Disorders, 4th Edition. Washington, DC, American Psychiatric Association, 1994

American Psychiatric Association: Diagnostic and Statistical Manual of Mental Disorders, 4th Edition, Text Revision. Washington, DC, American Psychiatric Association, 2000

Appellate Brief on Behalf of Defendant-Appellant Stephanie Wernick, 1–36, People v Wernick, 674 NE2d 322 (NY 1996)

Attia E, Downey J, Oberman M: Postpartum psychoses, in Postpartum Mood Disorders. Edited by Miller LJ. Washington, DC, American Psychiatric Press, 1999, pp 99–117

Barton B: When murdering hands rock the cradle: an overview of America's incoherent treatment of infanticidal mothers. Southern Methodist University Law Review 51:591–619, 1998

Brockington I: Infanticide, in Motherhood and Mental Health. Edited by Brockington I. Oxford, UK, Oxford University Press, 1996, pp 430–468

Brozovsky M, Falit H: Neonaticide: clinical and psychodynamic considerations. Journal of the American Academy of Child Psychiatry 10:673–683, 1971

Burgess AW, Holmstrom LL: Rape trauma syndrome. Am J Psychiatry 131:981–986, 1974

Commonwealth of Pennsylvania v Reilly, 549A2d 503 (Pa 1988)

Daubert v Merrell Dow Pharmaceuticals, Inc, 509 U.S. 579 (1993) d'Orbán PT: Women who kill their children. Br J Psychiatry 134:560–571, 1979

Ebert LB: Frye after Daubert: the role of scientists in admissibility issues as seen through analysis of the DNA profiling cases. University of Chicago Law School Roundtable, 1993, pp 219–252

Finnegan P, McKinstry E, Robinson GE: Denial of pregnancy and childbirth. Can J Psychiatry 27:672–674, 1982

Frye v United States, 293 F 1013 (DC Cir 1923)

Graham v State 547 SW2d 531 (Tenn 1977)

Green CM, Manohar SV: Neonaticide and hysterical denial of pregnancy. Br J Psychiatry 156:121–123, 1990

Hamilton JA: The issue of unique qualities, in Postpartum Psychiatric Illness: A Picture Puzzle. Edited by Hamilton JA, Harberger PN. Philadelphia, University of Pennsylvania Press, 1992, pp 14–32

Hamilton JA, Harberger PN, Parry BL: The problem of terminology, in Postpartum Psychiatric Illness: A Picture Puzzle. Edited by Hamilton JA, Harberger PN. Philadelphia, University of Pennsylvania Press, 1992, pp 32–40

Hickman SA, LeVine DL: Postpartum disorders and the law, in Postpartum Psychiatric Illness: A Picture Puzzle. Edited by Hamilton JA, Harberger PN. Philadelphia, University of Pennsylvania Press, 1992, pp 282–295

Hunter W: On the uncertainty of the signs of murder in the case of bastard children. Medical Observations and Enquiries 6:266–290, 1784

Infanticide Act, 2 Geo 6, ch 36 (Eng 1938)

Jacobsen T: Effects of postpartum disorders on parenting and offspring, in Postpartum Mood Disorders. Edited by Miller J. Washington, DC, American Psychiatric Press, 1999, pp 119–139

Katkin DM: Postpartum psychosis, infanticide, and criminal justice, in Postpartum Psychiatric Illness: A Picture Puzzle. Edited by Hamilton JA, Harberger PN. Philadelphia, University of Pennsylvania Press, 1992, pp 275–281

Kuhmo Tire Company, Ltd v Carmichael, 526 U.S. 137 (1999)

Kumar R, Marks M: Infanticide and the law in England and Wales, in Postpartum Psychiatric Illness: A Picture Puzzle. Edited by Hamilton JA, Harberger PN. Philadelphia, University of Pennsylvania Press, 1992, pp 257–274

Kaye NS, Borenstein NM, Donnelly SM: Families, murder, and insanity: a psychiatric review of paternal infanticide. J Forensic Sci 35:133–139, 1990

M'Naghten's Case, 8 Eng Rep 718 HL (1843)

Miller LJ, Rukstalis M: Beyond the "blues": hypotheses about postpartum reactivity, in Postpartum Mood Disorders. Edited by Miller J. Washington, DC, American Psychiatric Press, 1999, pp 3–19

Model Penal Code, § 4.01(1) (1985)

Murphy S: Assisting the jury in understanding victimization: expert psychological testimony on battered woman syndrome and rape trauma syndrome. Columbia Journal of Law and Social Problems 25:277–312, 1992

Oberman M: Mothers who kill: coming to terms with modern American infanticide. American Criminal Law Review 34:1–110, 1996

People v Doss, 574 NE2d 806 (Ill App 2d 1987)

People v Hampton, 746 P2d 947 (Colo 1987)

People v Lisnow, 151 Cal Rptr 621 (Cal App Dept Super Ct 1978)

People v Massip, 271 Cal Rptr 868 (Cal App 4 Dist 1990)

People v Newton, 87 Cal Rptr 394 (Cal Ct App 1970)

People v Taylor, 552 NE2d 131 (NY 1990)

People v Weinstein, 591 NYS2d 715 (NY Sup Ct 1992)

People v Wernick, 215 AD2d 50 (NY App Div 1995)

People v Wernick, 674 NE2d 322 (NY 1996)

Robinson PH: Criminal law defenses: a systematic analysis. Columbia Law Review 82:199–291, 1982

Robinson PH: Criminal Law Defenses, Vols 1–2. Minneapolis, MN, West Publishing Co, 1984

Robinson PH: A functional analysis of criminal law. Northwestern University Law Review 88:857–913, 1994

Saunders E: Neonaticides following "secret" pregnancies: seven case reports. Public Health Rep 104:368–372, 1989

Sneddon J: The mother and baby unit: an important approach to treatment, in Postpartum Psychiatric Illness: A Picture Puzzle. Edited by Hamilton JA, Harberger PN. Philadelphia, University of Pennsylvania Press, 1992, pp 102–114

Spinelli M: A systematic investigation of 17 cases of neonaticide. Am J Psychiatry 158:811–813, 2001

State v Skeoch, 96 NE2d 473 (Ill 1951)

Torrey M: When will we be believed? Rape myths and the idea of a fair trial in rape prosecutions. University of California Davis Law Review 24:1013–1071, 1991

United States v Freeman, 357 F2d 606, 618 (2d Cir 1966)

Walker L, Monahan J: Daubert and the reference manual: an essay on the future of science in law. Virginia Law Review 82:837–857, 1996

Wisner KL, Peindl K, Hanusa BH: Symptomatology of affective and psychotic illness related to childbearing. J Affect Disord 30:77–87, 1994

Chapter 9

Medical and Legal Dilemmas of Postpartum Psychiatric Disorders

Cheryl L. Meyer, Ph.D., J.D.
Margaret G. Spinelli, M.D.

. . . upon a trial in this country, where we are so happy as to be under the protection of judges, who by their education, studies and habits, are above the reach of vulgar prejudices, and make it a rule for their conduct to suppose the accused party innocent, till guilt be proved. With such judges, I say, there will be little danger of an innocent woman being condemned by false reasoning. But danger, in the cases of which we are now treating, may arise from the evidence and opinion given by physical people, who are called in to settle questions in science, which judges and jurymen are supposed not to know with accuracy. Many of our profession are not so conversant with science as the world may think; and some of us are a little disposed to grasp at authority in a public examination, by giving quick and decided opinion, where it should have been guarded with doubt; as character which no man should be ambitious to acquire, who in his profession is presumed every day to be deciding nice questions upon which the life of a patient may depend.

William Hunter, M.D., F.R.S.
Read to the members of the British Medical Society, July 14, 1783

Portions of this chapter are reprinted from Meyer CL, Proano TC: "Postpartum Syndromes: Disparate Treatment in the Legal System," in *It's a Crime: Women and Justice*, 2nd Edition. Edited by Muraskin R. Englewood Cliffs, NJ, Prentice-Hall, 1999. Copyright 1999, Pearson Education, Inc. Used with permission.

Postpartum disorders date to antiquity (Hamilton and Harberger 1992). Hippocrates described postpartum psychosis as "a kind of madness caused by excessive blood flow to the brain" (Meyer et al. 1999, p. 91; see also Cox 1988; Lynch-Fraser 1983). An eleventh-century gynecologist, Trotula of Salerno, suggested that postpartum blues resulted from too much moisture in the womb, causing the brain to fill with water, which was then involuntarily shed as tears (Mason-Hohl 1940).

It was not until the 1800s that physicians described postpartum syndromes in detail and began to theorize that there was a connection between physiological events and the mind (Hamilton 1989). Esquirol (1838) wrote the first review of 90 cases relating pregnancy and psychiatric disorders. In the group that had onset within several weeks or more after delivery, he noticed a high incidence of delirium, similar to our contemporary description, with acute onset of disturbances of perception and consciousness, disorganization, hallucinations, confusion, delusions, and marked changeability of mood.

In 1858, Louis Victor Marcé published the first textbook on postpartum disorders, *Traité de la folie des femmes enceintes* (Marcé 1858). In a sample of 310 cases of postpartum psychiatric illness, he identified psychiatric symptoms during pregnancy in 9% of cases; the symptoms manifested within the first 6 weeks after delivery in 58% of the cases and after 6 weeks in 33% of the cases. Although Marcé found no distinguishing features in the psychoses during pregnancy, he described unique qualities and characteristics of postpartum psychoses, which he identified as distinct from other psychoses. Marcé believed that wild mania followed by severe melancholia was a clue to specific organic mechanisms, which he termed "morbid sympathy." He suggested that "[t]he coexistence of the organic state raises an interesting question of pathologic physiology; one immediately asks if there exists a connection between the uterine condition and disorders of the mind" (Marcé 1858, pp. 7–8; quoted in Hamilton 1989, p. 326).

Marcé's book became the principal authority on which diagnoses of puerperal disorders were based. The identified diagnoses were generally accepted and repeatedly affirmed by other reported cases. Marcé's theory, derived from his clinical intuition, rests on the scientific knowledge of what today we describe as the hypothalamic-pituitary-ovarian (HPO) axis. He developed his theory prior to the discovery of the endocrine system, which supports the fact that the physiological mechanisms of reproduction communicate with chemical messengers of the brain through the biological cascade of events of the HPO axis (see Chapter 4: "Neurohormonal Aspects of Postpartum Depression and Psychosis").

In early twentieth-century America, thinking about postpartum disorders changed for unclear reasons, and the psychiatric community split over the existence of a formal diagnosis. The official word "postpartum" was stricken from the diagnostic psychiatric nomenclature (Hamilton and Harberger 1992) and was therefore not included in the first edition of the *Diagnostic and Statistical Manual of Mental Disorders* (American Psychiatric Association 1952).

Postpartum Psychiatric Disorders: The Medical Dilemma

The fourth edition of DSM, DSM-IV, includes the word "postpartum" as a modifier to diagnoses that occur within 4 weeks of childbirth (American Psychiatric Association 1994; a text revision, referred to as DSM-IV-TR, was published in 2000 [American Psychiatric Association 2000]). The exclusion of official diagnostic criteria is based on the determination that postpartum phenomenology is not demonstratively different from other mood and psychotic disorders (American Psychiatric Association 1994). Whether or not the postpartum disorders possess distinctive diagnostic features, these illnesses share both the same underlying neurohormonal pathogenesis and the precipitous event of childbirth. Wisner et al. (1994) suggest that the precipitous physiological event of hormone depletion is the underlying mechanism for the observed organic psychosis. The consistently described diagnostic picture includes delirium, impaired sensorium, and poor cognition. In addition, unusual perceptual experiences such as visual, tactile, and olfactory hallucinations are manifest, along with a picture of bizarre delusions and hallucinations (see Chapter 3: "Postpartum Disorders"). A pattern of waxing and waning sensorium and mood lability mimics the cycling pattern of bipolar disorder. This picture supports Kendell's findings of increased lifetime psychiatric admissions for affective psychoses in the immediate postpartum period (Kendell et al. 1987).

Postpartum psychosis presents as a psychiatric emergency. Whether mood changeability is associated with bipolar disorder or organic delirium, or both (see Chapter 3), this presentation may disarm even the psychiatric professional. Because moments of complete lucidity are followed by frightening psychosis for the new mother, the illness may go unrecognized and untreated. Out of shame, guilt, or a paranoid delusional system, the new mother may not share her bizarre thoughts and fears. Families may not offer necessary support or seek psychiatric intervention. It is in this context that acts of suicide and infanticide occur.

Acute Postpartum Syndromes and Infanticide

Infanticide, like postpartum illness, has occurred throughout history (Oberman 1996). In early centuries, justification for infanticide ranged from pagan sacrifice (Lagaipa 1990) to population control. When infanticide practices became increasingly common (see Chapter 1: "A Brief History of Infanticide and the Law"), societies adopted laws, and punishments became increasingly severe. In the seventeenth century, concealment of a murdered newborn became a capital offense. Penalties were more likely rendered to unmarried women using such methods as "sacking," in which a woman was placed in a leather sack with a dog, a snake, and a cock and thrown into the water (Brockington 1996; Oberman 1996).

Events took a turn in 1647, when Russia became the first country to adopt a more humane attitude toward infanticidal mothers. By 1881, all European states except England had established a legal distinction between infanticide and murder by assigning more lenient penalties to infanticide (Oberman 1996). In 1922, England passed the Infanticide Act (see Chapter 1 and Chapter 10: "Infanticide in Britain") making infanticide a less severe crime than homicide, with less severe punishment. By the end of the twentieth century, almost all Western societies had adjusted the penalty for infanticide (Brockington 1996). Through recognition of the unique biological changes of parturition, the charge of murder has been reduced, in most cases, to manslaughter. Psychiatric evaluation and treatment are the most frequent outcomes. The American judicial system makes no legal distinction between the murder of an adult and the murder of a newborn.

For the psychotic woman, decisions may be made by commanding voices in her head. Her actions may be the result of a paranoid and delusional belief system. Despite this psychotic state, the mother may not fulfill the legal definition of "insanity" as it is determined by the legal system (Meyer et al. 1999). Insanity is ascertained by additional factors, such as cognition, insight, and judgment (see Chapter 8: "Criminal Defense in Cases of Infanticide and Neonaticide"). For example, if the mother acts on command hallucinations, believing that she has no alternative to the directed behavior, the criteria for insanity may be fulfilled. On the other hand, if she had more observing ego capacity to resist command hallucinations, she may not fulfill the criteria for an insanity defense. The following vignette illustrates a case of postpartum psychosis linked to infanticide (Brusca 1990; Japenga 1987):

> T went from being an honor society member, her school's first female senior class president, and an athletic and sociable person to, later, being a

mother who drowned her second child, a 9-month-old son, in a bathtub. She claimed she heard voices telling her that her child was the devil. After T gave birth to her first child, she suffered hallucinations, panic, and obsessions. She attempted suicide by jumping out of a moving vehicle and then jumping from a 30-foot-high bridge, which led to psychiatric hospitalization. Unfortunately, when she became pregnant with her second child, her doctors told her to forget about her previous psychosis, saying that it would not happen again.

This case emphasizes the vital need for education as a method of prevention. How do women like T, invariably described as gentle and loving mothers, become"killers"? The following case vignette also exemplifies this paradox.

At 32, F was a middle-class immigrant woman who lived with her husband. F dated depressive symptoms to the 32nd week of pregnancy while she was on bedrest for premature labor. She became obsessed and guilt-ridden that she had harmed her baby. And despite a 36-week delivery of a healthy baby boy, her remorse worsened. By the tenth postpartum day, she was preoccupied by persistent auditory hallucinations of her baby's cry "as if something was smothering him." Neither her husband nor her sister could provide reassurance. She became sleepless and agitated and was obsessed by suicidal thoughts and dreams. Various calls for help were ignored or denied. F said she did not want to wake up. She told her husband, "If I hurt my baby please kill me." She asked her sister to take care of the baby if she died. F, a soft-spoken, gentle woman who frequently cared for her nieces and nephews exemplified the maternal image. Her calls for help did not alert her family.

F described the days before the death of her baby, J. On the evening of his nineteenth day and the last evening of his life, she and the family took pictures of J, perused the family album, and placed him in the crib. F woke to the sound of J's cry. She recalled, "I was outside . . . water in front of me . . . then sitting on a couch in the living room. I was not sure if I was sitting or actually sleeping. My husband asked, 'Where is the baby?'" F told him she left him in the pond.

F was charged with second-degree murder and taken to the county jail. F's attorney requested hospitalization for her psychotic client. The judge was not convinced of F's insanity and feared giving a "message that women can kill their babies and get away with it." After 6 weeks of incarceration and decompensation without medication, the judge granted a psychiatric hospital admission. Recognized only as a "killer," F's feet were shackled to her hospital bed. F pled guilty to manslaughter. She was remanded to a psychiatric facility for a 6-month observation period, then returned to her home country.

This case exemplifies how the dearth of available knowledge can mold the circumstances and shape the outcome of these cases. In particular, this vignette further emphasizes the need for education. Neither F nor her family had knowledge or understanding of postpartum illness. F's physician was not alerted to depression by her obsessive ruminations about her failure as a mother. F's husband and sister were unable to identify the problem. Her history as a warm and nurturing sister and wife overshadowed any concern voiced about harming her infant. The planned pregnancy and joy over the future were inconsistent with the thought of her as murderer.

Although her attorney pled for hospital admission, the court chose the county jail. Failure to educate our judicial system led the court to doubt an existing diagnosis. There were repeatedly missed opportunities for identification, intervention, and prevention of the tragic circumstances.

Chronic Mental Illness and Infanticide

A frequently ignored factor associated with infanticide is the role of chronic mental illness. Women with schizophrenia or severe bipolar disorder are often victims of unplanned and unprotected pregnancies. Although the data on pregnancy in women with schizophrenia are limited, a review by Tekell (2001) described the increase in stressors and the life events that contribute to the postpartum decompensation of women with schizophrenia. The danger of chronic illness is illustrated in the following vignette.

> At 29 years of age, M was charged with second-degree murder for throwing her 6-month-old infant from the eighth floor window of her apartment complex. Diagnosed with schizophrenia at 19, M had five previous psychiatric hospitalizations. She was compliant with medications throughout this recent and uneventful pregnancy. Two days postpartum, M was admitted to a psychiatric facility with florid psychosis and homicidal ideation toward her mother and the infant.
>
> Child protective services placed the infant under the care of M's mother, the custodial parent of her 7-year-old son because of homicidal threats and gestures after his birth. M's mother accompanied the infant back to their home state while M remained in the hospital.
>
> On the day before discharge, M was reported as psychotic, aggressive, and unpredictable but discharged to her home with her mother, who was encouraged to take M to the nearest hospital. There was no child service communication or intervention.
>
> On the day of her baby's death, while her mother was shopping, M remained home alone with her infant. She said that her baby "died" because she "twisted her body" out of her mother's arms and out of the window.
>
> M was arrested for murder and incarcerated for 4 years awaiting trial. She was found not competent to stand trial and admitted to a state psychiatric facility.

Unlike postnatal psychosis, with its precipitous onset, a history of schizophrenia itself signals prevention. Parent-infant programs with psychiatric services for mentally ill mothers are rare. M and her mother spoke little English. In addition, the stigmatization of the mentally ill in the general hospital setting may impair communication from antepartum to postpartum staff. The patient's limited cognitive capacities contributed to problems.

Insufficient mental health screening in antepartum clinics is also a factor in failed care. The breakdown in communication by professional child care organizations in this straightforward case was striking and led to tragic circumstances. In this case, child protective services did not communicate with M's home state for follow-up.

Use of Postpartum Syndromes in the Courts

Criminal Cases

A history of treatment for postpartum syndromes has been admitted into evidence in both criminal and civil courts (Meyer et al. 1999). Clearly, the use of postpartum syndromes in criminal cases has gained more publicity. This could be due to the nature of the crime or to the media frenzy that surrounds criminal cases involving the mental health of the defendant. The fact patterns of these cases are chillingly similar (Gardner 1990). Generally, the defendant has no prior history of criminal activity and often goes to great lengths to become pregnant. In other words, these are generally planned pregnancies and wanted children. In many cases, the woman may be experiencing delusions, perceiving the child as a source of evil. The murders are particularly gruesome—for example, running over the child with a car or throwing the child in an icy river. Afterward, the mother often has no recollection of the event and reports the child missing or kidnapped to the police.

In the United States, postpartum syndromes can become a part of criminal proceedings at several points, including evaluation of competency, pleading, and sentencing. For example, at the outset, the competency of the woman to stand trial could be at issue. However, most women are not experiencing postpartum effects at the trial. Moreover, this would probably be an ineffective defense strategy. Since the statute on murder never runs out, the defendant would likely remain in a treatment facility until competency is achieved in order for a trial to take place. A treatment facility may be an inappropriate place for most defendants who previously had a postpartum syndrome because postpartum syndromes are often transitory conditions.

More commonly, postpartum syndromes are used to attempt to exculpate or mitigate responsibility of a defendant. At issue is whether the defendant could have formed the requisite mental intent (*mens rea*) to commit murder. If someone was insane at the time of the act, her mental state may not rise to the appropriate level of intent, making conviction difficult. Since most of these cases are not federal cases, the jurisdictional criteria for legal insanity could be used. Each state has adopted tests (criteria) to determine whether particular components were also present at the time of the defense insanity (see Chapter 9).

Sentencing after the conviction can also be disparate. Because diagnostic guidelines for postpartum disorders are fuzzy, sentences vary from probation to life in prison or even the death penalty. Brusca (1990) reported that about half the women who raise postpartum psychosis as a defense are found not guilty by reason of insanity, one-fourth receive light sentences, and one-fourth receive long sentences.

The lack of clear diagnostic certainty limits the use of postpartum syndromes in criminal trials and creates further ambiguity in the criminal courtroom. Improved family and public education would likely change outcomes. In addition, language barriers affect these cases at every level, including the ability to report symptoms, interact with others in the community, and obtain legal representation, as well as the subtleties of reporting to professional expert witnesses.

Medical and Legal Dilemmas: Yates v. Texas

The difficulties described in this chapter are well illustrated in the case of *Yates v. Texas* (see "Introduction," this volume). Andrea Yates drowned her five children while suffering from a postpartum psychosis. Charged with capital murder and placed in the county jail (Yardley 2002), Mrs. Yates was treated with an effective regimen of antipsychotic medication. By August 3, 2001, her psychosis had lifted and she was found competent to stand trial on September 24, 2001 (CourtTV 2002).

The case of Andrea Yates must be viewed against the political and legal background of the Texas judicial system and Harris County jurisdiction. Harris County prosecutors have sent more people to death row than any other county in Texas, a state that has led the nation in executions. Harris County juries lead the country in death penalty verdicts. As Elaine Cassell (2002), professor of law and psychology and legal columnist for CNN, notes, "Texas's law is derived from the most restrictive legal insanity standard, the M'Naghten Rule—the defendant must prove failure *to know* the act was wrong. The law could hardly be narrower."

Yates pled innocent by reason of insanity to capital murder. The prosecution asserted that she knew right from wrong *at the time* of the killings because she called 911 and her husband *after* the killings. The responding officer said that when Yates answered the door, she was breathing heavily, with her hair and clothes soaked with water, and said, "I killed my kids." The defense maintained that she did not know right from wrong at the time of killings because she was in a psychotic state (Pies 2002).

"To know" right from wrong. Two well-respected and highly credentialed forensic psychiatrists testified as expert witnesses. The witness for the prosecution testified that Andrea Yates was responsible for the deaths of her children because she knew right from wrong at the time of the act (Grinfield 2002). The primary defense expert and several psychiatrists opined that Mrs. Yates was unable to know that the act of killing her children was wrong. The expert for the defense testified, "Even though she knew it was against the law, she did what she thought was right in the world she perceived through her psychotic eyes at the time" (CourtTV 2002). She thought drowning her four sons and her daughter was the only way to save them from hell. The prosecutor asked, "Even in the face of this cruel dilemma she knew it was a sin?" "Yes, she did," the expert replied.

This legal dilemma is described by Elaine Cassell (2002): "What constitutes 'knowing one's act is wrong' in this context? What is 'knowing'? Does 'wrong' mean, 'legally wrong' or 'morally wrong'? The statute does not explain, so the jury was left to apply the statutory language to the facts as it saw fit."

In an interview with the *Psychiatric Times* (Grinfield 2002), forensic experts questioned how witnesses for the prosecution and defense could interpret the insanity defense in polar opposite ways if they used the same facts and legal basis for interpreting the defense. Expert forensic psychiatrist and medical director of the American Academy of Psychiatry and the Law (APPL) addressed these concerns about the insanity defense: "we don't have any test to know which people do, can or can't follow those things [command hallucinations] . . . We are still left to sort of dealing with a certain degree of approximations in those answers" (p. 3).

He announced that APPL is scheduled to release its practice guidelines as an attempt to bring consistency to the evaluations of defendants who are mentally ill. These guidelines, titled Practice Guidelines for Forensic Psychiatric Evaluation of Defendants Raising the Insanity Defense, will assist forensic experts whose clients assert the insanity defense.

Although the guidelines may settle one problem, the quandary persists: Can we in psychiatry determine with certainty the ability to "know" right or wrong from the data? How reliable are retrospective accounts of a psychotic episode?

Retrospective recall is suspect under any circumstances in most disciplines. Moreover, psychosis is often associated with amnesia, particularly in postpartum-onset psychosis. How does one distinguish fact from fabrication or delusion?

The cognitive/disorganization psychosis. In Chapter 3, Wisner states, "The confused, delirium-like, disorganized clinical picture of postpartum psychosis has been observed and reported repeatedly." Wisner describes in detail her study of puerperal psychosis in which the most dramatic finding was cognitive/disorganization psychosis with impaired sensorium and orientation, memory, thought disorganization, and prominent cognitive impairment. This picture of acute-onset delirium was evidenced by cognitive examinations (such as drawings of clock faces and figures) and extensive laboratory evaluations.

Therefore, the expert witness who testifies for a woman with puerperal mental illness must have knowledge of the distinct presentation. Although postpartum disorders are not considered unique DSM-IV diagnoses, distinctive phenomenology is well described in the literature. The test of M'Naghten used to determine culpability is a test of cognitive (ability to know) capacity. By definition, a diagnosis of postpartum psychosis assumes impaired cognitive abilities. Therefore, the very factor (namely, cognition) used to determine culpability is pathognomonic for the illness itself.

Organic psychosis also implies the presence of a waxing and waning sensorium, a labile quality that is well documented (see Wisner, Chapter 3). Practitioners are cautioned about this erratic mental status and mood changeability, which make actions unpredictable and emphasize the need for caution when one is evaluating a psychotic mother who has an infant at home. A mother must be separated from the infant until the psychosis resolves. The very foundation of the Yates case was based on Mrs. Yates's mental state after the murders, a point that is mute in presentation of an ever-changing mental status.

The prosecution determined that Andrea Yates knew right from wrong because she called her husband and police *after* the event. This thinking suggests that we extrapolate backward then "predict" that she had an intact thought process. A call for help after the event is not indicative of a normal mental status during the event

The real challenge for psychiatry is to educate the legal profession and juries about the physiological underpinnings of postpartum disorders and other psychoses—to use the courtroom as a classroom to demonstrate our scientific and biologically based knowledge and expertise to the jury and, ultimately, to encourage verdicts based on facts.

The Yates case epitomizes the shortcomings of the American medical and legal institutions. Puerperal illness remains markedly understudied and underdiagnosed in the professional and lay populations.

Clear-cut diagnostic and legal guidelines for psychiatric illness associated with infanticide could likely assist our legal system with these cases. America's reluctance to distinguish postpartum disorders may lead to tragic outcomes for women in the family and society. Moreover, it results in disparate treatment for women in the legal system overall.

Civil Cases

Since rules of evidence are typically less strict in civil courts, postpartum syndromes are readily admitted into evidence during civil proceedings (Meyer et al. 1999). This has created a disparate situation wherein postpartum syndromes can be used to harm women in civil courts, such as through loss of custody, but are used inconsistently in criminal courts to mitigate their loss of liberty.

For example, in custody matters, the trial court has broad discretion. Mental health can generally be considered and weighted in relation to other factors in custody decisions. It is difficult to estimate how frequently the issue of postpartum syndromes is raised in custody cases, because undoubtedly many mothers abandon their pursuit of custody after the father makes clear his intention to make their mental health an issue. In addition, it is impossible to determine how persuasive postpartum syndromes are in judicial decisions, because trial court transcripts are often inaccessible and opinions are generally not formally written. In the infrequent event of an appeal, the court's opinion becomes more accessible.

If the father raises postpartum syndromes in custody cases, he generally asserts that the mother is an unfit parent because of her history of postpartum mental illness, even though the mother is not currently mentally ill and may have no other history of mental illness or unfit parenting. One of the first recorded cases using postpartum syndromes in custody cases was *Pfeifer v. Pfeifer* (1955):

> The father appealed an order that gave care, custody, and control of the child to the mother solely on the basis of her potential threat to the child because of her history of postpartum psychosis. When the couple separated, Kent, their child, went to live with his father and paternal grandparents. Ms. Pfeifer had recently recovered from postpartum psychosis and was trying to rebuild her life, but she had no home to offer Kent. Kent's grandmother became his primary caregiver. Mr. Pfeifer remarried and relocated, but Kent continued to live with his grandparents. Ms. Pfe-

ifer, who had also remarried, sued and eventually won custody of Kent. Mr. Pfeifer appealed the custody award, citing the mental instability of Ms. Pfeifer. At the time of the custody hearing the mother had suffered no symptoms of postpartum psychosis for 5 years and did not intend to have any more children.

On appeal, the father claimed there had been no change in circumstances warranting modification of the original custody award. The court held that

> the mother has remained in good mental health for more than two years without relapse; she has remarried, can offer the child a good home, and is willing to give up her profession to take care of him and her household. This change in the circumstance of the mother could in itself justify the change of custody ordered. Moreover, the father has also remarried and has moved out of the home of his parents to another neighborhood. The grandparents, with whom the child remained, have reached an age, which, notwithstanding their love and devotion, must make them less fit to educate a child of the age of Kent and compared to them, the mother has, if she is not unfit to have custody, certainly a prior claim to the child. (Pfeifer v. Pfeifer 1955)

This case was appealed on questions related to Ms. Pfeifer's mental status resulting from a brief episode of postpartum psychosis. Mr. Pfeifer's appeal was denied. This case is important for several reasons. First, it was not Mr. Pfeifer who would have retained custody but the grandparents. Second, Mr. Pfeifer had led Kent to believe his stepmother was his biological mother. The court felt this posed a danger that Kent would never learn the identity of his biological mother. Third, Ms. Pfeifer's marriage was important to the court because it represented stability; it is questionable whether the court would have awarded custody to Ms. Pfeifer if she had not remarried, even though the grandparents were becoming too elderly to care for the child. Fourth, Ms. Pfeifer had no intention of having any more children. Fifth, Ms. Pfeifer had not had any symptoms for 5 years. It would have been difficult to deny Ms. Pfeifer custody under these circumstances.

In contrast, consider the following case (In re the Marriage of Grimm 1989):

> Susan and Gary Grimm were married for 13 years and had three children. After the birth of each child, Susan suffered from postpartum depression and was hospitalized. During these hospitalizations, Susan phoned home daily to speak with her children and had personal visits with them. Following the last hospitalization, in 1985, the Grimms separated. During the separation, the children resided with their father, while the mother lived nearby and visited daily. Susan washed dishes, laundered and mended clothes, cooked for the children, and stayed with them at night whenever Gary was working.

The couple petitioned for dissolution and each sought sole custody of the children. Both were evaluated as excellent parents. However, it is clear that Susan Grimm's postpartum depression was an important factor in this custody award. Her treating psychiatrist was called to testify regarding her stability. No other testimony regarding the fitness of either parent was addressed. The court placed custody with Gary.

As in *Pfeifer v. Pfeifer* (1995), Susan Grimm had not been hospitalized for a long period prior to the custody hearing. In addition, Susan had been, and wanted to continue to be, actively involved with the children's lives. However, the court placed custody with Gary. Susan appealed and the appeals court reaffirmed the custody award. It is unclear why the Pfeifer and Grimm cases were decided differently.

In other civil matters, the court has refused to allow testimony regarding postpartum depression to be persuasive. For example, in a 1997 adoption appeal, a biological mother who had given her child up for adoption asserted that postpartum depression rendered her incompetent to consent to the adoption. The Tennessee Appellate Court stated:

> We do not dispute that [the mother] was probably depressed or emotionally distraught following this rather traumatic experience, but it is not unusual for there to be depression and distress following the birth of a child, even under the best of circumstances. If emotional distress meant that a parent was always incompetent to consent to an adoption, we would rarely have adoptions in this state. (Croslin v. Croslin 1997 at 10)

Similarly, in another case, the court did not find that postpartum depression invalidated a woman's competency to consent to a postnuptial agreement:

> Kim and Anthony L had a 1-year-old son when Kim gave birth to a daughter, Jill, who was premature and had to be returned to the hospital daily for a short time after her birth. Kim was caring for both children and preparing to return to work while still suffering from postpartum depression. Approximately 3 weeks after Jill was born, Kim had to be rushed to the hospital for severe hemorrhaging. Although she was not admitted to the hospital, the court acknowledged, "[i]t was obviously a very frightening and traumatic experience" (Latina v. Latina 1995 at 19). A few days after Kim was rushed to the hospital, less than 1 month postpartum, Anthony presented her with a postnuptial agreement. Regarding the effect of postpartum depression on Kim's capacity to consent, the Delaware Family Court stated:

> The break-up of a marriage never comes at a good time, and, as noted in many earlier opinions, usually separation agreements are signed in a highly charged atmosphere, thereby necessitating the precautions taken by the

Delaware courts to ensure the agreements' fairness. However, if the courts could set aside agreements based upon their being signed during the emotional turmoil of a marriage splitting up, no separation agreement would ever be permitted to stand. Although the court recognizes Wife was extremely distraught and probably feeling somewhat vulnerable when she signed the agreement, the Court finds that Wife signed more because she did not understand the implications of the agreement than because she was coerced. It should be noted that the second agreement was signed by Wife approximately six weeks after the first agreement, by which time Wife's postpartum depression and concern for Jill's health should have lessened. (Latina v Latina 1995 at 19)

The lack of a clear understanding associated with these cases underscores the obligation of psychiatry to educate the court about postpartum illnesses. These cases reflect the dearth of knowledge about these illnesses, which leads to inconsistencies in treatment. The fact that a disorder can be a key factor in one civil case but easily dismissed in another suggests a need for further clarification through improved research in order to resolve the continued dilemma for the medical and legal communities.

Medical and Legal Dilemmas

The medical and psychiatric communities share some responsibility for these discrepancies. First, there are no definitive postpartum diagnostic criteria. Second, the lack of criteria is compounded by legal ambiguities in the insanity laws and discrepancies in insanity criteria. When postpartum disorders are asserted in court, the validity and exculpatory capability of these disorders become the subject of dispute between experts.

Courts strive for bright lines, or clear criteria, on which to base decisions. Bright lines are difficult to achieve but reduce ambiguity and subjectivity and provide greater consistency and fairness in decisions. On the other hand, recognition of postpartum syndromes in the legal system could result in a slippery slope for the courts. For example, would a woman accused of child abuse now be able to assert postpartum syndromes as an exculpatory defense? Would the defense be available for other crimes, such as larceny or battery?

At first glance it appears that recognition of postpartum syndromes could lead to such unwieldy outcomes, but it is unlikely. First, this has not happened in other countries, where the postpartum defense is rarely used. Second, and more important, defendants with postpartum psychosis have committed very specific crimes with very specific victims. Also, the trigger is clearly due to one cause, pregnancy, and this cause is not likely to reoccur with such great frequency. Third, the danger is temporary. If anything, postpartum syndromes seem to have more specificity than already recognized defenses, such as posttraumatic stress disorder, and represent much less of a threat to the integrity of the legal system.

Courts could facilitate preventive action by the medical community if they would acknowledge the importance of postpartum syndromes in their opinions. The courts have been able to address this issue directly in cases involving insurance and disability claims for postpartum syndromes. As far back as 1964, a court was asked to determine whether postpartum syndromes represent a sickness or mental illness (Price v. State Capital Insurance Company 1964). If postpartum syndromes represent a sickness, the level of coverage under insurance and disability is generally expanded. Conversely, if they represent a mental illness, the coverage is generally restricted. The courts have routinely held that the cause of postpartum syndromes has not been proven to be physical and the treatment is generally psychological. Therefore, postpartum syndromes are excluded from coverage (Blake v. Union Mutual Stock Life Insurance Company 1990). The courts have also found that postpartum syndromes were outside the scope of pregnancy disability claims (Barrash v. Bowen 1988). The courts could address the issue of classification of postpartum syndromes in their opinions, which could facilitate a review of the status of these conditions by the medical and psychological communities as well as clarify insurance provisions.

Conclusion

Many women are reluctant to report symptoms of postpartum syndromes to health care professionals (Meyer et al. 1999). This reluctance to seek help for or even discuss postpartum syndromes makes early detection difficult. However, increased recognition of postpartum syndromes by the medical and psychological communities would certainly precipitate a debate on the impact of pathologizing normal processes in women on women's status overall. In addition, it could be argued that increasing the role of the psychological and medical community could increase the power these professions have over women.

It seems unlikely that recognizing postpartum syndromes could worsen the current situation for women. In fact, recognition of these conditions could actually benefit women. Recognition of pathology might actually be necessary in order for women to receive proper treatment, medical or psychological (Meyer et al. 1999). Without a clear pathology, health care providers might minimize women's syndromes, which then may go untreated. Therefore, pathology may be seen as a means to an end. Recognizing some postpartum syndromes as pathological and not others may decrease the overall level of pathology assigned to these conditions. The pathology of postpartum psychosis, which is a rare and serious disorder, may increase the distinction between this condition and less severe types of postpartum syndromes, which can be readily treated.

Some may argue that even seeing one type of postpartum syndrome as pathological does an injustice to women. In response to this argument, it is important to remember that women with postpartum syndromes are already being stigmatized. It is also important to realize that by increasing the recognition of postpartum syndromes, we can increase awareness of the context in which these conditions develop (Meyer et al. 1999). By increasing recognition of postpartum syndromes and acknowledging the social variables that contribute to them, we could provide women with the help they need, without viewing their conditions as inherently pathological.

Women should also be encouraged to actively participate in making decisions that affect their lives. A major concern is that women should not be identified as victims of their own biological changes. And yet, knowledge of the facts is, in and of itself, empowering. The search for scientific data and sanctioned diagnostic criteria should include a risk-benefit analysis. The benefit derived from recognition and equitable treatment under the law far outweighs the risk that women will be perceived as weak. The greatest risk is that women with these disorders will continue to suffer tragic consequences unless the potential benefits are met (Meyer et al. 1999).

References

American Psychiatric Association: Diagnostic and Statistical Manual: Mental Disorders. Washington, DC, American Psychiatric Association, 1952

American Psychiatric Association: Diagnostic and Statistical Manual of Mental Disorders, 4th Edition. Washington, DC, American Psychiatric Association, 1994

American Psychiatric Association: Diagnostic and Statistical Manual of Mental Disorders, 4th Edition, Text Revision. Washington, DC, American Psychiatric Association, 2000

Barrash v Bowen, 846 P2d 927 (4th Cir 1988)

Blake v Union Mutual Stock Life Insurance Company, 906 P2d 1525 (1990)

Brockington I: Motherhood and Mental Health. Oxford, UK, Oxford University Press, 1996, pp 430–468

Brusca A: Postpartum psychosis: a way out for murderous moms? Hofstra Law Review 18:1133–1170, 1990

Cassell E: FindLaw Forum: the Andrea Yates trial: did the jury do the right thing. CNN.com/LAWCENTER. Available at www.cnn.com/2002/LAW/03/columns/fl.cassel.Yates.03.18/. Accessed March 29, 2002

Cox J: Causes and consequences: the life event of childbirth: sociocultural aspects of postnatal depression, in Motherhood and Mental Illness, Vol 2. Edited by Kumar R, Brockington IF. London, Butterworth, 1988, pp 64–77

Croslin v Croslin, Tenn App Lexis 84 (1997)

Esquirol JED: Des maladies mentales consideres sous les rapports medical, hygienique et medico-legal, Vol 1. Paris, JB Bailliere, 1838

Gardner CA: Postpartum depression defense: are mothers getting away with murder? New England Law Review 24:953–989, 1990

Grinfield MJ: Mother's murder conviction turns insanity defense suspect. Psychiatric Times, June 2002, pp 1–5

Hamilton JA: Postpartum psychiatric syndromes. Psychiatr Clin North Am 12: 89–103, 1989

Hamilton JA, Harberger PN: Postpartum Psychiatric Illness: A Picture Puzzle. Philadelphia, University of Pennsylvania Press, 1992

In re the Marriage of Grimm, Minn App Lexis 143 (1989)

Japenga A: Ordeal of postpartum psychosis: illness can have tragic consequences for new mothers. Los Angeles Times, February 1, 1987, p 1

Kendell RE, Chalmers JC, Platz C: Epidemiology of puerperal pyschoses. Br J Psychiatry 150:662–673, 1987

Lagaipa SJ: Suffer the little children: the ancient practice of infanticide as a modern moral dilemma. Issues Compr Pediatr Nurs 13:241–251, 1990

Latina v Latina, Del Fam Ct Lexis 48 (1995)

Lynch-Fraser D: The Complete Postpartum Guide: Everything You Need to Know About Taking Care of Yourself After You've Had a Baby. New York, Harper & Row, 1983

Marcé LV: Traité de la folie des femmes enceintes, des nouvelles accouchées et des nourrices. Paris, J.B. Bailliere et Fils, 1858

Mason-Hohl E: Trotula, eleventh-century gynecologist. Medical Women's Journal 47:349–356, 1940

Meyer CL, Proano T, Franz J: Postpartum syndromes: disparate treatment in the legal system, in It's a Crime: Women and Justice. Edited Muraskin R. Englewood Cliffs, NJ, Prentice-Hall, 1999, pp 91–104

Oberman M: Mothers who kill: coming to terms with modern American infanticide. American Criminal Law Review 34:1–110, 1996

Pfeifer v Pfeifer, 280 P2d 54 (Cal App 1955)

Pies R: The Andrea Yates case: lessons from Euripides. Psychiatric Times, May 2002, pp 3–5

Price v State Capital Insurance Company, 134 SE2d 171 (Sup Ct 1964)

Tekell J: Management of pregnancy in schizophrenic women, in Management of Psychiatric Disorders in Pregnancy. Edited by Yonkers K, Little B. London, Arnold, 2001, pp 189–212

Wisner KL, Peindl KS, Hanusa BH: Symptomatology of affective and psychotic illnesses related to childbearing. J Affect Disord 30:77–87, 1994

Yardley J: Death penalty sought for mother in drownings of children. New York Times, August 9, 2001, A12

Chapter 10

Infanticide in Britain

Maureen N. Marks, D.Phil., C.Psychol., A.F.B.P.S.

> When a woman by any wilful act or omission causes the death of her child . . . aged less than a year, but at the time the balance of her mind was disturbed by reason of her not having fully recovered from the effect of giving birth to a child or by reason of the effect of lactation—the offence which would have amounted to murder is deemed to be infanticide and is dealt with and punished as if it were manslaughter.
>
> *Infanticide Act (1938)*

In England and Wales infants under 1 year of age are at much greater risk (about four times) of becoming victims of homicide than either older children or the general population (Marks 1996). This figure is based on official records of infant homicides, so the risk is probably an underestimate, because some infant homicides are never discovered—especially in cases when the infant was killed soon after delivery—and others are never recorded as such. For example, it is generally considered that at least 2%–10% of registered cot deaths are probably homicides (Emery 1985; Knowlden et al. 1985; Wolkind et al. 1993). The actual number of infants recorded as victims of homicide may seem relatively small—30–40 babies a year in England and Wales—but it is possible that these homicides are an extreme indicator of more widespread infant physical abuse that remains undetected.

A better knowledge of the background and causes of infant homicide may lead to possible prevention of infant homicides as well as infant abuse. However, research findings and reports in the scientific literature tend to be few and fragmentary, or alternatively anecdotal and speculative. There are inevitable difficulties in carrying out research with parents who have been involved in such tragedies.

In this chapter, I describe how legislation on infanticide differs in various parts of Britain and describe the outcomes of court proceedings in these systems. I also summarize current attempts to protect infants at risk.

Legislation on Infanticide

In England and Wales, a woman who has killed her infant under a year of age can be indicted for *infanticide* (see Chapter 1: "A Brief History of Infanticide and the Law"). The legislation that provides for this charge is contained in the Infanticide Act (1938). Alternatively, the woman can be charged with *murder* or *manslaughter*, as for any homicide offense, in terms of the more general Homicide Act (1957).

Thus, the term *infanticide* has a precise meaning in terms of this act. It applies to the killing of an infant under 1 year of age by its mother. There is no special legislation for fathers who kill their infants. Note, too, that the woman's mind must have been disturbed at the time of the offense, with the implication that this disturbance is in some way linked to childbirth and/or lactation.

The Infanticide Act, then, makes special and lenient provision for women who have killed their infant. This provision rests on two related assumptions: 1) childbearing disturbs the balance of a woman's mind, and 2) infanticide is likely a consequence of the mental instability associated with childbearing.

There has been ongoing debate in the United Kingdom about the advisability of retaining the Infanticide Act. Proponents of its abolition put forward a number of arguments (Payne 1995), including the following:

- There is no a priori reason why the killing of an infant should be considered as different from the killing of an older child or adult; to do so implies that infants are not being given equal status and hence equal protection by the law.
- In terms of infanticide legislation, "balance of the mind disturbed'" is taken to mean less of an abnormality than that usually required to substantiate a plea of diminished responsibility under Section 2 of the Homicide Act (1957).
- The medicalization of the offense ("disturbance of the balance of the mind . . . by reason of childbirth or lactation") is not justified because it

conceals the contribution of factors such as social and economic circumstances, inadequate knowledge about contraception, difficulties with child care, and so forth.

- The Homicide Act (1957), with its provision for diminished responsibility, has rendered redundant the need for separate infanticide legislation.
- Retention of the Infanticide Act encourages tolerance by society of the killing and harming of infants and inhibits an advance in understanding of the causes of such offenses.

These seductive arguments oversimplify the issues. To start with, many would argue that there *is* a difference between a parent killing his or her infant and an adult killing another adult. The relationship between a parent (especially the mother) and an infant has unique characteristics.

Epidemiological data suggest that infant homicides are different from other homicide offenses. For example, the rate of infant homicide in England and Wales appears to be unrelated to *positive* social changes associated with a decline in infant mortality, such as improved social and economic circumstances, nor has the rate of infant homicide fallen since the liberalization of abortion laws (Abortion Act 1967). Similarly, *negative* social changes associated with the steadily increasing rate of homicide observed in the population as a whole have not affected the incidence of infant homicide (Marks and Kumar 1993).

Proponents of abolition have noted with concern that the number of women found guilty of infanticide and imprisoned has decreased (Payne 1995). They suggest that judges' attitudes and hence sentencing are influenced by the relatively lenient framing of the British infanticide legislation. However, since the introduction of the Homicide Act (1957), there has been a steady decline in convictions for infanticide and a concomitant increase in convictions of some other homicide offenses (e.g., manslaughter or murder) (Marks and Kumar 1993; Parker and Good 1981). Individuals in the latter cases are more likely to be given prison sentences (Marks and Kumar 1993). Therefore, under existing legislation, the more serious infant homicide offenses are already associated with a conviction other than infanticide.

Rather than abolish the Infanticide Act, what is needed is research into the reasons that lead the prosecution to bring charges of murder, manslaughter, or infanticide. Further evidence to support this position comes from a comparison of England and Wales with Scotland. Homicide rates in Scotland in the general population are consistently higher than in England and Wales—19 per million per year (Scottish Office 1993) compared with 11 per million per year (Home Office 1997). In addition, Scottish legislation and judicial procedure differ from that of England

and Wales in many ways. In contrast to the law in England and Wales, Scottish legislation makes no special provision for maternal infanticide. A mother who kills her infant in Scotland will be charged with either murder or common law culpable homicide as for any other homicide offense. Mitigating factors, such as the defendant's mental state at the time of the death, will be taken into account as for any other homicide, as will her fitness to plead in the first place. However, there is no embodiment within Scottish law of causal links between childbirth or lactation, maternal mental illness, and infanticide.

So how do infanticide rates in Scotland compare with those observed in England and Wales? If more harsh legislation is a deterrent, then rates should be lower. If infant homicide is related to homicide generally, then rates would be expected to be higher. In an analysis of details obtained from the Scottish Office concerning all infants under 1 year of age who were recorded as the victims of homicide in Scotland during the period from 1978 to 1993, it was found that despite social, cultural, and legal differences between Scotland and England and Wales, rates of the offense, the characteristics of victims and perpetrators, and the patterning of both convictions and sentence were similar in the two regions (Marks and Kumar 1996). This suggests that the contribution of gross cultural, social, and legal factors to the occurrence of infant homicide may be less important than other, as yet unidentified, processes.

The infanticide legislation was designed primarily to protect *psychotic* mothers from the death penalty if they were convicted of killing their infants. Why, in principle, should one distinguish between them and non–psychotically depressed mothers (see Chapter 3: "Postpartum Disorders")? Very few depressed or psychotic women kill their infants, and we do not know the factors that render them more likely to do so. The causes of such relationship problems are unknown but may include a traumatic childhood and problematic adult social and family relationships, as well as some physiological dysfunction. However, at present, there is insufficient information available from appropriate systematic studies of the psychopathology of infanticidal parents to answer such questions.

In my view, the spirit of the Infanticide Act takes into account the unique psychological circumstances of giving birth to and then caring for a very young child, an abnormality of mind that is a feature of parenting. Charging every woman who kills her baby with murder and subjecting such women to the ordeal of a murder trial may increase the proportion that are sentenced to imprisonment. Abolition of the act is unlikely to result in a reduction in the number of infants killed or to facilitate research into the precursors of these crimes, nor is it likely to encourage the development of effective social policy to deal with the problem.

Neonaticide in Britain

About a quarter of all infant homicides in Britain are of infants within 24 hours of their birth (Marks 1996). The characteristics and causes of the homicide of these infants (neonaticide) are very different from those of the homicide of infants older than a day; it is therefore important to distinguish neonaticide from the homicide of infants or older children (see Chapter 6: " Neonaticide"). Unfortunately, few official records and epidemiological studies do so, and those that do tend to use different definitions of what constitutes a neonate—for example, up to 1 week of age or up to 1 month of age. This makes the interpretation of the data obtained difficult and comparisons between studies impossible.

Anecdotal reports and case note studies suggest that demographic features of neonaticides may also be different from those of homicides of infants older than a day. For example, compared with parents who kill older infants, neonaticidal mothers are more likely to be young (under 20), single, and still living at home with parents.

The infant's death is more likely to have resulted from inaction rather than the violent action that often characterizes the killing of older infants: nearly half die from neglect (Marks and Kumar 1993). Mothers who kill their neonates are treated comparatively leniently by the legal system in the United Kingdom. In a major proportion of cases, the mother is never indicted, and those who are usually receive infanticide convictions (Marks and Kumar 1993).

The most frequent observation about women who commit neonaticide is that the pregnancy had been denied (Brozovsky and Falit 1971; Green and Manohar 1990) (see Chapter 5: "Denial of Pregnancy"). This state of affairs is usually the consequence of an unconscious belief: if you don't think about it, then the pregnancy will, magically, disappear. Sometimes the woman does not seem to acknowledge even to herself that she is pregnant. In either case, the woman does not seek medical help and makes no preparation for the delivery. After the child is born and disposed of, the mother returns immediately to her normal daily life.

Pregnancy denial may be related to the fact that the biological manifestations of pregnancy sometimes become attenuated—for example, there may be reduced change in body contour, continuation of menstrual bleeding during pregnancy, and no complaints of pregnancy such as nausea or increased urinary frequency (Brozovsky and Falit 1971). The arrival of the baby is thus experienced as a traumatic shock and puts an end to the denial, and the woman is then confronted with the overwhelming fear that made the denial so necessary and effective in the first place.

A 20-year-old single woman had successfully concealed her pregnancy. She had a previous pregnancy that had also been concealed. This first baby had been delivered into a toilet at the parental home but had been rescued by one of the family and subsequently adopted. During her second pregnancy, the woman was able to convince her friends, family, and boyfriend who knew of the earlier concealed pregnancy that she was not pregnant. She "knew" she was pregnant, and yet when labor pains started (at term) she thought the pains were due to something she had eaten. She was alone at the time, and the infant was born into the toilet and subsequently died. (The cause of the infant's death was never fully established.) The mother placed the infant in a plastic bag and threw this into a nearby lake. The morning of the infant's delivery she returned to work complaining of a heavy period. The discovery of the infant by a passer-by set in train the inquiries, which led to the mother's arrest and trial. She was subsequently convicted of infanticide and sentenced to probation. The sentence included a treatment provision, namely, that she attend weekly psychotherapy for a year.

The key psychodynamic features of the therapy work with this woman involved addressing her denial of her underlying rage and murderousness and her unconscious guilt about these feelings. She was a "nice" girl—neat and tidy, compliant, hardworking, conscientious. She was always on her best behavior. Unpleasant thoughts and feelings she "put to the back of her mind." It was very difficult for the therapist to be in touch with her rage, despite the dead baby and despite, too, the violence of material brought to sessions. The latter included, for example, a car accident (hers), a suicide (a pregnant friend's), and a local boy's murder of his girlfriend. At times her rage and guilt formed an alliance, and she would do something violent to herself.

It became increasingly evident that the diagnosis of dissociative disorder given by the psychiatrist in his assessment for the court was accurate. This was exemplified not only in the way she was unable to experience her emotional life but also in her impact on the therapist, who knew there had been a dead baby but found this difficult if not impossible to keep in mind. A particularly concrete example of her capacity to dissociate occurred about halfway through the treatment. The patient worked in the catering industry. One day, during the course of her work that sometimes involved helping out with cooking when the restaurant was very busy, she noticed blisters on her hand and started to shake. She then realized she had inadvertently put her hand into the boiling oil she had been cooking with. She had not felt the pain of the burning until she had seen the blisters. The burns were serious and required hospital outpatient treatment, after which she went back to work. In the week preceding this event, a colleague had visited the work place to show people her new baby and the patient had held the baby.

She was persecuted with guilt, largely unconscious, that was to some extent addressed in the sessions. She would carry out menial tasks at work, such as cleaning the toilets, even though she was employed in a management role. She worked long hours for a pittance without complaining. She said this started when she was first charged: "I deserved to be the lowest of the low and now, well I feel bad if I don't." She believed she had "got away with murder" and lived with the constant fear of retribution. This fear of retribution was embodied in a recurring dream. In this dream she is in her bed, at home which is her mother's house. In her bedroom is a hatch to the loft. In the dream a man peers periodically out of the hatch. Sometimes there is a rope around her neck and he has the end of it. The man somehow gets her into the loft. He then removes bricks from the side of the house and takes her out through this hole. And there she is "nowhere." The man then replaces the bricks in the side of the house "without her in it." What is so terrifying for her about the dream is to be "nowhere." She thinks the dream is about the hangman—about her fear that "they are going to change their minds about prison."

I use this material, first, to illustrate the extent to which this patient resorted to the defenses of denial and dissociation and, second, to note how in the absence of sufficient punishment demanded by her super ego, she lived in fear of punishment and how, when her guilt became intolerable, she punished herself. A prison sentence may have relieved her of some guilt but may have made it more difficult for her to make her own restitution. She and the supportive partner whom she met during the year of her treatment now have a child. There are no concerns about this child being at risk.

The overrepresentation of women with dissociative disorder in studies of neonaticide mothers may be in part a consequence of not only their naïveté but also this particular form of defense. It may be that more mature, worldly, reality-oriented women are more able to successfully conceal an unwanted pregnancy and dispose of the newly delivered infant in such a way that it remains undiscovered.

Infanticide in Britain

Infants older than 1 day but younger than 1 year tend to be killed by either their mother or their father (see Chapter 2: "Epidemiology of Infanticide"). In the United States, in Florida, fathers and mothers are equally likely to be the perpetrator. Jason et al. (1983) analyzed national child (younger than 18 years) homicide data from the Federal Bureau of Investigation crime reporting system for 1976 through 1979. They found that mothers killed neonates and that slightly more fathers than mothers killed infants younger than 1 year. Likewise, in England and Wales (Marks and Kumar 1993) and Scotland (Marks and Kumar 1996), slightly more infants are killed by fathers than by mothers. In the England/Wales and Scotland studies, there was no interaction between sex of perpetrator and sex of victim: father and mothers were equally likely to kill boys or girls.

Infanticide is usually attributed to either mental illness or child abuse—

that is, the parent who has killed his or her infant is generally considered to be either "mad" or "bad." As discussed earlier, in England and Wales there is particular legislation that applies to a woman who has killed her child younger than 1 year (i.e., the Infanticide Act [1938]). Implicit in this legislation is the idea that childbirth may sometimes have a destabilizing impact on mothers' minds, that the infant homicide may have occurred under these unstable psychological conditions, and that, therefore, there may be a case for diminished responsibility for the crime. In contrast, in Scotland and in the United States, mothers who kill their children are charged as for any other homicide offense, with the possibility that the filicidal mother can plead diminished responsibility within the usual terms of each country's homicide legislation. Despite these differences in legislation, in most Western countries the younger the infant, the greater the likelihood that the offense will be attributed to some form of mental illness and the perpetrator will be convicted of a less serious offense and given a lighter sentence. This is particularly so for mothers who kill their infants.

In England and Wales, most mothers who kill their infants are convicted of infanticide and given probation sentences. In contrast, fathers who kill their infants are usually given prison sentences (Marks and Kumar 1993). Despite there being no infanticide act in Scotland, the outcome is similar. Most mothers who kill infants receive noncustodial sentences, either probation or hospital orders, and most fathers are sent to prison (Marks and Kumar 1996).

Public records provide limited information about the details surrounding these offenses, so it is difficult to know whether sentencing reflects the circumstances and severity of the crime. Data we obtained from the Scottish Office included a computer record of the motive for the offense. Mothers were usually recorded as having killed their infant because of their mental state, whereas the most frequent attribution given to fathers was that of rage (Marks and Kumar 1996). However, we were unable to determine how these motivations were ascribed and whether the difference between mothers and fathers was due to the circumstances surrounding the offense or to the effects of gender on the attributions about the causes of events.

Prevention

An important but difficult aspect in the management of maternal mental illness is that decisions about treatment have to take into account both the mother's and her infant's well-being. These decisions include judgments about immediate risk of harm to the infant as well as long-term judgments concerning the mother's ability as a parent that have to be balanced with the problems potentially resulting from overly intrusive care, which may impair the mother's natural and healthy bonding with her infant.

Another difficulty concerns the reluctance of mothers who are experiencing emotional problems to recognize the problems and then to feel it is safe to seek help for them. Many mothers feel they are not coping and that they have failed as mothers, and they sometimes fear that should their mental state become public they could lose care of their child. These concerns, as well as more general fears about "going mad" and being stigmatized, mean that women are often reluctant to have contact with psychiatric services. Offers of care, therefore, need to take into account the acceptability of the form of care delivery to the mother.

Strategies of treatment in the United Kingdom are influenced by the fact that peripartum women have close contact with obstetric, health visitor, and primary care services. This means that detection of cases and delivery of care are increasingly being carried out at the primary care level and that there is more psychiatric liaison with these groups in the provision of care for women with infants. Thus, in the United Kingdom, most mothers are cared for in the community with regular general practitioner and health visitor contact. A variety of services have been developed for mothers whose illnesses are more severe. These include psychiatric outpatient contact, day hospital care, and inpatient mother and baby units.

Obstetric Service

Parturient women are in repeated contact with obstetric services, and one way of targeting women who are depressed or at risk of becoming so is via these services. For example, at King's College Hospital in London, there is an obstetric-psychiatric liaison service that provides a psychiatric service to perinatal women who are identified at antenatal booking as having histories of mental disorder. Under this scheme, patients with current or histories of significant psychiatric illness (screened by midwives at antenatal booking) are offered an appointment with a psychiatrist and are then monitored by the psychiatrist at regular intervals during the pregnancy and postpartum.

Midwifery Support

Another response to the difficulty in providing accessible care has been the development of specialist midwifery services for high-risk women (Kumar et al. 1995). Continuity of care is thought to have a preventive role by providing social support to mothers, enhancing the likelihood of detection of prodromal symptoms, and improving successful follow-up care if referrals are made to other professionals (Briscoe 1986). There is evidence, too, that continuity of midwifery care may have direct beneficial effects. It has been shown to reduce postnatal "blues" (Odent 1984; see also Chapter 3, this volume), labor times, and obstetric complications in both mother and baby (Kennell et al. 1991; Klaus et al. 1986; Sosa et al. 1980), and it may also contribute to enhanced maternal postnatal mood. Indications are that this form of support is very popular with high-risk women.

Health Visitor Support

Health visitors (nurses who visit patients at home) have become increasingly involved in the detection of postnatal depression and in caring for women identified as depressed (Holden 1996), either in support groups (Pitts 1995; Romaine et al. 1995) or individually. Holden et al. (1989) demonstrated that weekly counseling sessions by trained health visitors are a successful treatment for postnatal depression. Women identified as having a postnatal depression were allocated to a control or a treatment group. Women in the treatment group received eight consecutive weekly visits from the health visitors. After 3 months, 69% of women in the treatment group, compared with 38% of the controls, had recovered.

Peer Group Support

Many women find it easier to seek help from nonprofessionals, such as can be obtained from peer-developed and -run self-help support groups. In Britain such organizations exist locally (e.g., Newpin in London) and at a national level (e.g., National Childbirth Trust, Association for Postnatal Mental Illness). Help provided includes *befriending*, whereby a member, usually a woman who has herself suffered postnatal mental illness, is introduced to the woman and becomes available to her for help and support as required; regular telephone chats with members; and support group meetings.

Mother-and-Baby Units

One response to the requirements of severely or psychotically depressed new mothers has been the joint hospitalization of both mother and baby, either to general psychiatric admission wards or to specialized mother-and-baby units. A preference for joint admission is based on the assumption that mother-infant separation is damaging to the burgeoning mother-infant relationship and may have deleterious consequences for the child's development (Bowlby 1969, 1973, 1980). It is thought, too, that the infant's presence may facilitate improvement in the mother's mental state and may even hasten her discharge. Few argue with the benefits of keeping mother and child together; however, intensive programs of community care for postnatally depressed mothers that have been developed as an alternative to admission are also effective (Oates 1988), as is community care in combination with day hospital support (Cox et al. 1993).

Conclusion

The younger the infant, the more likely the risk he or she will become the victim of homicide, and the younger the infant, the more likely the perpetrator will be a parent. Neonaticide is usually committed by mothers and is probably the least preventable of infanticides.

For children older than a day and younger than 1 year, a parent is the most likely perpetrator of infant homicide. Both mothers and fathers are at risk, although fathers may be slightly more likely to be, especially if the father is the main caregiver.

Child abuse fatalities appear to be the most frequent type of infanticide for younger infants. This usually involves a parent who is not severely mentally ill but whose parenting is, at least in some ways, inherently abusive to the infant.

As with assessing the risk of violence in psychiatric patients generally, there are difficulties in assessing the risk of infanticide in a mentally ill parent. Most parents with mental illness do not harm their children. When they do, the most frequent scenario involves a parent who is suicidal and who believes the child will also be better off dead.

One of the most important clinical developments in Britain the last decade or so has been the consequence of a shift in emphasis from parental rights to the rights of the child and parental responsibility in ensuring that these are adequately met. In the United Kingdom the passing and implementation of the Children Act (1989) has resulted in important changes in practice. The key feature of this act is that the welfare of the child is paramount: when there is conflict, the child's needs have priority over those of the parent.

There is always sympathy and concern for a woman who has a severe psychiatric disorder. Often she herself has been the victim of grossly inadequate parenting from which society failed to protect her. Under these circumstances, the woman's caregivers may find it difficult to keep both mother's and baby's sometimes conflicting needs in mind. A frequently expressed, and understandable, view is that all mothers need to be given a chance. A society that asserts and legislates for the primacy of the child's welfare ensures that it is the baby who is given a chance. This goal may be best achieved by offering therapeutic interventions aimed at helping a mother to better protect, care for, and understand her child—or, when necessary, through separation and safe and secure placement—rather than by introducing more punitive legislation.

References

Abortion Act 1967, 15 and 16, 2,c.87. October 27, 1967

Briscoe M: Identification of emotional problems in postpartum women by health visitors. BMJ 292:1245–1247, 1986

Brozovsky M, Falit H: Neonaticide: clinical and psychodynamic considerations. Journal of American Academy of Child Psychiatry 10:673–683, 1971

Bowlby J: Attachment and Loss, Vol I: Attachment. New York, Basic Books, 1969

Bowlby J: Attachment and Loss, Vol II: Separation: Anxiety and Anger. New York, Basic Books, 1973

Bowlby J: Attachment and Loss, Vol III: Loss: Sadness and Depression. New York, Basic Books, 1980

Children Act. London, Her Majesty's Stationery Office, 1989, C41

Cox JL, Gerrard J, Cookson D, et al: Development and audit of Charles Street Parent and Baby Day Unit, Stoke-on-Trent. Psychiatric Bulletin 17:711–713, 1993

Emery JL: Infanticide, filicide and cot death. Arch Dis Child 60:505–507, 1985

Green CM, Manohar SV: Neonaticide and hysterical denial of pregnancy. Br J Psychiatry 156:121–123, 1990

Holden J: The role of health visitors in postnatal depression. International Review of Psychiatry 8:79–86, 1996

Holden JM, Sagovski R, Cox JL: Counselling in a general practice setting: controlled study of health visitor intervention in treatment of postnatal depression. BMJ 298:223–226, 1989

Home Office: Criminal Statistics, England and Wales 1987–96. London, Her Majesty's Stationery Office, 1997

Homicide Act. London, Her Majesty's Stationery Office, 1957, C45

Infanticide Act, 2 Geo 6, Ch 36 (Eng 1938)

Jason J, Gilliland JC, Tyler CW: Homicide as a cause of pediatric mortality in the United States. Pediatrics 72:191–197, 1983

Kennell J, Klaus M, McGrath S, et al: Continuous emotional support during labor in a US hospital: a randomized controlled trial. JAMA 265:2197–2201, 1991

Klaus MH, Kennell JH, Roberson SS, et al: Effects of social support during parturition on maternal and infant morbidity. BMJ (Clin Res Ed) 293(6547): 585–587, 1986

Knowlden J, Keeling J, Nicholl JP: Post neonatal mortality. DHSS Report, London, Her Majesty's Stationery Office, 1985

Kumar R, Marks MN, Jackson K: Prevention and treatment of postnatal psychiatric disorders: the role of the midwife. British Journal of Midwifery 3:314–317, 1995

Marks MN: Characteristics and causes of infanticide in Britain. International Review of Psychiatry 8:99–106, 1996

Marks MN, Kumar R: Infanticide in England and Wales, 1982–1988. Med Sci Law 33:329–339, 1993

Marks MN, Kumar R: Infanticide in Scotland. Med Sci Law 36:299–305, 1996

Oates M: The development of an integrated community oriented service for severe postnatal mental illness, in Motherhood and Mental Illness. Edited by Kumar R, Brockington IF. London, Wright, 1988, pp 133–158

Odent M: Birth Reborn. London, Souvenir Press, 1984

Parker E, Good F: Infanticide. Law Hum Behav 5:237–243, 1981

Payne A: Infanticide and child abuse. Journal of Forensic Psychiatry 6:472–476, 1995

Pitts F: Comrades in adversity: the group approach. Health Visitor 68:144–145, 1995

Romaine S, Jones A, Watts T: Postnatal depression: facilitating peer group support. Health Visitor 68:153, 1995

Scottish Office: Statistical Bulletin: Criminal Justice Series. Edinburgh, Government Statistical Service, 1993

Sosa R, Kennell JH, Klaus MH, et al: The effect of a supportive companion on perinatal problems, length of labor, and mother-infant interaction. N Engl J Med 303:597–600, 1980

Wolkind S, Taylor EM, Waite AJ, et al: Recurrence of unexpected infant death. Acta Paediatr 82:873–876, 1993

Part **IV**

Treatment and Prevention

Chapter 11

How Could Anyone Do That?

A Therapist's Struggle With Countertransference

Anonymous

> The analyst contributes to the working alliance by . . . consistent emphasis on understanding and insight, . . . and by compassionate, empathic, straightforward, and nonjudgmental attitudes.
>
> *R. R. Greenson (1988)*

I first heard of this neonaticide when a television reporter called me to comment on the news of the mother's arrest. My response was not horror or sadness, I confess, but annoyance. Why, as an expert on postpartum depression, do I get these baby-killing calls from the media? Am I on a Rolodex somewhere that says "infanticide, postpartum depression, what's the difference, call her"? As is my policy on these once- or twice-a-year calls, I explained to the reporter that I couldn't possibly comment on the mental health or illness of an individual I've never seen. I was annoyed because I'm sick of hearing neonaticide linked to postpartum depression. How many depressed new mothers decided to stay sick, I wonder, sure that asking for help will raise their fitness as safe caregivers?

The author is a reproductive psychiatrist, psychodynamic psychotherapist, and a faculty member in a large academic medical center. In view of the publicity of this case, the author has chosen not to reveal her identity and geographical location in order to protect the confidentiality of the patient.

It had been a bad year for neonaticide, with several highly publicized cases scattered across the country. The reporter didn't want to take no for an answer. "Okay," she said, "I know the prom queen thing was partly about being too young, but this one's a 21-year-old, a junior in college." My reply was who can ever understand how a mother could ever do that? My response—how could anyone do that—didn't distinguish me from any other mother hearing of neonaticide, and this sent the reporter on her way.

The next I heard of Julie was several months later, when a colleague from another city called to refer her to me for psychotherapy while Julie was free on bail pending trial. My colleague had conducted a forensic evaluation for the defense and recommended that Julie receive treatment.

I refused.

I had heard this colleague lecture on neonaticide and knew that she had collected more clinical data on the phenomenon than anyone else in the field. I understood her explanation—a transient dissociative state in which the overwhelming shock of a denied and disastrous pregnancy caused a temporary loss of reality testing. As a fellow psychiatrist demystified of motherhood, I had the greatest respect for her work and admired her dedication to these most hated mothers. But I could not imagine finding the empathy to treat someone who had committed neonaticide. I explained this to her: my countertransference was going to be insurmountable, I knew it already. Like the reporter, she wouldn't take no for an answer. Trust me, you will find the compassion. She was certain that I would be able to help her, and besides, she said, if you can't, who can?

The circumstances leading up to the neonaticide were both typical—the patient was from an extremely conservative immigrant background in which unwed pregnancy was an unimaginable disaster—and atypical. She had been raped shortly before the pregnancy, possibly resulting in the pregnancy, and that too had been kept secret, almost as shameful in her family as voluntary intercourse. Given the rape, denial and dissociation were recently employed defenses against reality too painful for consciousness.

We made a deal: I would see the patient once or twice and decide whether I thought I could overcome my bias and work with her in psychotherapy.

It took a few months for her to call for an appointment. When she did finally come for an evaluation, it took approximately 5 minutes for me to want to bring her home with me. I went from distaste to rescue in an instant. I believe my initial countertransference to Julie (as opposed to my media-enhanced idea of who Julie must be) was like what I typically experience with "lost kittens." I know that I agreed to see her for evaluation because of the rape: she had some claim on victimhood and didn't just belong to my imagined group of young women too narcissistic to deal with pregnancy.

Julie was accompanied by her mother, who, though stylishly and contemporarily dressed, was extremely traditional at home. As I called Julie from the waiting room, her attentiveness to her mother was immediately obvious. It was the first crack in my assumption that only a raging narcissist could commit neonaticide, and this deference would come to be the major focus of our work together. Julie dressed nicely for her appointment—a typical looking young adult in every way but with this old fashioned respect for the doctor.

She told me her story in bits and pieces, looking like a deer caught in the headlights, and I was sunk. Nothing about Julie was remotely narcissistic: no self-pity, no rage at others, no indifference, no self-aggrandizement. There was no hint of borderline personality disorder either: she was a former honor student, a state-ranked athlete, and a woman with many solid and stable interpersonal relationships.

Julie told me in the first appointment that she was coaching children's sports. That she was allowed to work with small children in an affluent, educated community that has known her all her life and that knows of the infant's death gave her the tiniest fragment of self-respect. She never verbalized what it was like to be vilified, so hated in the media that even a psychiatrist who should know better thinks she's a monster, but she alluded to it frequently. "Some parents didn't want me to teach their kids at first, but my old coach stood by me and now I teach them all." This was her haven: here, alone, she was a loving and giving adult, a safe caregiver of children.

She could not imagine what was happening to her: How could she be charged with murder? How could she protect her parents from this shame? How could she believe what is said about her to be true?

Julie was largely amnestic for the events surrounding the death of her infant, and she related details as told to her. Her present awareness was profoundly affected by the circumstance of facing murder charges: she didn't remember the delivery, and her patchy dissociative recall was influenced by a pathologist retained by her lawyer, a prominent expert who alleged, in contradiction to the official autopsy, that the infant had not been delivered alive. This was balm for Julie, a way to maintain the sense of herself as a fundamentally good person.

She did clearly understand that she had not recognized her own pregnancy. (Neither had her roommates, her coach, or her fellow college athletes who saw her disrobed or in trim athletic outfits throughout the school year.) Her clothing size had never changed, and she believed that she had continued to menstruate throughout the year.

In the course of her treatment, the major focus was her extremely obedient relationship with her mother. On bail, facing a possible life sentence, Julie was permitted a curfew of midnight, despite the fact that her social peers would typically not begin a Saturday night evening until 10 P.M. Julie was aware that as the first born, she was the one expected to conform most to the rules of her mother's culture, while her younger sister was permitted marginally more freedom. Julie allowed her mother to decide which college she would attend, deferred to the expectation that she would date (and presumably marry) a man from her parents' culture, and planned, as instructed, to return after college to work in the family business. Throughout the trial preparations, Julie reported her mother's belief that Julie's current predicament was the direct result of her failure to accept her mother's advice to remain more dutiful.

In some ways, the most difficult countertransference reaction I had was my own reaction to Julie's extraordinary deference to her mother. No psychiatrist hasn't worked with the nonassertive patient, but it was deeply distressing to witness Julie's repeated compliance with the expectations of another world. I would find my thoughts drifting to the countless expressions of autonomy that my own children take for granted, the challenging of the "rubber rules," the gray zone between the firm no's and the softer maybe's that characterize the daily interactions of American parents and their children. Julie had no rubber rules, no maybes. There were no details too small to require parental approval and no challenging of parental authority. Rules and parental decisions were law.

My wish to rescue Julie, her kittenhood, was very similar to that which I often feel when treating adolescents in highly critical and "scapegoating" families. I was shocked by what sounded like a relentless use of shaming as a means of establishing authority. I understand that we only "see" our patients' families through their eyes, without the parents' input, but time after time, Julie would describe interactions that she recognized as emotionally painful but not as either ill-intentioned or even inappropriate. She seemed most able to recognize shame and control in her mother's approach to her sister, and a major task of her time on bail was helping her sister to do what Julie had not done: determine which college she would attend despite her parents' choice of another college. She would occasionally work to convince her mother to allow her younger sister an extra hour of curfew or to receive phone calls from a boy deemed unsuitable. Julie's vicarious autonomy was, truthfully, endearing.

At times, I wanted to scream at her: just say no! I would have imaginary conversations in my head in which I would ask her exactly what did she think would happen if she just stayed out dancing—with girlfriends—until 2 A.M. one morning? Didn't she realize the absurdity of surrendering reasonable freedom when she was probably going to prison? But my reaction would have compounded her sense of shame, multiplied her own sense of betrayal that she would even share such family secrets with me. I would have been another shaming, controlling mother telling her that what she was doing (obeying) was all wrong, not the way of my culture, not the way that would make me proud of her.

Over time, we were able to speak about Julie's American self caught in a traditional family. I believe that merely probing her mother's ways—calling her dorm room literally every morning and every evening, scrutinizing every unexpected absence, for example—validated her sense that she was not "bad" for wanting more freedom.

Already virtually boundaryless, Julie was raped shortly before her pregnancy. (Through most of my treatment with her, she believed that the rape had resulted in the pregnancy, a fact disconfirmed shortly before our sessions ended when it was discovered that the DNA analysis indicated that her boyfriend had been the father.) Julie showed more reticence to discuss the rape than perhaps any other victim I've treated, with tremendous resistance to recalling any detail. This, too, failed to meet my preexisting stereotype: I expected that she would rationalize the neonaticide on the basis of victimhood. She simply never went there, in part due to the severity of her posttraumatic stress disorder and phobic avoidance.

Instead, we discussed the rape as a secret that she could neither know nor let her parents know prior to her arrest. She never considered telling her parents that she had been raped. She anticipated that her mother would blame her for the rape, which indeed seemed more likely than not. She also feared upsetting her mother, who, I came to believe, was tortured by anxiety and unhappiness. If there was one reason Julie could state for her obeisance, it was to protect her mother from becoming distressed. Her description of the family dynamics suggested that her father and her sister also labored to keep her mother from discovering painful information.

Not surprisingly, her pregnancy would have been a disastrous knowledge for Julie and her mother. Julie was able to explore the reasons her pregnancy was unknowable to her, why her body and mind cooperated in keeping Julie from consciously recognizing that she was pregnant. In part, her American self—the one who voluntarily became sexually active at the age of 19—was split from her traditional self, who would remain a virgin until she married with parental approval. She had developed a compartmentalization of her American self. Born and raised in the United States, Julie had an identity at school, in her sports, and in her work with children who were American, a culture valuing autonomy and independence. She watched her peers rebel over issues large and small but lived her life as a traditionalist, one who remained childlike and undifferentiated by the cultural norms of her citizenship.

In my work with Julie, I sought integration of her experiences and compartmentalized selves. Ironically, she experienced herself as shameful when she had so much as a rebellious thought about which television program to watch but seemed almost clueless as to why she was charged with a crime. I doubt that my disapproval of a family environment that forbids its members to seek comfort following rape or unanticipated pregnancy was entirely hidden from her. But I believed that she also understood that I honored her traditional self as much as I did her American self. Had I insisted that she be a "typical" young American adult, or had I criticized her parent's values, I do not believe she would have remained in psychotherapy.

I also believe that my own personal experience with a close family member who married an immigrant from a very similar culture was useful in managing another countertransference obstacle, that of too readily accepting "it's just the way it is with my people." I've witnessed first hand the struggle of a strong maternal authority seeking to maintain traditional family relationships with a daughter married into an American family that values autonomy and individuation from parental sovereignty. It would have been easy to "excuse" Julie's denial of pregnancy, with its disastrous consequences, as "cultural" and to see her solely as a victim of cultural conflict. Often, when I would gently inquire as to what she wanted, felt, and experienced internally in described interactions with her mother, she would claim deference as "just the way it is" in families of her ethnicity. I believe my experience watching a healthier struggle with old versus new ways helped me to challenge the assumption that there was simply no other choice except protecting her mother from her American self and deferring to her parents' views.

In the background of treatment was the constant threat of incarceration and a murder trial. The reality of threats to her safety and integrity deeply affected my work with her, especially in terms of her posttraumatic stress disorder. I usually find that the reexperiencing and retelling of the trauma, while therapeutic in detoxification and necessary for reintegration, lead the patient to feel worse before she feels better. I was acutely aware of the need to treat Julie with kid gloves: to help her be as strong as she could possibly be in the face of the anticipated trial. She had overwhelming decisions to make: should she go to trial, testify on her own behalf, or accept a plea bargain? I feared that opening the extraordinarily painful memories of her rape, necessary in my view for healing, might risk decompensation and literally harm her. For almost a year, the trial was on again and off again, so I was never certain whether a wound opened one week could be healed were a trial to start suddenly. I generally chose to support rather than confront defenses. At times, I felt confident that this was the proper course; at other times, I feared that I was at best missing opportunities and at worst accepting her fragility and immaturity as fact.

The single most painful emotional reaction I had to working with Julie turned out to have nothing to do with my response to her actions but rather my firsthand look at what I continue to see today as the grave injustice done by the legal system to her. Like many psychiatrists, I realize that at one level the criminal justice system is flawed—too many of us have seen the sociopath succeed in feigning insanity as a defense while the patient with floridly psychotic schizophrenia is incarcerated rather than treated. But I also believed that the system would do right—that while punishment was far more likely than not, mercy and justice would temper her fate.

In part, my belief that she would receive reasonable and just legal treatment was based on ongoing resolutions to other highly publicized neonaticide cases across the country. In the course of our work together, several defendants were convicted and sentenced to imprisonment that, although significant, was clearly based on the complexity of these young women's circumstances. They were sentenced as troubled young adults with a potential for rehabilitation, not as monsters or willful child murderers. I hoped and believed that Julie would be similarly treated, especially since there was doubt about whether the infant was even living at birth, and she had highly capable legal representation.

Unfortunately, Julie's particular circumstances placed her in an especially vulnerable legal position. For one thing, the local prosecutor where the case occurred was a high-profile elected official, and the political value of this particular prosecution was significant. But most important, the local law had been recently changed to criminalize "child endangerment," which carried a mandatory 25-year sentence. In a mock trial, in which Julie "testified," the mock jurors reported that although they did not believe she had committed manslaughter, they "compromised" on child endangerment, since she had not called 911 at the time of the delivery, even if the infant was indeed dead already. As would have happened at a bona fide trial, the mock jurors were not permitted to know that such a conviction would result in a mandatory 25-year sentence. When debriefed, they were reportedly shocked at such an outcome.

Once the mock jury had "convicted" her of child endangerment, Julie's lawyer immediately advised her to plea bargain, because it was the sole charge, which would have allowed a judge no sentencing discretion. The risk that a jury would convict her of the seemingly "lesser" charge of child endangerment left Julie at too great a risk. In the next few weeks, Julie's attorney negotiated a plea bargain of 10 years, with a minimum of 5 years served. This was more than double the time to be served in any of the comparable cases that had been in the public eye. The prosecutor and judge allowed Julie an additional 7 months until reporting for sentencing.

That she was to serve 5 years, deferred by 7 months, made it very clear to me that her sentence was retribution. A judge or prosecutor who believed that Julie posed a risk to a child would not have reasonably allowed her to remain free for 7 months following conviction.

Ironically, I started my work with Julie anticipating antipathy. I imagined that she would fail to take personal responsibility—that she would expect me to see her as a victim of circumstances who couldn't be held accountable. Instead, I myself came to see her as a victim of circumstances, a young woman who experienced a great personal tragedy, one far more complex in origin than I would have imagined.

But greater still, I believe that Julie has suffered a social tragedy, becoming one of many victims of our cultural need to idealize pregnancy. As a culture, we regularly project ambivalence about parenting on highly publicized "bad mothers": cocaine addicted women, abusive parents, mothers who abandon toddlers—all serve to receive our hateful impulses and to simplify the complexity of the nature of the parent-child relationship. When we think about Susan Smith driving her children into the lake, Marie Osmond with postpartum depression handing her seven children to a housekeeper while she drives up the California highway, or the high school student who delivers her infant in the bathroom then goes back to the prom, we quench our thirst for reassurance that we are, will be, and were raised by unambivalently loving parents. Collectively, we ask, how could anyone do that, and we are comforted by the certainty that we could not.

My initial reaction—"How could anyone do that?"—in retrospect seems to have fed my own unconscious appetite for rejecting "bad mothering" impulses. I believe I did not want to know the answer to the question. As psychotherapists, we regularly are given privileged access to pain. We are witnesses to the complexity of human behavior. The answer—what chain of life circumstances, what psychological and social factors could culminate in such a great tragedy—is, not surprisingly, painful.

Chapter 12

The Mother-Infant Relationship

From Normality to Pathology

Pamela Meersand, Ph.D.
Wendy Turchin, M.D.

I made a quilt to keep my family warm. I made it beautiful so my heart would not break.

Sara Ruddick (1980)

Academic and clinical interest in the mother-infant relationship has intensified in the last 25 years, giving rise to a burgeoning research literature as well as new psychotherapies. When D. W. Winnicott (1965, p. 55), the famous psychoanalyst and pediatrician, asserted that "there is no such thing as a baby" outside the context of a mother-child dyad, it was considered a radical notion. Developmental research in the 1980s and 1990s confirmed Winnicott's vision of infancy: the importance of a healthy mother-baby attachment for social, emotional, and even cognitive functioning in later childhood became widely recognized and today is considered common knowledge.

Mother-infant interaction, with all its complexities, cannot be examined in isolation. Contemporary thinking places the dyad in an intricate system of parental, child, and social/environmental factors, all in dynamic interplay; multiple relationships and circumstances wrap around the pair, impacting mother and child at each stage of development (Emde 1991; Sameroff 1993). Risks to mother-infant relations may arise anywhere in the system as a result of maternal psychopathology or history of trauma, in response to severe environmental stress, or as a result of problems in the "fit" between maternal personality and infant temperament.

Selma Fraiberg coined the now-famous phrase "ghosts in the nursery" to describe those painful, early memories that haunt all mothers as caring for their infants stirs up old longings and fears (Fraiberg et al. 1975). Importantly, as research from multidisciplinary perspectives has elaborated those "ghosts," demonstrating specific variables that place mothers and infants at risk, new interventions have kept pace. Parent-infant psychotherapy, a psychodynamic treatment that improves mother-child attachment, has shown exciting potential for reducing child abuse and neglect. As clinicians become more skilled in the early identification of high-risk mothers, preventive psychotherapy can be offered in the antenatal period and continued during those critical first months of life.

In this chapter, we aim to arm the reader with information relevant to early identification of risk and prevention of tragic outcomes, such as child maltreatment and infanticide. The spectrum of mother-infant relations, from normal to pathological, is described from both theoretical and clinical perspectives. First, we briefly review those aspects of psychoanalytic and attachment theory most relevant to current thinking about vulnerable dyads. Next, we examine the complex components of mother-child interaction in both favorable and high-risk circumstances; clinical vignettes are used to highlight the reactions of various mothers to the mother-infant situation, with an emphasis on vulnerable dyads. Lastly, we discuss parent–infant psychotherapy and explore the potential of treatments for addressing attachment disorders.

Although attachment is a lifelong process, and treatment may be mutative at any point in the life span, we focus here on the earliest months of life, when the infant is most vulnerable and the mother is in the throes of adjusting to parenthood. The discussion is largely limited to the relationship between infant and mother; despite a growing body of evidence that fathers and even nonfamilial caregivers provide crucial early influences, most available research limits itself to mothers and their babies.

The Mother-Infant Dyad in Psychoanalysis and Attachment Theory: A Historical Review

Psychoanalytic Perspectives

In striking contrast to current thinking, early psychoanalytic views of infancy placed little emphasis on maternal behavior. With the publication of his famous *Three Essays on the Theory of Sexuality*, Freud (1905/1953) presented a vision of infancy driven by biology: development was seen as dominated by progressive phases of psychosexual organization. The infant's first relationships were inextricably tied to physical drives, such as hunger; Mother could achieve importance in the eyes of her baby only through the role of need-satisfier (Freud 1915/1957). Melanie Klein (1935, 1946) revised this view, suggesting that the newborn is relationship-seeking from the start. However, like Freud, she believed that biological predispositions—in the form of innate, unconscious fantasies—dominated the infant's early experience, relatively unaffected by maternal availability and responsiveness.

It was Winnicott, versed in infant observation from his practice as a pediatrician, who brought the maternal figure to life. Despite obvious struggles to position himself within the tradition of both Freud and Klein, Winnicott posed the radical idea that instinct alone does not govern infancy and that the ordinary and countless daily interactions between mother and child form the context in which the child's mental and emotional life develops. Mother's behavioral responses, personality, and attitudes toward her baby were considered to have a crucial impact on development. Winnicott described the mother's special state of mind during pregnancy and early infancy—"the primary maternal preoccupation"—as one of exquisite sensitivity to the needs of her baby. "The mother, through identification of herself with her infant knows what the infant feels like and so is able to provide almost exactly what the infant needs in the way of holding and in the provision of an environment generally" (Winnicott 1965, p. 55).

Winnicott and his contemporaries—most notably W. R. Bion and Margaret Mahler—were formative for current thinking about both healthy and pathological early development. For Winnicott, the infant's mental representations of self and others unfolded within the context of the mother's supportive presence, or her "holding environment." The "transitional object"—that much-cherished first doll or blanket that brings comfort much in the same way that the mother does—is a sign of the emotionally nourished infant's capacity to internalize the mother's love, even without her physical presence (Winnicott 1971). When the infant is forced to make elaborate accommodations to a demanding or hostile caregiver in order to maintain her love, a "false self" (Winnicott 1965) develops in which the child forfeits his or her own spontaneous needs and wishes. Bion's (1970) concept of good mothering assumed the capacity to contain the infant's discomforts and distresses. Mother's calm, timely responses allow the baby to achieve a gradual tolerance of previously overwhelming experiences, such as hunger; unempathic, ill-timed, or hostile maternal responses deprive the infant of the growing capacity to regulate negative internal states. In Mahler's theory of psychological development (Mahler et al. 1975), the mother's evenhanded acceptance of the infant's complex needs and demands allows the baby to achieve beginning independence without the paralyzing fear that he or she will lose the mother's love.

Importantly, the work of these clinician-theorists encouraged psycho-analysts to move beyond a focus on the infant's instinctual, intrapsychic life. All were keen observers of mother-child interaction and saw the dyadic relationship, rather than the individual infant, as the crucial entity; this view laid the groundwork for the current practice of parent-infant psychotherapy, in which mother and child are treated together rather than as separate units.

Contributions From Attachment Theory

After World War II, Renee Spitz's (1945, 1946) pioneering studies of orphaned babies showed the dramatic effects of maternal deprivation. Reared in institutions after the loss of their parents, these infants first exhibited angry protest; despair set in, and they stopped growing, developing, and exploring their environment. Depression, apathy, and even death resulted. These findings surprised many psychoanalysts who believed that infants were incapable of "true" attachment and mourning.

John Bowlby was heavily influenced by Klein and others who viewed infants as innately relationship-oriented. He drew from ethology, most notably Harlow's important demonstration that mother-deprived infant rhesus monkeys suffered long-lasting social deviance. Postulating a biologically based "attachment behavioral system" for human infants, Bowlby suggested that babies are programmed from birth to seek proximity to their mothers. Sucking, crying, and clinging behaviors designed to elicit the mother's interest and maintain closeness to her were seen as manifestations of attachment (Bowlby 1969, 1973, 1980). Separation from the mother was hypothesized to cause severe distress.

Bowlby viewed attachment as an overarching system that organized infant behavior and development. Like other psychoanalysts, he believed that infants develop mental representations of relationships, which he called "internal working models"; however, he rejected the Kleinian notion that these representations were deeply influenced by unconscious fantasy and asserted instead that real-life, daily experiences with the mother determined the infant's concepts of self and others. Laid down in the first months of life, internal working models were carried forward to influence relationships throughout the life span. The well-parented infant would develop positive representations in which the mother was viewed as a "secure base" from which to venture forth and explore the world; optimism and self-efficacy would be applied to future relationships with caregivers, peers, and teachers. By contrast, infants who lacked early empathic mothering would come to view others as disappointing and even hostile and would see themselves as helpless and unwanted. These less-fortunate babies would approach future relations with avoidance or aggression.

Continuing Bowlby's work, Mary Ainsworth studied the development of consequences of early mother-infant interaction. In their landmark study of 26 mother-child pairs, Bell and Ainsworth (1972) demonstrated that effective maternal response to infant crying—particularly close physical contact—was associated with decreased crying at the end of 1 year. Moreover, a mother's overall sensitivity and responsiveness—her ability to read her baby's cues, her capacity for timely response, and a positive attitude toward physical contact—was found to predict a "secure" mother-child attachment at the end of the first year of life (Ainsworth et al. 1978). For the first time, an empirical study had confirmed the critical role of maternal behavior.

Ainsworth and collaborators delineated three attachment categories, which are now familiar to most child researchers and clinicians. The predominant category, *secure attachment*, was characterized by babies who explored comfortably with the mother present, evidenced concern when she left the room, and showed relief and pleasure on her return. *Avoidant attachment* was exhibited by babies who failed to show distress when left alone with the stranger and who generally ignored their mothers. *Resistant attachment* described infants who were greatly stressed by separation and failed to be comforted by the mother on her return. Main and Solomon (1986) added a fourth category, *disorganized attachment*, to describe the behavior of babies who show a disoriented, incoherent response to the stress of separation.

These classifications, easily applied to research, brought attachment theory into the forefront of empirical work in early child development, a position it has enjoyed for more than 20 years. Secure attachment has been shown to predict good developmental functioning in all areas: higher levels of symbolic play (Slade 1987), positive attitude toward problem-solving tasks (Matas et al. 1978), competent peer relations (Pastor 1981), positive adjustment to school (Sroufe 1983), and lower chances of psychopathology such as disruptive behavior problems (Greenberg et al. 1993).

Recent attachment studies have pointed the way to early identification of high-risk mothers. This research owes much to the seminal work of George, Kaplan, and Main (1985), who identified three styles of adult attachment: *secure*, achieved by those adults who present balanced, integrated views of relationships; *dismissing*, characterized by a tendency to diminish the importance of others; and *preoccupied*, typified by over-involvement with unsatisfying past relationships. Research has demonstrated continuity between attachment status in infancy and patterns of relating in early adulthood (Waters et al. 2000). Numerous studies in the 1980s and 1990s linked a mother's attachment style to her baby's attachment status at 1 year: the secure, dismissing, and preoccupied maternal styles corresponded to secure, avoidant, and ambivalent child styles, respectively (Main et al. 1985). Demonstrating the use of the antenatal period for early identification and prevention, Fonagy and colleagues (1991b) predicted mother-infant quality of attachment at age 1 year from their assessment of mother's relational style during pregnancy.

Current Views

Current influential theorists integrate concepts from both attachment and psychoanalytic theory, also drawing on the vast research in infant cognitive and emotional development. Written from his unique vantage point as both a developmentalist and a psychoanalyst, Daniel Stern's *The Interpersonal World of the Infant* (1985) stirred wide interest in infancy and offered a new way of looking at the first few months of life. Postulating that even newborns possess a rudimentary sense of a separate and cohesive self, Stern proposed that very young infants accrue emotionally laden memories of interactions with mother that lay the groundwork for mental representations of self and other. Developing motor, language, and other cognitive skills combine with ongoing interpersonal experience, and the infant develops increasingly complex, integrated notions of the interpersonal world.

Peter Fonagy, a well-known psychoanalyst, suggests that a mother's capacity to contemplate her own and her child's thoughts and feelings—called *reflective self-functioning*—may be key in the intergenerational transmission of attachment styles (Fonagy et al. 1991a). Mothers with low reflective self-functioning are seen as incapable of viewing the world through their infants' eyes; they are typically concrete, hostile, and unempathic. Their infants, in turn, fail to develop age-appropriate social abilities.

Current thinking about maternal psychopathology draws from notions of internal representations from both psychoanalytic and attachment theory. In their studies of child maltreatment, Crittenden and Ainsworth (1989) suggested that abusive mothers have mental models of relationships that feature conflict, control, and rejection. Their children tend to develop patterns of interaction that feature passive compliance or resistance. Neglecting mothers are characterized by models of helplessness in relation to others; they experience emptiness and depression as dominant emotions. Neglected children, having learned that they cannot effectively elicit maternal response, tend to become clingy and demanding or depressed and defeated.

Most recently, additional evidence from neurobiology supports the critical role of early mother-infant interaction in optimal child development. Studies of Romanian orphans, reared in institutions with minimal human contact, have linked early maternal deprivation with brain abnormalities, which are thought to have far-reaching consequences for later social, emotional, and cognitive functioning (Nelson and Bosquet 2000). Fully consistent with Spitz's (1945, 1946) observations of war-orphaned infants in the 1940s, these current findings support major tenets of both object relations and attachment theories. The modern techniques of neuroscience may provide the most compelling evidence to date that, as Winnicott declared, there is "no such thing as a baby" without a mother.

Early Mother-Infant Relations: The Beginnings of Secure and Disordered Attachments

Transactional Model of Risk

Ainsworth's landmark studies, summarized earlier, provided empirical support for the importance of maternal sensitivity in the first months of life. Since then, a great deal has been learned about the intricate components of dyadic interaction. Daniel Stern and T. Berry Brazelton, a noted pediatrician, conducted a microanalytic study of mother-child interaction, documenting the moment-by-moment interchanges in the dyad. Reciprocal, rhythmic patterns of mutual attention and arousal were described as part of the typical face-to-face play behavior of mothers and their infants (Brazelton et al. 1974; Stern 1974). In positive circumstances, these subtle precursors of childhood turn-taking and even adult conversational patterns serve as the building blocks of the secure mother-infant attachment.

The transactional approach to child development suggests that ordinary mother-infant interaction can be disrupted by a number of factors in the "parent-child-environment system" (Cicchetti 1989); these factors, which impinge on the dyad, interrelate in complex ways. Environmental distress, maternal psychopathology, or difficult child characteristics can disrupt the fine-tuned adjustments that typify maternal behavior. A depressed and isolated mother may be preoccupied with her own thoughts and therefore less available to read her infant's cues; paired with a fussy, premature newborn, that same mother may become defeated or angry, finding the baby's cries unbearable.

Using the transactional model for assessing risk of child abuse and neglect, Cicchetti and Rizley (1981) categorize variables that impinge on the dyad into two domains: *potentiating* factors stress the dyad and increase risk for problems, whereas *compensatory* factors protect against attachment disorders. When potentiating factors are present in several domains (e.g., maternal depression in addition to infant prematurity and poverty), the result is a dyad at risk for insecure attachment and even child maltreatment. In contrast, an abundance of compensatory factors, such as adequate financial resources and a history of close family relations, contribute to a positive attachment outcome; these may even help ameliorate the presence of one or two difficult conditions, such as infant illness.

Although the transactional model attempts to account for a wide range of variables in the biological and environmental spheres, not all factors are necessarily accorded equal weight, and there is no cookbook method for assessing level of risk. For example, Halpern (1993) suggests that poverty is a particularly devastating factor that wreaks havoc with childrearing, causing parents to become preoccupied with their difficult circumstances and to suffer an undermined sense of efficacy about their lives in general. Many clinicians working with high-risk families consider social isolation to be a key factor in risk for child maltreatment; Pianta and colleagues (1989) suggest that "psychological processes involved in mothers' ability to engage in interpersonal relationships serve a central causal role in maltreatment" (p. 245). On the positive side, a factor such as treatment may override numerous potentiating ones. Erickson et al. (1992) suggest that a trusting relationship with a therapist may function as a protective factor, providing a high-risk mother with new ways of viewing herself and others. The success of parent-infant psychotherapy with extremely high-risk dyads—those with severe environmental stressors as well as maternal psychopathology—suggests that treatment may buttress healthy attachment in even the most dire circumstances.

Pregnancy: A Critical Time for Assessment of Risk

Describing the enormous psychological requirements of successful adjustment to pregnancy, Cohen and Slade (2000) include 1) a dramatic reorganization of the woman's own identity within the context of her marriage and society; 2) the ability to view her child as part of her and yet ultimately separate from herself; and 3) the creation of an internal representation of the baby that includes negative affects but is primarily loving and joyful. These involve all aspects of the pregnant woman's personality: memories of early experiences with her own mother, conscious and unconscious fantasies about herself and others, and the capacity for self-reflective functioning as described by Fonagy—that is, the ability to "hold two minds in her mind: her own changing sense of self alongside her fluctuating and intense affects and the reality of her baby, both part of and apart from her" (Slade and Cohen 2000, p. 30).

Stern (1995) and Benedek (1959) view motherhood as a unique developmental phase. Maternity is seen as providing the opportunity for forward development via new identities and the reworking of old relationships and conflicts. In *The Motherhood Constellation*, Stern (1995) suggested that "with the birth of a baby, especially the first, the mother passes into a new and unique psychic organization" (p. 171). However, women who are too burdened by unresolved past conflicts may not be able to accept the new role as parent; early trauma and the lack of stable, internal representations of relationships to others may impede the joy and excitement that typically balance the fears and anxieties of new motherhood. As early as the antenatal period, she may dread or even deny her impending maternity (see Chapter 5: "Denial of Pregnancy"). After birth, if the mother fails to achieve a sense of parenting competence or is burdened by her own early traumatic experiences, motherhood may instead become a time of deep conflict and despair.

The following clinical description of a 22-year-old pregnant woman who is at very high risk illustrates the impact of traumatic history and psychiatric disorder on the attitudes and expectations of the antenatal period:

> K, a young woman with a history of both physical and sexual abuse in childhood, was referred for treatment during the last trimester of her third pregnancy. During two previous pregnancies, both of which had resulted in low-weight babies who were ultimately removed from her care for failure to thrive syndrome, she had steadfastly denied she was pregnant through the first two trimesters, even in the face of obvious physical signs. Now, 32 weeks' pregnant with her third child, her refusal to plan for or even think about the baby caused her obstetrical team extreme pessimism about her ability to parent the next infant.
>
> K had suffered from untreated anorexia and bulimia since adolescence and appeared gaunt. Introducing herself to the therapist, she cheerfully exclaimed, "I never know I'm pregnant until it's practically over. I think it's best that way not to think about the thing too much." She was preoccupied with fears of gaining weight and openly described her plans to "trick" her midwife into thinking she was gaining weight "so that Nosy Nellie'll leave me alone about gaining." Asked if she had thought about the consequences of her poor nutritional status for herself and the infant,

she replied: "If the baby's small, it'll be quieter." She refused to discuss the father, select a name for the baby, or in any way prepare herself or her home (a small room, where she lived as a boarder) for the infant's arrival. Otherwise cheerful and outgoing, she grew listless and apathetic when the subject of the child was raised. When the therapist realistically stated her fears that this infant, too, would be removed from K's care, the young woman shrugged, although her eyes grew teary at the mention of her first two children.

Despite her refusal to discuss the infant, K's fears and fantasies were revealed through her reports of intensely vivid dreams wherein alien invaders took over her body, distorting it and ultimately causing her death. The first time her therapist suggested that this might be the way she viewed the baby, she was shocked; gradually, however, she revealed that she did, in fact, think of the baby much as she thought of food: getting it out of her body was her only goal. She was horrified by the very idea of pregnancy, of having "a thing growing inside me, who knows how big it could get." With few memories from her own childhood, and all of them unpleasant, K could barely imagine herself parenting an infant: her own mother had failed to protect her from a dangerously volatile, alcoholic stepfather.

The therapist continued to state her own concerns in a forthright, nonjudgmental manner, making clear that it seemed K could barely care for herself, let alone for a newborn. At the young woman's request, she accompanied K to the next maternity appointment, and for the first time K showed some interest in the midwife's educational efforts. Concrete discussions about childbirth and about the needs of newborns helped K see the pregnancy as real and graspable; this allowed for some fantasies about the child. As she began to imagine herself with the newborn, K showed interest in her impending maternity for the first time. Although her nutritional status remained poor and she had great difficulty picturing herself as a mother, she was able to engage in some basic planning for the birth: a crib, some clothing, and finally a name was chosen.

This young woman experienced the growing fetus as such an intolerable threat to her bodily and emotional integrity that for many weeks she could not acknowledge her pregnancy (see Chapter 5). As in Pollack and Percy's (1999) description of mothers who deny pregnancy, K viewed the developing child as a persecutory, invasive intruder. After the infant girl's birth, acknowledging that she had felt a tiny suspicion about being pregnant from the start, K vaguely recalled the magical idea that if she denied the pregnancy long enough, the fetus would "go away somehow—maybe die, maybe just sort of fade." Some months later, she admitted that her rage toward the fetus was so great she feared she might kill the child after birth; fear of her own homicidal impulses (which had probably been acted on, albeit in a somewhat less direct fashion, by her complete failure to nourish her first two infants) contributed to her need to avoid knowledge of her pregnancy.

K's therapist and her maternity team made sure that intensive, comprehensive services were provided at birth: daily home visiting by a preventive agency and parent-infant psychotherapy with her existing clinician three times per week functioned as a way to monitor the infant's safety as well as to support K in her growing desire to mother her baby. For the first time K accepted treatment for her eating disorder, and individual, psychiatric treatment for her was added on shortly after the birth. Although an informal assessment of attachment at 1 year showed a clearly avoidant style on the part of the infant, the child was healthy and well developed. Extensive services helped this mother care for her daughter's basic needs and avoid yet another foster care placement.

Over 40 years ago, Bibring (1959) recommended psychotherapy for women who could not achieve an adequate emotional adjustment to pregnancy. Without the benefit of modern research, he recognized that acute distress or apathy in the antenatal period placed the infant at risk. Today, research has confirmed Bibring's notions, demonstrating that a woman's attitude toward her pregnancy and her notions about her future child predict later mother-infant attachment status. The growing body of clinicians trained in assessment of high-risk mothers and schooled in the principles of parent-infant psychotherapy make real the possibility of truly early intervention.

Temperament and Mother-Infant "Goodness of Fit"

From the first moments of birth, the infant brings his or her own unique style to the mother-child relationship. The well-known researchers on temperament Chess and Thomas (1986) proposed nine dimensions of temperament: activity level, rhythmicity of biological functions, intensity of affective reaction, predominant mood, persistence, approach-withdrawal in novel situations, adaptability to changes in routine, sensory threshold, and distractibility when upset. Infants were then classified according to three patterns: "easy" infants were cheerful, followed predictable biological routines, and adapted easily to novel circumstances; "difficult" babies had predominantly negative mood and intense reactivity; "slow to warmup" infants were low in activity and withdrawing in new situations. These researchers found that temperamental patterns were consistent over a number of years; for example, infants classified as having "difficult" patterns were shown to have a higher risk of behavioral difficulties years later when they entered school (Chess and Thomas 1986; Thomas and Chess 1977).

Although Chess and Thomas believed that temperament had biological roots—a position endorsed by most theorists—they emphasized the interplay of constitution and environment. "Goodness of fit" (Thomas et al. 1968), the match between the infant's temperament and the mother's personality, was seen as crucial. For example, the mother of a very intense, active baby may be either thrilled or overwhelmed by his behavior; one mother may find her child a smart, inquisitive explorer, whereas another may fear he is going to be impulsive and difficult to handle. One adolescent mother with a history of conduct disorder described her motorically advanced 7-month-old as "a future juvenile delinquent." The following case example of a young, first-time mother with very adequate emotional and environmental resources serves as an illustration:

> Mike kicked constantly in utero. His mother, J, an industrious and vivacious lawyer who cheerfully looked forward to her 6-month maternity leave, happily anticipated an active newborn. Active he was; however, she was baffled and upset by how hard he was to soothe. Mike would cry for hours at a time for much of the day. J was exhausted from trying to calm him. She would rock him, sing to him, and walk him all around the house. Frustrated and overwhelmed, she questioned her own competence and even her decision to have a child. At the worst moments, in tears, she found herself feeling angry at Mike, as well as at her husband, who failed to provide any relief from infant care. She called her pediatrician and began to describe her desperation. The doctor examined the infant, determining that he was healthy but easily overstimulated.
>
> The pediatrician suggested that J try making smaller and simpler gestures to comfort him. J began to sing more quietly to Mike, making sure that the rest of the apartment was quiet. She began to move more slowly and with smaller motions, even though this did not naturally fit with her own active style: she loved to dance vigorously with him. Mike responded to her changes: he began to quiet down for longer periods of time and to seem more content. J found that she, too, was becoming calmer, and it became easier to read the infant's signals. Although he remained difficult to soothe throughout infancy and had fierce tantrums by 15 months, J felt she had at least some capacity to help him calm down.

The scenario may have been completely different had it involved a mother with significant psychopathology, perhaps burdened by her own history of trauma. High-risk mothers, who often have distorted perceptions about their babies, may interpret temperamentally derived behaviors as intentional and designed to upset them. For example, one single, socially isolated mother with paranoid tendencies described that each time her fussy baby cried, she was certain the newborn was wailing out her disappointment over having an inadequate mother. Feeling accused and defeated, she avoided the baby more and more, which of course led the infant to even greater distress and more crying bouts.

J was able to realize that her anger was irrational, even in the midst of being upset and frustrated, and took steps to get help. A more defensive mother might become extremely angry at the infant, unswerving in her belief that the baby meant to undermine her parenting competence. A vicious cycle might ensue, wherein the mother, feeling more and more overwhelmed, failed to seek the support of others, such as a pediatrician, who might help shed a more realistic light on the situation. The result could be severe isolation, neglect of the baby, or even abuse when the mother could no longer bear to listen to the child's cries (see Chapter 1: "A Brief History of Infanticide and the Law").

Emotion Regulation and the Role of Maternal Psychopathology

Both attachment theorists and psychoanalysts recognize the mother's crucial role in helping the infant gradually learn to tolerate and integrate various emotional experiences. Abundant studies that illustrate the youngest infant's capacity to "read" and respond to human facial expressions suggest that from birth, the infant is impacted by the emotional reactions of those responsible for his or her care. The sense of shared emotional states is a critical dyadic development. Affective sharing in the first few months of life takes place largely through face-to-face interactions; more sophisticated forms of sharing develop with the infant's increasing cognitive and motor capacities. At 9 months, joint attention serves as a way to share interesting, pleasurable experiences as mother and infant look first at an interesting toy and then at each other. Examining their mother's facial expressions, infants of this age follow her cues about whether or not an unfamiliar situation is safe or threatening. As language develops, verbal communication becomes a rich, complex way for mothers and babies to share their experiences.

Maternal depression is a particularly challenging condition for infant development and for infant-mother attachment. Postpartum depression, affecting about 15% of women (Seifer and Dickstein 2000), occurs at a time when mothers are already stressed by the need to adjust to newborn feeding schedules, lack of sleep, and the general household disruption that inevitably comes with a new baby. Increased irritability, listlessness, poor concentration and difficulty focusing on the baby, lack of pleasure in the infant as well as in the overall environment, and lack of efficacy and self-esteem are typical complaints (see Chapter 3: "Postpartum Disorders").

In her often-cited study, Tiffany Field (1984) showed that infants as young as 3 months respond to maternal mood and are adversely affected by depressed mothers: they themselves develop passive, depressed styles of interacting. When mothers with normal mood were asked to feign depression (i.e., assume a sad face, decrease their responsiveness), their infants manifested clear signs of distress, with gaze avoidance, negative affect, and decreased vocalizations. In an earlier study, Brazelton et al. (1975) found that even 6-week-old infants showed distress and avoidance when their mothers were asked to "act" withdrawn and depressed (Brazelton et al. 1975). Furthermore, in her study of postnatal depression and infant development, Murray (1992) found that maternal depression predicted higher rates of insecure attachment at 18 months of age.

When the mother functions as a "container," as Bion proposed, she correctly reads her infant's expression of emotion, allows herself a spontaneous reaction to it, but then responds in a timely and helpful manner. For example, confronted with a frequently hungry and very distressed, crying newborn, the containing mother will experience both the infant's desperation and her own sense of exhaustion and frustration; her manifest reaction, however, is one of calm and sympathy, and she quickly arrives with the desired milk. With an older, verbal baby she may label the affect state, encouraging his or her ability to symbolize and communicate emotions. Appropriate, empathic responding in the face of boredom, frustration, and irritation is a complex task for any mother; for a woman with little ability to control her own emotions or who is emotionally constricted herself, it becomes an impossible demand.

According to Fonagy and colleagues (1995), mothers with low reflective self-functioning fail to provide effective emotional support and guidance for their infants. Describing the chilling impact of a frightening or withdrawn mother on the young child's capacity to develop shared mental states, they state, "In cases of an abusive, hostile, or simply totally vacuous relationship with the caregiver, the infant may deliberately turn away from the object because the contemplation of the object's mind is overwhelming, as it harbors frankly hostile or dangerously indifferent intentions toward the self" (p. 257).

> S was a bright, articulate, but emotionally constricted 25-year-old mother who wore a fixed smile on her face; her expression did not change when she discussed sad or distressing material. An extensive psychiatric history included three significant suicide attempts in adolescence, with lengthy hospitalizations. As a young child, her alcoholic parents had counted on her to provide care for several younger siblings. Her role as caregiver had commenced at age 5 years, when her parents would often leave her and her siblings alone in the evenings. She recalled being required to execute household duties in a cheerful manner. Although she denied any memory of physical abuse, she remembered that protestations or complaints of being tired were met with severe disapproval and verbal threats by the par-

ents. Removed from her parents' home at the age of 12, she was separated from her siblings and placed in a group setting.

Mothering her infant daughter was extremely challenging for S. She could not tolerate any expression of negative emotion from her infant. Although Lily was placid and content from birth, even her occasional cries for food were overwhelming for S. However, this mother denied ever feeling irritated or frustrated by the demands of motherhood. She described the infant as a "joy" and a "gift from God," claiming that she had never found any undertaking as rewarding as parenthood. A demonstration of their interaction was provided, 2 weeks into treatment, when Lily had just turned 3 months of age.

At one point in the session, the infant began to cry softly. S assumed a fixed expression, avoiding eye contact with the girl, and began to hum to herself. She busied herself cleaning up toys they had been playing with. When the baby's crying escalated, S began to sing. At the point of Lily's greatest distress, S maintained a fixed expression and sang a loud, jovial-sounding tune without emotion. The therapist suggested that S pick up the child. S cooperated but stated oddly, "She loves my singing; it makes her happy." She seemed not to notice the distress of the infant at all. Apparently satisfied with being held, Lily ceased crying. When the therapist later asked S about her reaction to the crying, the mother looked puzzled; it was clear that she had only a hazy memory of the entire interaction. Only after many sessions was the therapist able to point out to S that she was unable to cope with Lily's distress; together they began to acknowledge, label, and respond to the infant's cries.

S's own early history of severe neglect, a condition she had been forced to accept cheerfully, made it impossible for her to tolerate her baby's expressions of distress: the old, repressed longings and rage evoked by her infant's cries were simply unbearable. She responded by enlisting well-entrenched, formerly adaptive patterns—namely, dissociating herself from powerful, negative affects. This completely prevented S from responding empathetically to Lily. Her inability to acknowledge Lily's and her own unhappiness, in addition to her unconscious resentment about once again assuming the caring role, led to severely misattuned responses to the infant's communications.

Psychotherapy, which ultimately helped S link previously disowned emotional reactions to events, was instrumental in allowing her to achieve more appropriate responses to her baby.

Maternal Perceptions and Attitudes

Even before their first pregnancy, mothers engage in fantasies about their children. Fears, wishes, and expectations, deeply influenced by their own childhood experiences, are brought to mothers' first infant interactions. Mothers with traumatic histories and serious psychopathology often manifest persistent, distorted ideas about their babies: unrealistic developmental expectations, inappropriate notions about the infant's thoughts and feelings, and projections from unhappy past relationships may dominate their every reaction to their child.

Alicia Lieberman (1992), a well-known infant researcher, describes how babies become unwitting partners in their mothers' unresolved psychological conflicts. First, the mother projects onto her child an unresolved emotional experience; second, she pressures the child to comply with the projection (e.g., she may make clear the unspoken threat that maternal attention and approval are contingent on certain behaviors); and third, the child accepts and identifies with the maternal expectation. Inhibition of exploration, recklessness, and precocious competence in self-protection may result when infants are the focus of maternal projections (Lieberman and Pawl 1990).

> B, a bright and outgoing 17-year-old first-time mother with a history of sexual and physical abuse, became suicidal during pregnancy on "learning" (from the guesses of friends) that she was likely to give birth to a girl; she described despairing of her child's future, because "girls are always victims." After giving birth to a healthy male infant, whom she immediately described as "macho," she expressed deep pleasure in his fisted hands: "He's ready to fight." When a nurse commented that all newborns hold their hands in the fisted position, she seemed deflated. Several weeks later, B noted that little Michael was bicycling with hands and feet and proudly reported to her therapist that he was "a tough guy," and "going to ride a motorcycle, like his father." The home-visiting nurse noted that B played aggressively with the infant, jabbing at him with plastic toys to the point where the child seemed to wince, as well as avert his gaze and cry; this made the mother laugh, and she persisted with her "game."
>
> B's interest in promoting what she perceived as a masculine attitude intensified as the infant gained motor capacities. At 6 months, she was eager to "help him practice walking" and spent many hours holding him up by his hands as he attempted to move his legs. She encouraged all sorts of physical play, generally ignoring him if he was subdued. She spoke proudly of his "attitude" and declared that he "wasn't going to take anybody's bullshit."
>
> Aside from her obvious pleasure in his physical activities, however, B showed little actual interest in the baby and did not seem to know much about him. He was primarily cared for by the maternal grandmother, who complained that B spent most of her time pursuing her relationship with the child's father. B clearly knew little about her infant's likes and dislikes; could not describe aspects of his temperament other than to note, laughing, that he was "mean"; and did not seem to know how to interact with him unless she was teaching him a motor task or engaging in roughhouse play.
>
> When the child was approaching his first birthday, B was referred for psychotherapy. By gradually pointing out B's investment in the boy's mascu-

linity and her tendency to equate him with other significant male figures, B's therapist was able to bring some of these processes to B's consciousness, placing them more under her control. To encourage her interest in all aspects of her son's personality and his developmental skills, the therapist sat with B, and together they observed and commented on the boy's activities. B was surprised to discover certain things about her son—for example, his fascination with picture books; she commented, "He's like me in some ways; I used to love to sit with a book."

This young woman held rigidly dichotomous views about males and females: men and boys were associated with her volatile and abusive stepfather, while females of all ages were seen as unhappy victims. Even the commonplace features of her infant son's physical development were interpreted as signs of a tough, masculine attitude. As the baby became a more active partner in the relationship—that is, at around 9 months, when joint attention and social referencing behaviors emerged—she found ways to communicate her pleasure in active behavior and her expectations that he would follow in the steps of his father, an adolescent delinquent whom she both admired and feared. For example, she would quickly intrude upon any quiet behaviors (e.g., when he would sit and handle toys) in order to engage him in motor activities; she was not dissuaded from this even when he would cry from obvious displeasure in being interrupted. Even when he was about to fall asleep, she would often jostle and awaken him.

Over time, this infant protested less and less his mother's aggressive interferences. Complying with maternal projections, he was an early walker and an athletic risk-taker as a toddler. As in Lieberman's (1992) notion of distortion in secure base behavior, he showed a reckless disregard for safety in his approach to the environment. However, along with winning maternal approval, his "macho" behaviors placed this infant in a bind: his mother also began to grow angry with him, seeing him as defiant and uncontrollable.

The Role of Fathers

Research on the role of fathers lags far behind that of mothers, and paternal influences are only beginning to emerge as critical. Fathers can complement solid mothering or compensate for maternal weaknesses; during difficult periods of adjustment, such as the postpartum weeks, the father can play a crucial role both in his support to the mother and through his direct care for the newborn. Moreover, the quality of the couple's relationship may figure importantly in the severity and chronicity of maternal depression (Campbell and Cohn 1997). Through their naturally more rigorous manner of play, fathers provide rich and diverse emotional experiences for infants (Crockenberg and Leerkes 2000). The next few years should shed increasing light on the direct and indirect impact of fathering on early child development.

Parent-Infant Psychotherapy: The Earliest Intervention

Development of a Treatment for High-Risk Dyads

On the basis of years of work with high-risk mothers and their neglected or abused children, Selma Fraiberg (1980) formulated a new treatment in which the infant's physical presence was a crucial part of the session. Mother and infant would interact together, displaying their typical patterns of behavior; the therapist would use these interchanges as meaningful points to begin her exploration of the mother's memories and attitudes. Fully compatible with attachment theory's emphasis on the intergenerational transmission of attachment styles, this innovative treatment also drew heavily from psychoanalytic concepts: interpretation of the mother's responses to her infant aimed at elucidating underlying, often unconscious issues and anxieties. Ultimately, Fraiberg (1980) sought to "free infants from the distortions and displaced affects engulfing them in parental conflict" (p. 70).

Following Fraiberg's seminal work with high-risk dyads, numerous forms of parent-infant psychotherapy were developed. Stern (1995) noted that all these forms share the following characteristics: they are generally brief (3–12 sessions), they focus on promoting a positive working relationship with the mother, and they concern themselves with impacting those maternal beliefs and attitudes that are enacted in day-to-day mother-infant interaction. The treatments vary in whether they emphasize concrete interactions or symbolic representations; accordingly, some will provide straightforward advice and information, whereas others work via the method of psychoanalytic interpretation.

As described by Stern (1995), the parent-infant therapist selects from among the various features the dyad displays—awkward interactions, inappropriate maternal expectations, difficult infant temperament—and chooses one as his or her immediate clinical focus. Through this "port of entry," the therapist approaches the parent-infant system and begins to work. Depending on the clinical presentation, the therapist may choose the maternal representations, the infant's behavior, the parent-child interaction, or his or her own reactions as the initial entry point for intervention.

A parent-infant psychotherapist who seeks improved mother-infant interaction as her major goal would likely select the mother's overt behavior as the port of entry. For example, a mother who does not read her infant's initial bids for face-to-face contact, waiting until the child's attention has waned, may experience defeat and disappointment when the baby finally gets around to responding. The parent-infant specialist points out her delay and helps her discern the subtle, initial overtures of her low-keyed baby. The therapist may or may not also explore the mother's feelings and associations around the issue of the infant's approaching her and the failure of the baby to respond to her awkward sense of timing. Changes in the mother's gestures toward the baby often lead to changes in infant responsiveness; ultimately, improvement might occur at a deeper level (i.e., in the mother's internal representations of how she sees herself and her child). In this case, the parent may begin to experience herself as more competent and effective, as well as needed and wanted by her infant.

Lieberman and colleagues (1991) hypothesized that anxious attachment results primarily from "affective dysynchronies between mother and infant"; their practice of parent-infant therapy sought to increase maternal empathy and responsiveness. These researchers designed an eclectic approach for high-risk Mexican mothers with severe social and economic stressors. Weekly home visitors hoped to improve attachment by encouraging mothers to function as a secure base for their children and sought to decrease environmental stress by concrete interventions (e.g., help with job training, English skills, housing). Dyadic improvements included increased maternal empathy, less avoidance and resistance on the part of children, and more cooperative, harmonious mother-child interactions.

Drawing on principles of attachment theory and psychoanalysis, Erickson and colleagues (1992) developed a home-based psychotherapy program that sought to promote healthy parent-infant relationships for high-risk dyads. These authors emphasize the establishment of a positive therapeutic relationship as a potential way for mothers to develop new working models that reflect an increase in self-esteem and trust in others. Insight is described as critical in fostering change: "by making the unconscious conscious, by facilitating the parent's thinking about what was previously automatic or unthought, the therapist hopes to give the parent greater control over actions" (p. 500). Benefits of parent-infant treatment included decreased maternal depression and anxiety and improved maternal responsiveness to the infants.

Research on the effectiveness of parent-infant psychotherapies is promising, although limited. One well-known evaluation of brief mother-infant psychotherapy (Cramer et al. 1990) compared the efficacy of two very brief treatments. The first, an interpretive psychotherapy, approaches mother-infant disturbances by identifying a "focal symptomatic interactional sequence." No direct advice or instruction on how to interact is provided to mothers. The second form of treatment is based on "interaction guidance," a parent-infant psychotherapy created by Susan McDonough for families with severe social/environmental stressors who are difficult to engage in treatment (McDonough 1993). Videotape technology is used to highlight and then reinforce maternal strengths, emphasizing the positive aspects of her interaction with her infant.

Cramer and his team hypothesized that the interpretive therapy would have more influence on internal and unconscious representations, whereas interaction guidance would tend to impact actual behavior. Results support the notion that behavior and representations are interconnected: differences in outcome for the two approaches were minimal. Both were effective in improving behavior (increasing maternal sensitivity and responsiveness) and in changing maternal perceptions of herself and her infant (mothers began to see their infants as more affectionate and themselves as calmer and more competent). Positive changes were still evident 6 months after termination. Overall, the results suggested that parent-infant psychotherapy has potential as a "major agent of change" (Cramer et al. 1990).

Early Identification and Evaluation of High-Risk Dyads

The antenatal period is the ideal point for early intervention. Guided by the transactional model, clinicians can evaluate level of risk on the basis of a pregnant woman's various social and emotional assets and vulnerabilities. For example, an adolescent with a history of conduct disorder, living in deep conflict with her own parents, would be considered at risk for forming an unhealthy relationship with her baby; should she also display hostile attitudes and unrealistic expectations toward her unborn child, concern about future abuse and neglect would be raised. A modified version of parent-infant psychotherapy, in which the pregnant woman and the "imagined and expected" baby are the dyad, can then be provided. Standard parent-infant psychotherapy can be initiated at birth, when the mother's first reactions to the baby can be incorporated into the treatment.

Interviews and questionnaires developed by attachment theorists over the last 20 years have been enormously helpful in guiding the identification of high-risk dyads. Many infant specialists use a brief separation-reunion paradigm to assess mother-infant attachment style; avoidant, ambivalent, or disorganized styles are easily discerned. Additionally, it is now widely accepted practice to assess the mother's other relationships, both past and present. History of trauma or relational instability suggest that she may encounter difficulty establishing a secure attachment with her infant.

Conclusion

Both psychoanalytic and attachment theories have molded current thinking about mothers and infants, uniting in the view that early mother-infant interaction is formative for development. Moreover, mothers' psychological functioning is seen as the key to dyadic success, although contributions from the infant, family, and the larger social milieu are critical. Although typical mothers are seen as specially equipped to meet their infant's needs, the demands of motherhood are formidable: women must discern the cues of preverbal infants; respond in a timely and empathic manner, even when overwhelmed and exhausted; and rework those inevitable old fears and anxieties that arise in the day-to-day mother-infant situation. Severe problems in attachment may result when mothers are overburdened by history of trauma, psychiatric illness, distorted ideas, or emotional constriction. It remains for future research to elaborate the role of fathers and other caregivers who may have significant influence on mother and child.

Parent-infant psychotherapy uses mother-infant interaction as the window to those unconscious maternal thoughts and feelings that ultimately determine an infant's attachment security. This promising new form of treatment seeks to make the mother's "ghosts in the nursery" more accessible, resulting in improved interactions as well as in deeper change at the level of mental representation. As mother-infant treatment becomes more widely used and researched, its effectiveness for avoiding tragic outcomes such as child abuse and infanticide can continue to be assessed.

References

Ainsworth M, Blehar MC, Waters E, et al: Patterns of Attachment. Hillsdale, NJ, Erlbaum, 1978

Bell S, Ainsworth M: Infant crying and maternal responsiveness. Child Dev 43: 1171–1190, 1972

Benedek T: Parenthood as a developmental phase. J Am Psychoanal Assoc 7:389–417, 1959

Bibring G: Some considerations of the psychological processes in pregnancy. Psychoanal Study Child 14:113–121, 1959

Bion WR: Attention and Interpretation: A Scientific Approach to Insight in Psychoanalysis and Groups. London, Tavistock, 1970

Bowlby J: Attachment and Loss, Vol I, Attachment. New York, Basic Books 1969

Bowlby J: Attachment and Loss, Vol II: Separation: Anxiety and Anger. New York, Basic Books, 1973

Bowlby J: Attachment and Loss, Vol III: Loss: Sadness and Depression. New York, Basic Books, 1980

Brazelton TB, Koslowski B, Main M: The origins of reciprocity: the early mother-infant interaction, in The Effects of the Infant on Its Caregiver. Edited by Lewis M, Rosenblum LA. New York, Wiley, 1974, pp 49–76

Brazelton TB, Tronick E, Adamson L, et al: Early mother-infant reciprocity, in Parent-Infant Interaction. Edited by CIBA Foundation. Amsterdam, Elsevier, 1975, pp 137–154

Campbell SB, Cohn JF: The timing and chemistry of postpartum depression: implications for infant development, in Postpartum Depression and Child Development. Edited by Murray L, Cooper PJ. New York, Guilford, 1997, pp 165–197

Chess S, Thomas A: Temperament in Clinical Practice. New York, Guilford, 1986

Cicchetti D: How research on child maltreatment has informed the study of child development, in Child Maltreatment: Theory and Consequences of Child Abuse and Neglect. Edited by Cicchetti D, Carlson V. New York, Cambridge University Press, 1989, pp 377–431

Cicchetti D, Rizley R: Developmental perspectives on the etiology, intergenerational transmission, and sequelae of child maltreatment. New Dir Child Dev 11:31–55, 1981

Cohen L, Slade A: The psychology and psychopathology of pregnancy: reorganization and transformation, in Handbook of Infant Mental Health, 2nd Edition. Edited by Zeanah C. New York, Guilford, 2000, pp 20–37

Cramer B, Robert-Tissot C, Stern D, et al: Outcome evaluation in brief mother-infant psychotherapy: a preliminary report. Infant Mental Health Journal 11:278–300, 1990

Crittenden P, Ainsworth MDS: Child maltreatment and attachment theory, in Child Maltreatment: Theory and Consequences of Child Abuse and Neglect. Edited by Cicchetti D, Carlson V. New York, Cambridge University Press, 1989, pp 432–463

Crockenberg, S, Leerkes E: Infant social and emotional development in family context, in Handbook of Infant Mental Health, 2nd Edition. Edited by Zeanah C. New York, Guilford, 2000, pp 60–90

Emde RN: The wonder of our complex enterprise: steps enabled by attachment and the effects of relationships on relationships. Infant Mental Health Journal 12:164–173, 1991

Erickson MF, Korfmacher J, Egeland B: Attachments past and present: implications for therapeutic intervention with mother-infant dyads. Dev Psychopathol 4:495–507, 1992

Field T: Early interactions between infants and their postpartum depressed mothers. Infant Behavior and Development 7:517–522, 1984

Fonagy P, Steele M, Steele H, et al: The capacity for understanding mental states: the reflective self in parent and child and its significance for security of attachment. Infant Mental Health Journal 12:201–218, 1991a

Fonagy P, Steele M, Steele H: Maternal representations of attachment during pregnancy predict the organization of infant-mother attachment at one year of age. Child Dev 62:891–905, 1991b

Fonagy P, Steele M, Steele H, et al: Attachment, the reflective self, and borderline states, in Attachment Theory: Social, Developmental and Clinical Considerations. Edited by Goldberg S, Muir R, Kerr J. Hillsdale, NJ, Analytic Press, 1995, pp 233–278

Fraiberg SH: Clinical Studies in Infant Mental Health: The First Year of Life. New York, Basic Books, 1980, p 70

Fraiberg SH, Adelson E, Shapiro V: Ghosts in the nursery: a psychoanalytic approach to the problem of impaired infant-mother relationships. Journal of the American Academy of Child Psychiatry 14:387–422, 1975

Freud S: Three essays on the theory of sexuality (1905), in The Standard Edition of the Complete Psychological Works of Sigmund Freud, Vol 7. Translated and edited by Strachey J. London, Hogarth Press, 1953, pp 123–243

Freud S: Instincts and their vicissitudes (1915), in The Standard Edition of the Complete Psychological Works of Sigmund Freud, Vol 14. Translated and edited by Strachey J. London, Hogarth Press, 1957, pp 109–140

George C, Kaplan N, Main M: The Adult Attachment Interview. Unpublished manuscript, University of California at Berkeley, 1985

Greenberg MT, Speltz ML, DeKlyen M: The role of attachment in the early development of disruptive behavior problems. Dev Psychopathol 5:191–213, 1993

Halpern R: Poverty and infant development, in Handbook of Infant Mental Health. Edited by Zeanah C. New York, Guilford, 1993, pp 73–87

Klein M: A contribution to the psychogenesis of manic-depressive states. Int J Psychoanal 16:145–174, 1935

Klein M: Notes on some schizoid mechanisms. Int J Psychoanal 27:99–110, 1946

Lieberman A: Infant-parent psychotherapy with toddlers. Dev Psychopathol 4:559–574, 1992

Lieberman A, Pawl J: Disorders of attachment and secure base behavior in the second year of life: conceptual issues and clinical intervention, in Attachment in the Preschool Years. Edited by Greenberg MT, Cicchetti D, Cummings EM. Chicago, IL, University of Chicago Press, 1990, pp 375–398

Lieberman A, Weston D, Pawl J: Preventive intervention and outcome with anxiously attached dyads. Child Dev 62:199–209, 1991

Mahler M, Pine F, Bergman A: The Psychological Birth of the Human Infant: Symbiosis and Individuation. New York, Basic Books, 1975

Main M, Solomon J: Discovery of a new, insecure-disorganized/disoriented attachment pattern, in Affective Development in Infancy. Edited by Brazelton TB, Yogman M. Norwood, NJ, Ablex, 1986, pp 95–124

Main M, Kaplan N, Cassidy J: Security in infancy, childhood and adulthood: a move to the level of representation. Monogr Soc Res Child Dev 50(1–2):66–106, 1985

Matas L, Arend R, Sroufe LA: Continuity in adaptation in the second year: the relationship between quality of attachment and later competence. Child Dev 49:547–556, 1978

McDonough S: Interaction guidance: understanding and treating early infant-caregiver relationship disturbances, in Handbook of Infant Mental Health. Edited by Zeanah C. New York, Guilford, 1993, pp 414–427

Murray L: The impact of postnatal depression on infant development. J Child Psychol Psychiatry 33:543–561, 1992

Nelson C, Bosquet M: Neurobiology of fetal and infant development: implications for infant mental health, in Handbook of Infant Mental Health, 2nd Edition. Edited by Zeanah C. New York, Guilford, 2000, pp 37–59

Pastor D: The quality of mother-infant attachment and its relationship to toddler's initial sociability with peers. Dev Psychol 17:326–335, 1981

Pianta R, Egeland B, Erickson MF: The antecedents of maltreatment: results of the Mother-Child Interaction Research Project, in Child Maltreatment: Theory and Consequences of Child Abuse and Neglect. Edited by Cicchetti D, Carlson V. New York, Cambridge University Press, 1989, pp 203–253

Pollack P, Percy A: Maternal antenatal attachment style and potential fetal abuse. Child Abuse Negl 23:1345–1357, 1999

Ruddick S: Maternal thinking. Feminist Studies 6(2):342–367, 1980

Sameroff A: Models of development and developmental risk, in Handbook of Infant Mental Health. Edited by Zeanah C. New York, Guilford, 1993, pp 3–14

Seifer R, Dickstein S: Parental mental illness and infant development, in Handbook of Infant Mental Health, 2nd Edition. Edited by Zeanah C. New York, Guilford, 2000, pp 145–161

Slade A: The quality of attachment and early symbolic play. Dev Psychol 23:78–85, 1987

Spitz R: Hospitalism: an inquiry into the genesis of psychiatric conditions in early childhood. Psychoanal Study Child 1:53–73, 1945

Spitz R: Anaclitic depression: an inquiry into the genesis of psychiatric conditions in early childhood. Psychoanal Study Child 2:313–342, 1946

Sroufe LA: Infant-caregiver attachment and patterns of adaptation in preschool: the roots of maladaptations and competence, in Parent-Child Interactions and Parent-Child Relations in Child Development (Minnesota Symposia on Child Psychology, Vol 16). Edited by Perlmutter M. Hillsdale, NJ, Erlbaum, 1983, pp 41–83

Stern D: Mother and infant at play: the dyadic interaction involving facial, vocal and gaze behaviors, in The Effect of the Infant on Its Caregiver. Edited by Lewis M, Rosenblum LA. New York, Wiley, 1974, pp 187–213

Stern D: The Interpersonal World of the Infant. New York, Basic Books, 1985

Stern D: The Motherhood Constellation. New York, Basic Books, 1995, p 171

Thomas A, Chess S: Temperament and Development. New York, Brunner/Mazel, 1977

Thomas A, Birch HG, Chess S: Temperament and Behavior Disorders in Children. New York, New York University Press, 1968

Waters E, Merrick S, Treboux D, et al: Attachment security in infancy and early adulthood: a twenty year longitudinal study. Child Dev 71:684–689, 2000

Winnicott DW: The Maturational Processes and the Facilitating Environment. New York, International Universities Press, 1965

Winnicott DW: Playing and Reality. London, Tavistock, 1971

Chapter 13

The Promise of Saved Lives

Recognition, Prevention, and Rehabilitation

Margaret G. Spinelli, M.D.

Dear Dr. Spinelli,
I have read your report on neonaticide. . . . I believe my case fits with the cases outlined in the report.

I have been charged with criminally negligent homicide and have just begun my sentence of 1–3 years here at ——.

I am writing to you to ask if you have any programing recommendations. It has been suggested that I complete an anger management program while I am here. I was hoping that you may have some suggestions as to the type of programing I may require for rehabilitation.

The anger management was suggested by programing because the case charge is criminally negligent homicide. The case itself was not looked into by anyone who programs inmates.

I have the ability to take other programs that I think may be helpful to me. There are programs for other crimes here[,] but I have yet to find anything rehabilitating for myself.

I may have overlooked a program. Please respond[,] as I ask for your help.
Thank you,
G

Letter from a woman in prison

As this chapter signals conclusion, I remind the reader of this book's original intent. Future research and education pertaining to infanticide are paramount, particularly because early intervention, and thus prevention,

may easily be achieved. I address this deficiency by returning to the typology and associated details of infanticide described by the distinguished
contributors to this book and repeat Oberman and Meyer's warning (see
Chapter 1: "A Brief History of Infanticide and the Law") that there is no
singular cause for infanticide. Because mothers who kill their infants are
not a homogenous group, prevention must be multifactorial.

Unlike other types of murder, infanticide has known and identifiable
precipitants, namely, pregnancy and childbirth. Women come to us in obstetrician's offices, antenatal clinics, and well-baby centers. We meet their
families and children. They complete questionnaires and attend interviews
with physicians, nurses, and social workers. How do we miss the warning
signs of potential tragedy?

This chapter is about women and infants at risk—about recognizing
clues, hearing unspoken messages, and establishing communication with
vulnerable mothers. While I describe assessment tools to identify depression or assess potential for fetal abuse, child maltreatment, or infanticide, I
also emphasize our relationships with mothers as our most important tools
for identification, intervention, prevention, and treatment. I also describe
self-help organizations, associations for professional and lay members, a
pen pal network of women serving prison sentences for infanticide, and
other vehicles and opportunities for prevention and treatment.

Mother-Infant Attachment

The continuum of mother-infant interaction disorders ranges from delayed
attachment to infanticide (Robinson and Stewart 1993). Approximately
10% of new mothers will experience delayed attachment to their infants.
Another 1% will have negative or hostile thoughts about their newborns.
Although child abuse is also on the continuum of poor attachment, infanticide is the ultimate failure of bonding (see Chapter 12: "The Mother-
Infant Relationship"). Although mother-infant attachment disorders are
most often described in the postpartum period, they may be detected,
and therefore explored, during gestation to facilitate the resolution of
hostile feelings before delivery. In essence, the antenatal period is the
paramount time for prevention.

Selma Fraiberg (1980) coined the phrase "ghosts in the nursery" to describe the process through which unresolved conflicts in a parent's childhood may resurface in the parent-infant relationship (Scott 1992). The
mother's preexisting conflicts, centered on unmet dependency needs or
on an ambivalent internalized image of herself as mother, may be exacerbated by the event of childbirth (see Chapter 12).

During pregnancy, a woman redefines her relationship with her own parents. Depending on early relationships, some antepartum women may develop ambivalent or even hostile feelings toward their pregnancy and the fetus that they carry. The anticipated maternal role may cause the woman to reevaluate her relationship with her own mother, and old conflicts may surface.

When Bonding Fails

The process of bonding between mother and infant begins during pregnancy and continues through infancy and beyond. Because the growing relationship between mother and fetus has its roots in the mother's early experiences, these experiences may predict the success or failure of this relationship. If pregnancy is a developmental state, as Benedek (1959) suggested, then it makes sense that difficulties like conflicts, traumas, or psychological stumbling blocks encountered along earlier paths of development may cause a woman to experience pregnancy as a time of turmoil. If a mother is stuck at a particular phase of her own development, the bonding process is interrupted.

The mother's awakened "ghosts in the nursery" may generate love or hostility that shape her interaction with her infant (see Chapter 12). The predictive nature of the bonding process provides a template for early intervention, which has the potential to reverse pathological interaction and prevent sequelae such as abuse or infanticide.

Throughout normal pregnancy, the emotional attachment between mother and infant grows (Pollock and Percy 1999). The mother develops an elaborate internalized image of the fetus, a process conceptualized by Rubin (1984) as "binding in"—the fetus becoming part of the self.

This early antenatal attachment is predictive of the postnatal bond and may, in fact, determine the potential for later child abuse or even infanticide. Most murdering mothers have histories shaped by chaos, abuse, violence, and dysfunction. A history of childhood maltreatment is the most consistently reported characteristic of abusive parents (Korbin 1986)—an intergenerational cycle prevalent among women who are imprisoned for killing their children.

Women with a history of childhood sexual or physical abuse or both are more likely to experience suicidal ideation during pregnancy (Farber et al. 1996). Childhood abuse is also associated with the likelihood of previous suicide attempts, and childhood sexual abuse often results in reproductive conflicts (Friedman 1996). The trauma of abuse can become an organizer for future development and conflict, merge with wishes and inhibitions, and affect adult behavior and neuroses.

Pregnancy can reawaken a mother's memories of past sexual traumas and shame about body image and changes, and feelings like grief and anger may be manifested as suicidal ideation or infanticidal ideation (Farber et al. 1996). Her feelings of vulnerability, helplessness, and despair associated with the newborn may elicit unbridled rage toward the infant.

Dietz et al. (1999) discovered a dose-response relationship between unintended pregnancies in adulthood and a history of abuse or family dysfunction. Because women with unintended pregnancies are more likely to be young and lacking in adequate support systems, they possess all the risk factors for child abuse and necessitate close monitoring, early assessment, and intervention. Similarly, certain character traits (e.g., aggression, isolation, and suspicion), drug or alcohol abuse, and poor social supports are also indicators of potential violence against children (Korbin 1989). In sum, women's early histories are a most important predictor of outcomes during their pregnancies.

The Myth of Maternal Bliss

Historically, pregnancy has been freighted with a mythic social expectation that it is a time of well-being, even bliss, for women. However, recent data demonstrate a 10% prevalence of antepartum depression (Gotlib et al. 1989; O'Hara et al. 1990). The fact that postpartum depression is the outcome for one-half of women who are depressed during pregnancy (Graff et al. 1991) emphasizes the need for and benefit of early intervention (Evans et al. 2001). Although fetal abuse implies a direct assault such as punching or hitting the abdomen (Kent et al. 1997), it also includes seemingly passive actions such as substance abuse. In addition to poor appetite, weight loss, and poor compliance with prenatal care, the depressed pregnant woman is at greater risk for using nicotine, drugs, and alcohol (Scott 1992), further underscoring the potential for fetal abuse in these women.

Women at Risk

Postpartum Risks

A dearth of information and education for new parents and families explains undiagnosed and untreated puerperal mental illness. In addition, postpartum psychosis is abrupt and unexpected; it has a labile quality that is misleading and confusing. A mother experiencing postpartum psychosis may appear well at one moment and quite psychotic at the next (see Chapter 3: "Postpartum Disorders").

In contrast, postpartum depression has an insidious onset. If psychotic symptoms arise, they may be subtle and invasive, lacking the manic quality of acute postpartum psychosis. The secret paranoid nature of delusion may also inhibit self-disclosure.

Although childbirth itself is a signal for postpartum illness, society's expectation that the transition from pregnancy to mothering will be smooth and joyful can produce denial of any unpleasant events associated with childbirth. Because the new mother is expected to be unfailingly happy, the stigma of mental illness is even more pronounced at this time in a woman's life. Not surprisingly, she often keeps secret any thoughts and feelings of guilt and failure she has experienced.

A mother with postpartum psychosis can be ashamed and confused by her murderous thoughts, and thus her thinking is not easily detectable to others. Her own observing ego attempts to keep hallucinations at bay. Alternatively, a paranoid delusional system may prevent disclosure by threat, as illustrated by the following case:

> An obstetrician referred to me patient A, who had florid psychosis on postpartum day 3. The psychiatrist recommended that A go to the university hospital emergency room. During A's evaluation, she told the emergency room psychiatric resident that she had no intention of harming herself, her infant, or anyone else. The psychiatric resident, planning discharge, called the outpatient psychiatrist to arrange a visit for the next day. The psychiatrist insisted that A be admitted because she was psychotic and had an infant at home. The attending psychiatrist equally adamantly insisted on discharge. But just before A was discharged, she attacked her brother as he entered the emergency room, making the professional discussion moot and A's admission mandatory.
>
> A remained on the psychiatric unit for 2 weeks. She received neuroleptics but no mood stabilizer, despite her hyperreligiosity and manic presentation. When A was discharged, she revealed to the treating psychiatrist a secret delusional system that she had not disclosed to anyone during her 14-day hospitalization. She reported a delusional theme circumscribed around the number 3: Her labor lasted for 3 hours, her infant was 3 days old, and there were 3 delusional personae (or witches) demanding that she kill herself, her mother, or her new infant. When A attempted to stab herself with scissors, her mother phoned A's obstetrician.

No inquiries directed at uncovering a delusional scheme were made of A before her discharge and resumption of care of her infant. The failure to detect A's delusional scheme could easily have led to tragedy, underscoring the need for medical and psychiatric professionals to query infanticidal ideation sensitively, yet persistently.

While doing so, the clinician should be aware that obsessional intrusive thoughts to harm the infant might also arise in the setting of postpartum depression (Wisner et al. 1999; see also Chapter 3). Unlike psychotic symptoms, these obsessions are ego-dystonic thoughts of harming the infant that create tremendous stress for the mother; they must be differentiated from those that pose a danger to the infant.

Wisner et al. (1994) described the biopsychosocial model of postpartum illness as a classification of symptoms with a common presentation. Interestingly, their contemporary description and diagnostic classification are in agreement with the work of the earliest researchers in the field, including Marcé (1858) and Esquirol (1838). Wisner's group identified the phenomenology and organic presentation of postpartum psychosis through clinical interviews and standardized objective mood and cognitive testing. They described the waxing and waning presentation, indicating the need to evaluate infanticidal ideation very carefully, because a mother may appear well then rapidly deteriorate (see Chapter 3).

A family or personal history of mood disorders is the most important clue to early prophylaxis of postpartum depression. Psychopharmacological intervention before or after delivery is responsible for a large decrease in the risk of recurrence and is described elsewhere in this book (see Chapter 3). Stewart et al. (1991), Cohen et al. (1995), and others have demonstrated this model of prevention in clinical trials.

The therapist or physician working with childbearing women faces the unique challenge of treatment and prevention during a time of psychological and developmental transition. Such ports of entry as mother-infant interaction or family relationships may provide clues to the mother's mood and well-being. It is imperative to evaluate her interaction with the infant as well as any suicidal or infanticidal ideation. Concerns should be addressed through couple and family intervention.

Treating mothers at risk also carries potential complications. Postpartum psychosis is a medical emergency. Hospitalization is imperative because of the unpredictable and labile quality of mood and likely paranoid delusional system. Additional concerns include providing family education and addressing concerns for the infant's well-being.

Early Trauma as Risk

Although infanticide and suicide are extreme outcomes of postpartum depression and psychosis, mothers with postpartum mood disorders are also at high risk for child maltreatment. Children of depressed mothers are more withdrawn and irritable and have significant behavioral problems such as sleep and eating disorders, frequent temper tantrums, and, when the effects of lower socioeconomic status exacerbate the situation, delayed language development (Murray 1992). Because the depressed mother is unable to respond to infant cues or provide warmth and acceptance (Biringen and Robison 1991), early development is marked by insecure attachment behavior.

The depressed mother has several risk factors for consideration (Table 13–1). Her increasing frustration and her inability to soothe the infant may cause her to view the infant as hostile. Infant behaviors such as those mentioned above may in turn elicit hostile feelings from the mother towards the infant. Halpern (1993) suggests the presence of one or two difficult conditions, such as infant illness, poverty, or difficult personality, intensifies hostile feelings in the mother. Certain social or environmental factors, such as poverty, are particularly conducive to escalating hostile or even murderous feelings on the part of the mother.

Table 13–1. Risk assessment for pregnant women

Family/personal history of depression of other psychiatric illness
   Antepartum depression
   Previous postpartum depression
   Bipolar disorder
Childhood trauma
Home violence (past or present)
Substance abuse
Poverty, less education, young age
Increased number of children
Child illness
Poor or hostile antenatal attachment
Poor support system or unavailable partner
Edinburgh Postnatal Depression Scale > 10

In their case series of women who killed their children, Haapasalo and Petäjä (1999) found that 63% of the women had a history of child abuse. The mother with hostile or angry feelings or a history of abuse suffered at the hand of her own mother will likely be overwhelmed by the stirrings of hostile feelings aroused by her infant's crying and neediness (see Chapter 12: "The Mother-Infant Relationship").

For example, colic and intractable crying are common triggers for child abuse. Levitsky and Cooper (2000) examined the impact of colic on emotional state of mothers in 25 mother-infant pairs. Explicit aggressive thoughts and fantasies were reported by 16 (70%) of the mothers, while 6 (26%) admitted to thoughts of infanticide during a colic period.

Denial as a Risk for Neonaticide

A woman who denies her own pregnancy is at risk for a host of problems, the most serious being neonaticide (see Chapter 6: "Neonaticide"). These women, usually young, often fail to manifest symptoms of pregnancy and fail to attend prenatal clinics, a situation frequently complicated by their families' collusion in denying the pregnancy.

The term *denial of pregnancy* implies the problem in identifying risk (see Chapter 5: "Denial of Pregnancy"). However, when compiled, scattered reports in the literature reveal a similar picture of precipitant signs, symptoms, and personal and family history. Therefore, early identification of the described presentation provides signals for prevention.

In cases of neonaticide following denial of pregnancy, retrospective accounts hinting at trouble surface, almost without fail. Teachers report having recognized a difference in the young woman's mood and a drop in grades. Family physicians may have actually diagnosed pregnancy but failed to follow up. Professionals, relatives, and other people known to the young woman invariably substantiate missed opportunities for intervention, as demonstrated in the following case:

> C appeared to her co-workers to be pregnant, although she denied this. Staff from C's employer's Employee Assistance Program literally escorted her to prenatal clinic visits. Although C went along with this, she continued to disavow her pregnancy—even in the face of evidence like the fetal image on her sonogram. When one day C returned to work no longer pregnant, the staff became alarmed and alerted the police to their suspicions. Regrettably, C's infant was already dead.

If C's denial of her pregnancy had been recognized earlier as a potential danger, a timely psychiatric referral may have saved her baby's life.

By and large, things are not much better in the schools, because teachers are generally not well educated about adolescent mood disorders. A depressed child is rarely bothersome and causes few problems in the classroom. Usually quiet, withdrawn, and isolated, he or she attracts notice only when the depression precipitates misconduct, truancy, or tragedy.

Neonaticide is associated with denial of pregnancy (see Chapter 5), dissociative symptoms, dissociative hallucinations, depression, and suspicion of early trauma in isolated, rigid family structures (Spinelli 2001). To ignore the existence of this prodrome is to abandon hope of reaching and educating parents, teachers, and health professionals. If we identify the precipitants associated with neonaticide, we can construct treatment strategies and devise prevention and rehabilitation programs and methods. Treatment strategies include individual and family psychotherapy, prenatal care, mobilization of support systems, adoption alternatives, and parenting programs. Prevention includes educating health providers, teachers, and parents to identify early signs.

Fathers, Families, and Recovery

Rehabilitation for the mother recovering from postpartum psychosis includes psychopharmacology education and compliance, psychoeducation, engagement of support systems, and psychotherapy. Because the shock and precipitous onset of postpartum disorder affect the entire family, the family must also be rehabilitated. Couple and family interventions are vital and should include psychotherapy and psychoeducation as well as interventions for other children. The conjugal balance that has been perturbed by postpartum mental illness can be restored by crisis treatment focused on the postpartum problem (Lalive and Manzano 1982). If the balance is incompatible with integration of a child, long-term treatment is advised.

Childbirth is a developmental stage for the entire family. Couple therapy is effective for new parents as they adapt to new roles and replace fantasized parenthood with real life (Apfel and Handel 1999). In addition, it provides the opportunity to identify paternal pathology, which may challenge the relationship.

Implications for family therapy are supported by O'Hara's (1985) report that depressive symptom severity decreased and marital satisfaction improved when rated at intervals during pregnancy and the postpartum period. In addition, Marks and colleagues (1996) demonstrated that women with histories of postpartum illness with supportive husbands are less likely to relapse.

Postpartum depression organizations can also offer a valuable experience for the new mother and father. Through group, individual, and family support, other mothers who have experienced puerperal psychiatric illness can support the new mother through her recovery. These organizations have expanded to include fathers support networks and Web sites for shared experience.

After the Tragedy

Little information exists about fathers who have experienced the tragedy of infanticide. In my case sample of 17 neonaticides (see Chapter 6), only two women identified the baby's father. In all others, the relationship was denied or described as a one-time experience. The theme of secrecy and denial remained through arrest, trial, and incarceration. The two identified fathers remained supportive, although they colluded in the denial of pregnancy despite a continued sexual relationship. Both fathers were approached by the prosecution to testify against the woman but refused. Generally, fathers were not expected to share responsibility for the infant's death. In one case that was not part of my series, the father had an active role in the infant's demise and received a sentence similar to the mother's (Callaway 1999).

Women who have killed an infant during a psychotic episode are frequently married, some with small children. In cases familiar to me, husbands were strikingly supportive, often sharing responsibility and blame for neglecting cries for help and failing to recognize signs of potential tragedy. Life becomes fraught with court appearances, media exploitation, and years of incarceration. Sustaining a relationship in the face of such tragedy remains an enormous challenge, as illustrated by the following case ("Postpartum: Beyond the Blues" 1989):

> S killed her 4-week-old infant son during a postpartum psychotic episode. S had suffered a severe depression after her 5-year-old daughter's birth. Her husband and family were unsympathetic and angry. They asked why she had become pregnant if she was so unhappy with a child. When she conceived a second time, her doctor assured her that the depression would not recur.
>
> During the second postpartum episode, S remained silent, thinking, "I will hang on a little longer." She could not.
>
> S and her family were "confronted with the unthinkable" at her murder trial when she received an 8- to 20-year prison sentence. S's husband fought for his wife's release and worked to encourage a greater understanding of postpartum disorders through appearances on television and before the State Board of Pardons. "We must get K's mother home," he said. "It is not right to punish S so severely for something that has grown from family ignorance and denial. The disease itself is a monster. It comes from nowhere, takes the things closest to you and does not look back." Unfortunately, the parole board refused to moderate her sentence.

The Tragedy of the Yates Family: What Can We Learn?

A series of errors paved the way to the tragic events of June 20, 2001, when Andrea Yates drowned her five children (see "Introduction," this volume). I use these data not to add to the suffering of this family, but as a message of caution and hope for the future.

The following factors represent precipitants or missed opportunities for prevention.

Personal or Family History of Psychiatric Illness

Prior to the episode at the time of the drownings, Mrs. Yates had at least two previous postpartum episodes. She reported psychosis after her first birth. After John's (her fourth child's) birth in 1999, she was hospitalized twice for psychosis, each admission precipitated by suicide attempts. A family history of psychiatric illness was also reported.

Family Denial, Ignorance, or Fear of Stigma

Family members described Mrs. Yates as catatonic, noting that she stared for hours and scratched bald spots into her head. Mr. Yates said his wife was withdrawn because of her father's death, and he often minimized her illness despite her deterioration.

Poor Partner Support

A rigid belief system seemed to dominate the home and family. "Man is the breadwinner and woman is the homemaker," Rusty Yates told the prosecutor. His wife had 2 hours of personal time each week

Isolation

Andrea Yates home-schooled her children and had little interaction with neighbors and friends.

Increased Number of Children

Mrs. Yates had five children from 1994 to 2000.

Family and Child Services Intervention

During a 1999 hospitalization, Mrs. Yates reported to the staff that she was overwhelmed, living in a converted Greyhound bus with her growing family of four children (Yardley 2001). Mr. Yates told a social worker that he was training his sons, including the 3-year-old to use power drills. The social worker filed the report with Children's Protective Services, but the state agency declined to pursue the case.

Inadequate Psychoeducation

The couple was warned about recurrence of her postpartum illness. Mr. Yates explained that the couple would talk it over when she felt better and decided to have more children; however, early medical intervention during pregnancies would likely have prevented a recurrence of psychosis.

Inadequate Medical Education About Postpartum Disorders

The psychiatrist must understand that postpartum psychosis is a psychiatric emergency. The waxing and waning quality of psychosis makes behavior unpredictable. Psychotic mothers must be separated from their infants and children.

Poor Medical Management of Puerperal Psychosis

For unclear reasons, the treating psychiatrist discontinued Andrea Yates from antipsychotic medication. In general, she failed to receive an acceptable standard of medical care.

Stigma and Lack of Public Education

Her friend wrote in a journal that Andrea smelled like she had not bathed in days, paced "like a caged animal," and warned Mr. Yates (CourtTV 2002). A report to Child Services would have been warranted.

We as a society failed Andrea Yates. We share equal responsibility for the tragedy. Friends, neighbors, and family watched as Mrs. Yates continued to decompensate. The medical community failed to provide appropriate protection, social work assistance, and child services to a severely psychotic mother of five children. When the legal community and the state failed to appreciate the severity of her illness, they eliminated her last opportunity for appropriate treatment.

The Yates trial attracted national attention. The National Organization for Women and the American Civil Liberties Union held vigils during the trial. Advocates for the mentally ill blamed Texas law's narrow standards for the insanity defense. Other troubling issues—such as the quality of the insanity defense and the troubling nature of expert psychiatric witnesses whose opinions differed so remarkably—came to the forefront.

The case also aroused the attention of several mental health advocacy groups such as the National Depressive and Manic-Depressive Association and many organizations dedicated to postpartum disorders. They requested clarification of postpartum DSM-IV diagnostic criteria, improved medical education and guidelines for treatment, a greater understanding of a biopsychosocial model of postpartum disorders, education for families, identification of women at risk, and consideration of infanticide legislation.

After sentencing, the American Psychiatric Association made a public announcement on the insanity defense and mental illness ("APA Statement on the Insanity Defense and Mental Illness" 2002):

The American Psychiatric Association hopes that the Yates case will lead to broad public discussion of how our society and its legal system deals with defendants who are severely mentally ill. . . . reviews of insanity cases show that the more heinous the act, the less likely that an insanity plea will succeed, despite the disabling presence of severe mental illness.

Also, the standards for handling mentally ill defendants vary across jurisdictions. A mentally ill person tried for a capital offense in one state may be found "not guilty by reason of insanity," while another person with similar severity of mental illness tried in another state may be convicted.

Advances in neuroscience have dramatically increased our understanding of how brain function is altered by mental illness, and how psychotic illness can distort reality. . . . Unfortunately, public understanding has not kept pace with these advances.

A failure to appreciate the impact of mental illness on thought and behavior often lies behind decisions to convict and punish persons with mental disorders. . . . Prisons are overloaded with mentally ill prisoners, most of whom do not receive adequate treatment.

Defendants whose crimes derive from their mental illness should be sent to a hospital and treated—not cast into a prison, much less onto death row.

The fact that the insanity defense is nonexistent in some states and extremely limited in others speaks to our disregard for mental illness and the rights of those who suffer. Until we treat mental illness with the same dignity afforded to other illnesses, the course will remain unchanged. And when the next tragedy occurs, we will gasp in horror.

Treatment After Tragedy

Treating a woman who has killed an infant presents a formidable task for the therapist. A woman who has killed during a psychotic episode is remorseful and must work through her feelings of guilt and loss. It is imperative that the therapist work through his or her own countertransference in order to assist the patient through this time (see Chapter 11: "How Could Anyone Do That?"). Significant attention must be paid to suicidal ideation while including the family in treatment, if possible.

Countertransference feelings are more complicated with the young neonaticidal mother who denied her pregnancy. Their fragile, childlike personalities place significant limitations on treatment. A detached style, isolated affect, and *la belle indifférence* in the face of infant death and a murder trial can be a source of frustration for the therapist.

In all cases, the therapist must be mindful of potential legal involvement and seek guidance from appropriate sources. Documentation should be factual and accurate.

Screening Tools and Mood Assessment

The earliest intervention for mothers at risk takes place in the antepartum period. With recognition that antepartum screening is the best intervention strategy for identifying women at risk, the prenatal clinic is the optimum environment to use simple screening tools and objective mood scales. A number of reliable diagnostic and assessment tools are available to evaluate maternal mood and assess risks for neglect and abuse. Although these tools do not replace a diagnostic interview, they may facilitate collection of focused information. These measurements of maternal risk factors can be easily administered in the antenatal clinic, where women at risk can be identified in time for intervention.

Depression Rating Scales

The Edinburgh Postnatal Depression Scale (EPDS), designed to identify postpartum depression (Harris et al. 1989), is a timely and simple screen for antepartum changes. The EPDS includes only behavioral symptoms without somatic symptoms, which may be confused with the discomforts of pregnancy or the immediate postpartum state. The EPDS is a 10-point patient-rated scale translated into several languages that takes approximately 3 minutes to complete.

Beck and Gable (2000) devised a scale, the Postpartum Depression Screening Scale, that is a reliable and valid self-rated assessment of postpartum mood disorders. Items are exquisitely sensitive to what is experienced by mothers with postpartum depression. Additionally, the Peripartum Events Scale, developed by O'Hara et al. (1986), measures stressful life events that may precipitate peripartum mood disorders. The Peripartum Events Scale significantly correlates with antepartum and postpartum measures of depression and a woman's self-rating of problems with labor and delivery. The Antenatal Health Questionnaire queries prepregnancy emotional disturbances and identifies women likely to experience a postpartum mood disorder (Nordström et al. 1988). Finally, interventions such as interpersonal psychotherapy for antepartum depression have been used successfully to treat depression during pregnancy and prevent subsequent postpartum mood disorders (Spinelli 1997).

Early Maternal Attachment Scales and Abuse Potential

It is critical to address the risk of abuse potential before parenthood. Fonagy et al. (1991) found that the quality and style of maternal attachment can be predicted when the Adult Interview Scale is administered before birth.

Condon (1993), using the Maternal Antenatal Emotional Attachment Scale (MAEA), proposed a model of maternal antenatal attachment. The MAEA predicts four different styles, each representing a particular combination of underlying attachment dimensions and aggressive potential toward the fetus and the newborn (see Chapter 12: "The Mother-Infant Relationship").

The Child Abuse Potential Inventory (CAP) is designed to identify acute or potential physical child abusers. A study by Todd and Gesten (1999) demonstrated that the CAP was a useful and valid measure of personality characteristics common to abuse victims who have an increased potential to commit future physical abuse. The CAP is an excellent tool for identifying women at risk in order to treat underlying psychopathology.

Pregnant adolescents are more vulnerable to depression and child abuse by virtue of their youth, inadequate support systems, greater likelihood that the baby's father is absent, and conflicts over education. Efforts to include significant others in care are a priority, and parent-infant therapeutic care is a major foundation for prevention. Parent-infant psychotherapy and interventions such as Field's (1984) use of infant massage for depressed mothers are early interventions to reshape the mother-infant bond through early treatment (Erickson et al. 1992). A trusting relationship with a therapist may function as a protective factor and as a mechanism of developing parenting skills and attachment.

A Measure of Progress

Organizations dedicated to psychiatric disorders associated with childbirth and mother-infant health grew out of a fundamental need to recognize isolated and untreated women with depression and other psychiatric illnesses and prevent consequences ranging from impaired early mother-infant interaction to mortality.

The Marcé Society dates to the 1980s, when professionals in different disciplines were working on postnatal disorders (Glangeaud-Freudenthal 2001) but lacked a forum for sharing knowledge and ideas. Responding to this problem, Professors Channi Kumar and Ian Brockington of the United Kingdom and Professor James Hamilton of the United States founded an international society aimed at improving the understanding, prevention, and treatment of mental disorders related to childbirth. They named the society after the French physician Louis Victor Marcé, whose early work described the temporal relationship of mental disorders and childbirth (Marcé 1858).

The Marcé Society was officially launched during the first academic meeting on puerperal mental disorders, in Manchester, England, in 1980.

Since then, experts from around the world gather at biennial meetings to share state-of-the-art research and clinical knowledge. The society's focus has grown to include antepartum and postpartum disorders, mother-infant attachment, child abuse, and infanticide.

In the United States, women initiated a grass-roots movement in the 1980s to remedy the failure to identify postpartum disorders. Nancy Berthold, for example, after her own isolating and confusing experience of postpartum psychosis, organized women who had suffered from puerperal mood disorders into a group called Depression after Delivery (DAD). Today, DAD, a national group under the direction of Joyce Venis, R.N.C., provides individual and group support, professional referrals, and education for women and families with puerperal disorders (Venis 2000).

Under the umbrella of the Marcé Society, Jane Honikman founded Postpartum Support International (PSI) in 1987 to meet women's need for timely and relevant resources, information, and referral (Honickman 2000). Today, PSI members include representatives of self-help organizations and social support networks and individual professionals and experts in this field. Other international organizations under the PSI roof include the Postnatal Depression Support Association (South Africa), Meet a Mum Association (United Kingdom), and the Prenatal Association of Canada (PASSCAN). China, Denmark, Mexico, and 14 other countries have organizations under the PSI umbrella, as do 31 U.S. states (in addition to DAD, which is national).

In groups like DAD and PSI, members of diverse backgrounds and experience work together toward a shared goal of improved care for mothers and infants. Their membership rosters include laypeople—mothers, fathers, children, other relatives of affected families—and professionals—social workers, nurses, psychiatrists, obstetricians, pediatricians, and psychologists, to name a few. Such organizations function as a national and international postpartum referral and networking system. For example, PSI's Pen Pal Network Project, created in 1990, is an effort to connect women serving sentences for infanticide in U.S. prisons with one another and with PSI members. The network provides information and updates on the women, their parole status, clemency petitions, and sentence modifications, as well as ongoing education and group efforts to influence public policy and legislation.

In the realm of public policy advocacy, PSI claimed a victory with the passage of U.S. House of Representatives Resolution 163 (H-RES 163, October 10, 2000), The Postpartum Depression Resolution (U.S. Congress 2000). This resolution, co-sponsored by Representatives Jack Kingston (R-Ga.) and Lois Capps (D-Ca.), recommends that all hospitals and clinics provide departing new mothers, fathers, and other family members with information about postpartum psychiatric illness, including symptoms and treatment resources, and that the National Institutes of Health promote additional research on postpartum psychiatric illness.

Another recently passed bill demonstrates increased social awareness of the problem of abandoned infants. The Abandoned Infant Protection Act (House Bill 1616) (2000) provides that "no parent shall be prosecuted . . . for abandonment of an infant less than 15 days of age when that parent voluntarily delivers the infant to one of the following individuals and does not express an intent to return for the infant[:] . . . a health care provider . . . [,] a law enforcement officer . . . [,] a social services worker . . . [,] an emergency medical technician . . . [,] or any adult of suitable discretion who willingly accepts the infant."

A bill was recently introduced in the House of Representatives by Bobby Rush of the First District in Chicago, Illinois. Bill 2380, the Melanie Stokes Postpartum Depression Research and Care Act (June 28, 2001), has the goal of providing research on and services for individuals with postpartum depression and psychosis (U.S. Congress 2001). The bill is named for Melanie Stokes, a young mother who committed suicide while in the throes of postpartum depression (Venis 2001).

Although postnatal women generally have a low rate of suicide, those who develop severe postpartum illness are at high risk of suicide in the first postpartum year (Appleby 1998). Uncharacteristically for females, methods are violent and tend to peak in the first postnatal month.

Conclusion

Mothers characterized by certain socioeconomic factors, poor social supports, or mental illness are at significant risk of committing infanticide. To date, however, effective strategies for identification, intervention, and prevention are glaringly absent from the continuum of antenatal and postnatal care and services. The ability to detect antenatal and postnatal psychiatric illness more reliably and consistently than has been done historically holds the key to prevention.

Infanticide is not caused by a single factor (Haapasalo and Petäjä 1999). The complexity of factors related to the origins of the impulse to kill, whether individual, social, cultural, or developmental, must be acknowledged. Known precipitants include abuse, psychosocial complications, immaturity, isolation, marital problems, inadequate social supports, financial constraints, domestic violence, early trauma, parental chaos, and adult "motherless" motherhood (Simpson 2000). Because mothers are more likely to commit child homicide in the first year after childbirth, the mother's own identification with her child may be an important trigger for aggressive impulses. Other circumstances that increase vulnerability include social isolation, early loss, immigrant status, abandonment by a partner, and domestic violence. A striking aspect of many infanticide cases—suggesting, perhaps, an area for future study—is that the infant's father is rarely identified and rarely implicated in the act (Table 13–1).

As a major public health problem, postpartum psychiatric illness is predictable, identifiable, treatable, and, most importantly, preventable. Research methodology must be designed to substantiate a cluster of identifiable symptoms and precipitants on the basis of contemporary diagnostic criteria and the biopsychosocial model of psychiatry. Phenomenological studies will help identify symptoms in order to pave the way for treatment strategies, prevention, and rehabilitation. This primary method of prevention of postpartum psychiatric disorders and other sequelae of childbirth also provides secondary prevention by treating parents of children at risk. Adult psychiatric services should reach beyond the mother's mental state to the family as the focus of intervention (Scott 1992).

As I indicated at the outset of this book, my own professional involvement in infanticide cases in the judicial system spurred my belief that we, as a society, could do a far better job of preventing these tragedies. Just as I began by enjoining the reader to share in the admittedly difficult task of entering the minds of mothers who kill, I will close with a request.

I hope the reader who has journeyed through these chapters may now share the belief that infanticide is preventable. Developing effective interventions and preventions will, of course, require further study of the mental states of antepartum and postpartum women who are at risk to commit or have committed infanticide. Those of us who pursue the goal of prevention will be obliged to override any anger or revulsion we may feel with the compassion and courage to seek a more in-depth understanding of infanticide. The collective knowledge and experience of the contributors to this book suggest that, while we need to know more, we already know too much to look away any longer.

So I ask the reader who has come this far to take heart: the goal of saving lives through the prevention of infanticide is attainable. We are acquainted with mothers who may kill their babies, and perhaps some who have already committed child murder. We see them in hospitals and clinics and other settings; we interview them and their families; we know their stories and circumstances. What is required of us is to not look away but to communicate with and learn from these mothers. The great promise of understanding them better will play out in incalculable saved lives.

References

Abandoned Infant Protection Act, North Carolina General Assembly House, Bill 1616, May 18, 2000

APA Statement on the Insanity Defense and Mental Illness in response to the Andrea Yates case, by Richard K. Harding, M.D., President, American Psychiatric Association. Release No. 02-08, March 15, 2002

Apfel RJ, Handel MH: Couples therapy for postpartum mood disorders, in Postpartum Mood Disorders. Edited by Miller LJ. Washington, DC, American Psychiatric Press, 1999, pp 163–178

Appleby L, Mortensen PB, Faragher EB: Suicide and other causes of mortality after post-partum psychiatric admission. Br J Psychiatry 173:209–211, 1998

Beck CT, Gable RK: Postpartum Depression Screening Scale: development and psychometric testing. Nurs Res 49(5):272–282, 2000

Benedek T: Parenthood as a developmental phase: a contribution to the libido theory. J Am Psychoanal Assoc 7:389–576, 1959

Biringen Z, Robison J: Emotional availability in mother-child interaction: a reconceptualization for research. Am J Orthopsychiatry 61(2):258–271, 1991

Callaway B: Peterson asks for work release option. The Review of the University of Delaware 126(2):1, 1999

Cohen LS, Sichel D, Robertson LM, et al: Postpartum prophylaxis for women with bipolar disorder. Am J Psychiatry 152:1641–1645, 1995

Condon JT: The assessment of antenatal emotional attachment: development of a questionnaire instrument. Br J Med Psychol 66:167–183, 1993

CourtTV: Texas mom drowns kids. Available at http://www.courttv.com/trials/yates. Accessed March 2002.

Dietz PM, Spitz AM, Anda RF, et al: Unintended pregnancy among adult women exposed to abuse or household dysfunction during their childhood. JAMA 282:1359–1364, 1999

Erickson MF, Korfmacher J, Egeland B: Attachments and present: implications for therapeutic intervention with mother-infant dyads. Dev Psychopathol 4:495–507, 1992

Esquirol JED: Des maladies mentales consideres sous les rapports medical, hygienique et medico-legal, Vol 1. Paris, JB Bailliere, 1838

Evans J, Heron J, Francomb H, et al: Cohort study of depressed mood during pregnancy and after childbirth. BMJ 323:257–260, 2001

Farber EW, Herbert SE, Reviere SL: Childhood abuse and suicidality in obstetrics patients in a hospital-based urban prenatal clinic. Gen Hosp Psychiatry 18:56–60, 1996

Field T: Early interactions between infants and their postpartum depressed mothers. Infant Behavior and Development 7:517–522, 1984

Fonagy P, Steele M, Steele H: Maternal representations of attachment during pregnancy predict the organization of infant-mother attachment at one year of age. Child Dev 62:891–905, 1991

Fraiberg SH: Clinical Studies in Infant Mental Health: The First Year of Life. New York, Basic Books, 1980

Friedman S: Reproductive conflicts in incest victims: an unnoticed consequence of childhood sexual abuse. Psychoanal Q 65:383–388, 1996

Glangeaud-Freudenthal N: Towards a history of the Marcé Society. The Marcé Society Newsletter 11:5–6, 2001

Gotlib IH, Whiffen VE, Mount JH: Prevalence rates and demographic characteristics associated with depression in pregnancy and the postpartum. J Consult Clin Psychol 57(2):269–274, 1989

Graff LA, Dyck DG, Schallow JR: Predicting postpartum depressive symptoms and structural modeling analysis. Percept Mot Skills 73:1137–1138, 1991

Haapasalo J, Petäjä S: Mothers who killed or attempted to kill their child: life circumstances, childhood abuse, and types of killing. Violence Vict 14:219–239, 1999

Halpern R: Poverty and infant development, in Handbook of Infant Mental Health. Edited by Zeanah C. New York, Guilford, 1993, pp 73–87

Harris B, Huckle P, Thomas R, et al: The use of rating scales to identify postnatal depression. Br J Psychiatry 154:813–817, 1989

Honickman J: News from the postpartum support movement. Postpartum Support International Newsletter 11(4):2–4, 2000

Kent L, Laidlaw JDD, Brockington IF: Fetal abuse. Child Abuse Negl 21:181–186, 1997

Korbin JE: Childhood histories of women imprisoned for fatal child maltreatment. Child Abuse Negl 10:331–338, 1986

Korbin JE: Fatal maltreatment by mothers: a proposed framework. Child Abuse Negl 13:481–489, 1989

Lalive J, Manzano J: Beyond postpartum psychosis: the couple in question. Information Psychiatrique 57:633–645, 1982

Levitsky S, Cooper R: Infant colic syndrome—maternal fantasies of aggression and infanticide. Clin Pediatr 39:395–400, 2000

Marcé LV: Traité de la folie des femmes enceintes, des nouvelles accouchées et des nourrices. Paris, JB Bailliere, 1858

Marks M, Wieck A, Checkley S, et al: How does marriage protect women with histories of affective disorder from postpartum relapse? Br J Med Psychol 69:329–342, 1996

Murray L: The impact of postnatal depression on infant development. J Child Psychol Psychiatry 35(3):343–363, 1992

Nordström UL, Dallas JH, Morton HG, et al: Mothering problems and child morbidity amongst "mothers with emotional disturbances." Acta Obstet Gynaecol Scand 67:155–158, 1988

O'Hara M: Depression and marital adjustment during pregnancy and after delivery. American Journal of Family Therapy 13:49–55, 1985

O'Hara MW, Varner MW, Johnson SR: Assessing stressful life events associated with childbearing: the Peripartum Events Scale. Journal of Reproductive and Infant Psychology 4:85–98, 1986

O'Hara M, Zekoski EM, Philipps LH, et al: Controlled prospective study of post-partum mood disorders: comparison of childbearing and nonchildbearing women. J Abnorm Psychol 99(1):3–15, 1990

Pollock PH, Percy A: Maternal antenatal attachment style and potential fetal abuse. Child Abuse Negl 12:1345–1357, 1999

Postpartum: Beyond the Blues. Narrated by Susan Sarandon. Lifetime Series, WTLJ TV WBAL. New York, Sound One Corp, 1989

Robinson GE, Stewart DE: Postpartum disorders, in Psychological Aspects of Women's Health. Edited by Stewart DE, Stotland NL. Washington, American Psychiatric Press, 1993, pp 115–138

Rubin R: Maternal Identity and the Maternal Experience. New York, Springer, 1984

Scott D: Early identification of maternal depression as strategy in the prevention of child abuse. Child Abuse Negl 16:345–358, 1992

Simpson AIF, Stanton J: Maternal filicide: a reformulation of factors relevant to risk. Criminal Behaviour and Mental Health 10:136–147, 2000

Spinelli M: Interpersonal psychotherapy for depressed antepartum women: a pilot study. Am J Psychiatry 154:1028–1030, 1997

Spinelli MG: A systematic investigation of 16 cases of neonaticide. Am J Psychiatry 158:811–813, 2001

Stewart DE, Klompenhouwer JL, Kendell RE, et al: Prophylactic lithium in puerperal psychosis: the experience of three centres. Br J Psychiatry 158:393–397, 1991

Todd MK, Gesten EL: Predictors of child abuse potential in at-risk adolescents. Journal of Family Violence 14:417–436, 1999

U.S. Congress, House of Representatives, 106th Congr, 1st Sess: First house resolution bill on postpartum depression. October 10, 2000

U.S. Congress, House of Representatives, 107th Congr, 1st Sess: Melanie Stokes Postpartum Depression Research and Care Act, Bill 2380, June 28, 2001

Venis J: Heartstrings: Depression After Delivery Newsletter 10(1):1, 2000

Venis J: Written in memory of Melanie Stokes. Heartstrings: Depression after Delivery Newsletter 11(2):2, 2001

Wisner KL, Peindl K, Hanusa BH: Symptomatology of affective and psychotic illnesses related to childbearing. J Affect Disord 30:77–87, 1994

Wisner KL, Peindl KS, Gigliotti T, et al: Obsessions and compulsions in women with postpartum depression. J Clin Psychiatry 60:176–180, 1999

Yardley J: Despair plagued mother held in children's deaths. New York Times, September 8, 2001, A7

Index

*Page numbers printed in **boldface** type refer to tables or figures.*

Abandoned Infant Protection Act
(U.S.), 251
Abandonment, fears of, and
pregnancy denial, 88–89
Abuse. *See also* Child abuse
emotional, and pregnancy denial/
neonaticide, 112
fetal, 238
sexual, and reproductive conflicts,
112, 114, 237
ACTH. *See* Adrenocorticotropic
hormone
Adam Bede (Eliot), 81
Addiction, and pregnancy denial, 83,
91
Adolescence, pregnancy in
denial of, 90
risks associated with, 249
Adrenocorticotropic hormone
(ACTH), 70
Affective denial of pregnancy, 82–84,
91
Age
of infant, and risk of homicide, 195
of perpetrators of infanticide, 24–25
of perpetrators of neonaticide, 90,
135, 189
of victims of infanticide, 23, **24**

Ainsworth, Mary, 213, 214, 215
Alto do Cruzeiro (Brazil), 120
child death in, 121–125
Amazon, Brazilian, infanticide in, 126
American Academy of Pediatrics, 29
on SIDS, 27
American Academy of Psychiatry and
the Law (APPL), 175
American Civil Liberties Union, 246
American Psychiatric Association
recognition of postpartum
disorders by, 147
Yates case and, 246–247
Amitriptyline, use during breast-
feeding, 49
Amnesia, intermittent, in neonaticide,
107, 110
Amygdala, 66
Ancient cultures, infanticide in, 4–6
Anemia, vs. postpartum depression,
47
Antenatal Health Questionnaire, 248
Anthony, Susan B., 105
Antidepressants, use during breast-
feeding, 49–50
Anxious attachment, causes of, 227
APPL. *See* American Academy of
Psychiatry and the Law

Arabia, female infanticide in, 5
Arson, infant deaths caused by, **22**
Assault, infant deaths caused by, 21, **22**
Assessment. *See* Evaluation
Assisted/coerced infanticide, **11,** 12
Attachment
    adult styles of, 214
    mother-infant. *See also* Mother-
      infant relationship
      antenatal assessment of, 249
      assessment of, 228
      categories of, 213
      disorders of, 236–238
      early treatment of problems in,
        249
      importance of, 209
      intergenerational transmission
        of, 226
      psychotherapy for improving,
        210
      sources of problems in, 229
Attachment theory, 212–214
Automatism. *See* Involuntary act
    defense
Autoscopy, in pregnancy denial/
    neonaticide, 109
Avoidant attachment, 213

"Baby blues," vs. postpartum depres-
    sion, 41
Babylonian civilization, 4
Bariba (West African people), infanti-
    cide practiced by, 126
"Bastardy infanticide," 7
Battering, and infant deaths, 21, **22**
Befriending, of mothers at risk, 194
Benin, People's Republic of
    (West Africa), infanticide in, 126
Berthold, Nancy, 250
Bion, W. R., 211
Bipolar disorder
    acute-onset postpartum psychosis
      as, 42–43
    postpartum admission for women
      with, 39

risk of recurrence for, 54
    thyroid dysfunction and, 68
    use in legal defense, 148, 149–150
Birth. *See* Labor and delivery
Birth defects, cultural responses to,
    125–127, 128
Birth order, as risk factor for infanti-
    cide, 24
Bowlby, John, 212
Brain
    abnormalities of, early maternal
      deprivation and, 215
    basic structure of, 66
    neurochemicals in, and depression,
      65–66
Brain stem, 66
Brazelton, T. Berry, 215
Brazil
    infant death in, high expectancy of,
      121, 124
    mother love in, 121–123
    selective neglect in, 121, 123
    tolerance of difference in, 127
Breast-feeding
    during antidepressant therapy,
      49–50
    during antipsychotic therapy, 52–53
    during estrogen therapy, 74
Brief psychotic disorder, use in legal
    defense, 148
Britain
    infanticide in, 191–192
    infanticide legislation in, xvi, 16,
      137, 186–188
    history of, 7–8, 9
    neonaticide in, 189–191
    prevention of infanticide, 192–195
Brockington, Ian, 249
Bromocriptine, manic symptoms after
    treatment with, 46

Calcium homeostasis, disorder of,
    46–47
Canada, infanticide legislation in, xvi,
    137

CAP. *See* Child Abuse Potential
Inventory
Capps, Lois, 250
Carbamazepine, use during breast-
feeding, 52
Cassell, Elaine, 174, 175
Catechol O-methyltransferase
(COMT), 67
Catholic Church, and infanticide,
6
Chaldean civilization, 4
Chavez, Linda, 10
Child abuse
absence in traditional societies,
128, 129
by fathers, xx–xxi
history of
and pregnancy outcomes, 112,
237–238
and risk for mother-infant
relationship, 241
infant deaths caused by, 21, **22**
infanticide related to, **11**, 13, 195
risk of
assessment of, 216, 248–249
postpartum disorders and, 240
in SIDS cases, 27
triggers for, 241
Child Abuse Potential Inventory
(CAP), 249
Child death. *See* Infant death
Childbearing. *See also* Labor and
delivery
and risk for psychiatric morbidity,
36, 186. *See also* Postpartum
psychiatric disorders
"Childbirth Under X" (France), 101
Children Act of 1989 (Britain), 195
China, female infanticide in, 5–6
Christian society, medieval, infanticide in, 6–7
Circadian rhythms, disruption in labor
and postbirth, 42
Civil cases, use of postpartum
syndromes in, 177–180

Clomipramine, use during breast-
feeding, 49
Cognition, with pregnancy denial/
neonaticide, 88, 112
Cognitive-behavioral counseling, for
postpartum depression, 47–48
COMT. *See* Catechol O-methyltrans-
ferase
Condemned infant syndrome, 124–125
Confucian doctrine, and female
infanticide, 5
Constantine (Roman emperor), 6
Contraceptives, oral, and postpartum
disorder symptoms, 63
Cortex, brain, 66
Corticotropin-releasing hormone
(CRH)
in "fight or flight" response, 70
during pregnancy, 45
Cortisol
levels of, in postpartum depression,
70–71
as stress hormone, 70
Countertransference problem, 202,
247
Couple therapy, 243
CRH. *See* Corticotropin-releasing
hormone
Crime, infanticide as, xv
Criminal cases
infanticide, 140–141
neonaticide, 138–140
types of defense in, 141–146, **142**
use of DSM in, 146–151
use of postpartum psychosis in,
problems of, 9–10, 140
use of postpartum syndromes in,
173–177
Cultural conflict, and pregnancy
denial/neonaticide, 205–206
Cultural norms, 12, 13
infanticide as rejection of, 4
Culture(s). *See also* Sociocultural
factors
ancient, infanticide in, 4–6

Culture(s) *(continued)*
  medieval Judeo-Christian,
    infanticide in, 6–7
  traditional
    absence of child abuse in, 128,
      129
    infanticide in, 125–126
Custody cases, use of postpartum
  syndromes in, 177–178
Custody loss, previous, and pregnancy
  denial, 89
Cuts/stabbing, infant deaths caused
  by, **22**

DAD. *See* Depression after Delivery
Daubert test, 157, **157**
  for neonaticide syndrome,
    161–162
*Daubert v. Merrell Dow Pharmaceuti-
  cals, Inc.*, 158–160
Death. *See* Infant death; Infanticide;
  Neonaticide
Defense, criminal law
  types of, 141–146, **142**
  use of DSM in, 146–151
  use of postpartum syndromes in,
    173–177
Defense attorney, guidance for,
  134–135
Delivery. *See* Labor and delivery
Delusions
  identification of, 239
  in postpartum mental illness, 136,
    173
Denial of pregnancy. *See* Pregnancy
  denial
Depersonalization, in pregnancy
  denial/neonaticide, 109
Depersonalization disorder, use in
  legal defense, 148–149
Depo-Provera, and postpartum
  disorder symptoms, 63
Depression
  antepartum, 238
  brain-body relationships in, 68–75

etiology of, theories of, 65
major
  and obsessions, 40–41
  in postpartum period, 38,
    39–40
  symptoms of, 39–40, **40**
  use in legal defense, 148,
    149–150
minor, in postpartum period, 38
neurochemical factors for, 65–66
postpartum
  vs. "baby blues," 41
  cortisol levels and, 70–71
  evaluation for, 47
  health visitors in treatment of,
    194
  hormonal contribution to,
    45–46, 70–71
  and infant development,
    221–222, 240–241
  insidious onset of, 239
  lack of full recognition of, 147
  obsessional thoughts in, 41,
    44–45, 240
  prevalence of, 36
  prevention of, 50–51, 240
  risk for recurrence of, 54
  screening for, 54, 248
  support organizations for, 243
  thyroid illness and, 47, 69–70
  treatment of, 47–51, **48**
  and pregnancy denial, 92
  in women, 65
Depression after Delivery (DAD),
  250
DES. *See* Dissociative Experiences
  Scale
Desipramine
  for postpartum depression, **48**
  use during breast-feeding, 49
Deterrence
  harsh infanticide laws and lack of,
    188
  as rationale for punishment, 14–15
Dexamethasone resistance, 71

Diagnostic and Statistical Manual of Mental Disorders, 4th Edition (DSM-IV), 147
  postpartum-onset specifier in, 38, 147–148, 169
  use in criminal defenses, 146–151
Dietz, Park Elliott, 10
Diminished capacity defense, 143
  depersonalization disorder and, 149
  psychotic disorder and, 150
  requirements for, **142**
Disability requirement, for criminal defense, 146
  using DSM to satisfy, 146–151
Dismissing attachment, 214
Disorganized attachment, 213
Dissociation
  during birth experience, pregnancy denial and, 85
  in neonaticide, 107, 109–110, 202
Dissociative disorder
  in neonaticide perpetrators, 190, 191
  and pregnancy denial, 113
  use in legal defense, 148
Dissociative Experiences Scale (DES), 107, 110–111, 116
Dissociative psychosis, in neonaticide, 110
Dopamine
  chemical precursor of, 66
  estrogen and levels of, 72
  neurotransmitters, 65
  psychiatric symptoms associated with, 66
  receptors, and mental status changes, 74–75
Doss, Ms., 138–139
Dowry system, and female infanticide, 5
Doxepin, use during breast-feeding, 49
Drowning, infant deaths caused by, 21, **22**

DSM-IV. *See Diagnostic and Statistical Manual of Mental Disorders*, 4th Edition

Early identification. *See* Identification
Eating disorders, and pregnancy denial, 92
Edinburgh Postnatal Depression Scale (EPDS), 54, 248
Education
  and infanticide prevention, 171
  maternal, and risk for infanticide, 25
Electroconvulsive therapy, for postpartum psychosis, 51
Eliot, George, 81
Emotion regulation, maternal psychopathology and, 221–223
Emotional abuse, and pregnancy denial/neonaticide, 112
England. *See also* Britain
  "poor law" of 1576, 7
EPDS. *See* Edinburgh Postnatal Depression Scale
Esquirol, Jean-Etienne, 8
Estradiol
  in postpartum depression, 45
  in postpartum psychosis, 51
Estrogen
  postpartum effect of, 73
  receptors in brain, 72
  and regulation of neurotransmitter activity, 66, 68
  therapy, for postpartum disorders, 45, 51, 52, 55, 73–74
  withdrawal, psychosis after, 46
Ethnography, 120
Eugenics, and infanticide, 4, 5, 128
Europe. *See also* Britain; France
  medieval, infanticide in, 6–7
Evaluation. *See also* Identification
  of child abuse risk, 216, 248–249
  of infanticide risk, 195
  of mother-infant attachment, 228, 249

Evaluation *(continued)*
of parenting behavior, 98–99
for postpartum disorders, 47
of pregnant women, 216–219,
228, **241**
Evans-Pritchard, E. E., 125
Evidence
admissibility of, tests of, **157,**
157–160
novel scientific, 157
syndrome, 155, 156–157
Expert testimony, vs. syndrome
evidence, 156
Exposure, and infanticide, 5

Family dynamics
with infanticide, 245
with pregnancy denial/neonaticide,
107, 111, 114, 189, 204–206
Family planning, pregnancy denial
and, 99
Family therapy, 243
Fathers
child abuse by, xx–xxi
infanticide and, 243–244, 245, 252
infanticide by, xx, 191, 195
sentencing for, 192
and pregnancy denial, 244
role of, 225–226
Federal Rule 702, 160
Federal Rules of Evidence, 158, 159
Fetal abuse, 238
Fetal death registrations, 26–27
Fetus, violent fantasies toward, 89–90,
94
Field, Tiffany, 221
"Fight or flight" response, 70
Filicide, xx
perpetrators of, 44
Fluoxetine
for postpartum depression, 47–48,
48
use during breast-feeding, 50
Fonagy, Peter, 214
Fraiberg, Selma, 210, 226, 236

France, pregnancy laws in, 101
Freud, Sigmund, 115, 211
Frye test, 157, **157**
for neonaticide syndrome,
161–162
Frye v. United States, 158

Gamma-aminobutyric acid (GABA),
68
General deterrence, as rationale for
punishment, 14
"Ghosts in the nursery" (Fraiberg),
210, 236
Gingrich, Newt, 10
Gonadal hormones, alterations in, and
postpartum disorders, 46, 72–73
Gonadotropin-releasing factor, 71
Greece, ancient, 4
Gregor, Thomas, 126
Grimm, Susan, 178–179
Guilt
neonaticide and, 190–191
in postpartum psychoses, 42

Hallucinations
dissociative, in neonaticide, 107,
109
vs. obsessions, 40
in postpartum mental illness, 136,
141
Hamilton, James, 73, 249
Harlow, Harry, 212
Health visitors, and treatment of
postpartum depression, 194
Hinckley, John W., Jr., 144–145
Hippocampus, 66
Historical perspective
on infanticide, xvi, 4–9
on infanticide legislation, in
Britain, 7–8, 9
"Holding environment," 211
Homicide, infanticide treated as, 134
Homicide Act of 1957 (Britain), 186,
187
Honikman, Jane, 250

Hormones. *See also specific hormones*
  and mood disorders in women, 64
  in postpartum depression, 45–46,
    70–71
  in postpartum psychosis, 46
  and regulation of brain chemicals,
    68
  in women, 64, **69**
Hospitalization
  involuntary, with pregnancy
    denial, 100–101
  in mother-and-baby units,
    194–195
  for postpartum psychosis, 240
House of Representatives Resolution
  163 (H-RES 163), 250–251
Hypercalcemia, vs. postpartum
  psychosis, 47
Hypothalamic-pituitary-adrenal
  (HPA) axis, 70–71
Hypothalamic-pituitary-ovarian
  (HPO) axis, 71–75, 114
  in pseudocyesis, 115
Hypothalamic-pituitary-thyroid
  (HPT) axis, 68–70
Hypothalamus, 66
Hysterical pregnancy (pseudocyesis),
  114–115
Hysterical psychosis, 115

ICD-10. *See International Classification of Diseases*, 10th Revision
Identification. *See also* Evaluation
  missed opportunities for, 171–172
  of mother-infant disturbances,
    228–229
  of postpartum depression, 54, 248
  of postpartum psychosis, need for
    training in, 43
  of pregnancies at risk, 216–219,
    228, 237–238
  of pregnancy denial, 96, 242
  screening tools for, 248–249
  of women at risk, 44, 213–214,
    238–243

Illegitimacy, and infanticide, 6–7
Imipramine, for postpartum
  depression, **48**
India, female infanticide in, 5
Infant(s). *See also* Mother-infant
  relationship
  maternal projections on, 224–225
  psychoanalytic perspectives on,
    210–211
  temperament of, 219
Infant death. *See also* Infanticide;
  Neonaticide
  causes of, 21–23, **22**
  in Northeast Brazil
    acceptance of, 124–125
    mother love and, 121–122
Infanticide. *See also* Neonaticide
  clinical considerations in, 136–137
  historical perspective on, xvi, 4–9
  legal treatment of. *See*
    Jurisprudence; Laws
  perpetrator characteristics, 20,
    24–25, 195, 203
  prevalence of, 19, 25, 27–28
  prevention of. *See* Prevention
  rate of, social conditions and, 187,
    188
  reporting of, 20–23
  risk factors for, 23, 24–25, 28,
    251–252
  typology of, 10–13, **11**
  as ultimate failure of bonding, 236
Infanticide Act of 1922/1938 (Britain),
  xvi, 9, 137, 170, 186, 192
  criticism of, 186–187
  support for, 188
Insanity, criteria for, 170
Insanity defense, 143–146
  American Psychiatric Association
    on, 246–247
  concerns about, 175
  depersonalization disorder and,
    149
  postpartum psychiatric disorders
    and, 140–141, 174

Insanity defense *(continued)*
  psychotic disorder and, 150
  requirements for, **142**
  successful use of, 140
Insecure attachment
  causes of, 227
  postpartum depression and, 241
  types of, 213
Intellectual deficits, and pregnancy
  denial, 91
Interaction guidance, for mother-
  infant disturbances, 228
International Classification of Diseases,
  10th Revision (ICD-10), 38
Interpersonal abandonment, fears of,
  and pregnancy denial, 88–89
Interpersonal psychotherapy (IPT),
  for postpartum depression, 47,
  48
Interpretive psychotherapy, for
  mother-infant disturbances, 228
Interventions. *See* Identification;
  Prevention; Treatment
Interviews
  in diagnosis of postpartum
  disorders, 44, 62–63
  forensic psychiatric, 106
Involuntary act defense, 143
  depersonalization disorder and,
  148–149
  requirements for, **142**
IPT. *See* Interpersonal psychotherapy
Irish of West Kerry, infanticide
  practiced by, 125–126
Isolation
  and pregnancy denial, 93
  and risk for child abuse, 216
  and risk for infanticide, 245

Jurisprudence, infanticidal. *See also*
  Criminal cases; Laws
  in Britain, xvi, 7–8, 9, 16
  international comparisons of, xvi
  in United States, xvi, 9, 14–16, 134
  grave injustices in, 207–208

infanticide court cases, 140–141
neonaticide court cases,
  138–140
use of postpartum syndromes
  in, 173–177

Kingston, Jack, 250
Klein, Melanie, 211, 212
Knowledge deficits, and pregnancy
  denial, 91
Kumar, Ramesh (Channi), 249

Labor and delivery
  disruption of circadian rhythms in,
  42
  pregnancy denial and experience
  of, 85, 110
Laws. *See also* Jurisprudence
  infanticide
    in Britain, xvi, 7–8, 9, 137,
    186–188
    in Canada, xvi, 137
    harsh, lack of deterrent effect
    of, 188
    in United States, xvi, 9, 137–138
  pregnancy, in France, 101
Lieberman, Alicia, 224
Limbic (reptilian) brain, 66
Lithium, for postpartum psychosis, 51
Loss of child, previous, and pregnancy
  denial, 89
Luteinizing hormone, 72

MAEA. *See* Maternal Antenatal
  Emotional Attachment Scale
Mahler, Margaret, 211, 212
Major depression
  and obsessions, 40–41
  in postpartum period, 38, 39–40
  symptoms of, 39–40, **40**
  use in legal defense, 148, 149–150
Maltreatment. *See* Child abuse
Mania, in postpartum period, 38
Manic depression. *See* Bipolar
  disorder

MAO. *See* Monoamine oxidase
Marcé, Victor Louis, 8, 249
Marcé Society, 249–250
Marital status, of neonaticide
  perpetrators, 135, 189
Massip, Sheryl, 9, 10, 15, 141
Maternal Antenatal Emotional
  Attachment Scale (MAEA), 249
McDonough, Susan, 228
Media, and infanticide cases, 14
Medical model, of infanticide, 8–10
Mehinaku Indians, infanticide
  practiced by, 126
Melanie Stokes Postpartum
  Depression Research and Care
  Act (United States), 251
Mental illness, maternal. *See also*
  specific illnesses
  effects on offspring, 53–54,
    221–222, 240–241
  and emotion regulation, 221–223
  infanticide related to, **11**, 13,
    172–173
  postpartum. *See* Postpartum
    psychiatric disorders
  and pregnancy denial, 91–92
Middle Ages, infanticide in, 6–7
Midwifery services, for high-risk
  women, 193–194
M'Naghten test, 145, 163, 174
  defense based on psychotic
    disorder and, 149–150
  postpartum psychosis and, 176
Model Penal Code (MPC)
  defense based on psychotic
    disorder and, 150, 151
  and insanity defense, 145–146
Monoamine oxidase (MAO), 67
  estrogen and levels of, 72
Monoamines. *See* Neurotransmitters
Mood disorders. *See also* Bipolar
    disorder; Depression
  neurochemical factors for, 65–66
  in postpartum period, 38–39
  in women, 63–64

Mother(s). *See also* Mother-infant
    relationship; Motherhood
  age of
    and risk for infanticide, 24–25
    and risk for neonaticide, 90,
      135, 189
  education of, and risk for
    infanticide, 25
  high-risk
    identification of, 213–214,
      238–243
    responses to infant's
      temperament, 220
  infanticide/neonaticide committed
    by. *See* Perpetrators
  love for child. *See* Mother love
Mother-and-baby units, in Britain,
  194–195
Mother-infant relationship, 209–229
  attachment theory of, 212–214
  current views on, 214–215
  disorders in, 236–238
  early evaluation of, 228–229
  emotion regulation in, 221–223
  maternal perceptions and attitudes
    and, 223–225
  psychoanalytic perspectives on,
    210–212
  risks to, 209–210
    transactional model of,
      215–216
    temperament and "goodness of fit"
      in, 219–221
Mother love
  ambiguities of, 122–123
  child death and, 121–122
  perspectives on, 123–124
Motherhood
  demands of, 229
  as developmental phase, 217
  social norms governing, 12, 13
    infanticide as rejection of, 4
MPC. *See* Model Penal Code
Mull, Dorothy and Dennis, 126
Murder, vs. infanticide, 170

National Depressive and Manic-
    Depressive Association, 246
National Organization for Women,
    246
Neglect
    infant deaths caused by, 21, **22,** 189
    infanticide related to, **11,** 12–13
    risk of, transactional model for
        assessing, 216
    selective
        in Northeast Brazil, 121, 123
        suppression of, 129
    in SIDS cases, 27
Neonaticide, 12
    ascertainment problems for, 26–27
    biopsychosocial model of, 113–116
    in Britain, 189–191
    clinical findings in, **107,** 107–112
    court cases in United States,
        138–140
    depersonalization in, 109
    dissociation in, 107, 109–110, 202
    family dynamics with, 107, 111,
        204–206
    incidence of, 23, **24**
    perpetrator characteristics, 20, 90,
        135–136, 189
    pregnancy denial and, 12, 81, 93, 94,
        105, 108–109, 136, 152, 189
    psychodynamic paradigm of,
        115–116
    recurrence of, 95
    risk for, pregnancy denial and,
        242–243
    sociocultural factors for, 92, 101
    systematic investigation of,
        105–117
    in typology of infanticide, **11**
Neonaticide syndrome
    alternative diagnoses for use in
        legal defense, 148
    case illustration of, 151–154
    lack of recognition of, 147
    legal acceptance of, determination
        of, 161–162

Neurotransmitters
    deficiency of, and negative mood
        states, 65
    mechanism of action, 66–67, **67**
    psychiatric symptoms associated
        with, 66
Newborns
    with birth defects, cultural
        responses to, 125–127, 128
    maternal killing of. See Neonaticide
Norepinephrine
    chemical precursor of, 66
    estrogen and levels of, 72
    in "fight or flight" response, 70
    neurotransmitters, 65
Norms governing motherhood, 12, 13
    infanticide as rejection of, 4
Nortriptyline
    for postpartum depression, **48**
    use during breast-feeding, 49, 50
Novel scientific evidence,
    admissibility of, 157–160
Nuer (African people), infanticide
    practiced by, 125

Obsessions
    definition of, 40
    in major depression, 40–41
    in postpartum depression, 41,
        44–45, 240
Obsessive-compulsive disorder, in
    postpartum period, 38
Obstetric/gynecological factors, and
    pregnancy denial, 92
Obstetric services. See also Prenatal
    care
    and identification of pregnancy
        denial, 97–98
    and prevention of infanticide, 193,
        239
Oral contraceptives, and postpartum
    disorder symptoms, 63
Organizations, support, 243, 249–
    250
Osmond, Marie, 208

Panic disorder, in postpartum period, 38

Para potens, end to, 6

Parent-infant psychotherapy, 210, 226–229
  effectiveness of, research on, 227–229
  groundwork for, 212
  success of, 216, 219

Parenting
  assessment and rehabilitation of, 98–99
  after denied pregnancy, 94–95, 98

Paroxetine
  for postpartum depression, **48**
  use during breast-feeding, 50

Participant observation, 120

Passive behavioral style, and pregnancy denial, 91

Peer group support, 194

Peripartum Events Scale, 248

Perpetrators
  of filicide, 44
  of infanticide, 20, 195, 203
    age of, 24–25
    therapy for, 247
    as victims, xv
  of neonaticide, 20, 135–136
    age of, 90, 135, 189
    dissociative disorder in, 190, 191
    therapy for, 190, 201–208

Personality disorders, in postpartum period, 39

Pervasive denial of pregnancy, 84–85

Pfeifer v. Pfeifer, 177–178

Pharmacological treatment
  for postpartum depression, 47–50, **48**
  for postpartum psychosis, 51, 52–53

Population control, infanticide as method of, 4–5

Postpartum Depression Resolution (U.S. Congress), 250–251

Postpartum Depression Screening Scale, 248

Postpartum-onset specifier, in DSM-IV, 38, 147–148, 169

Postpartum psychiatric disorders, 35–55, 134. *See also* Depression, postpartum; Psychosis, postpartum
  acute, and infanticide, 170–172
  biological considerations in, 45–47, 61–76
  clinical phenomenology of, 39–45
  definitions of, 37, 38
  diagnosis of, 44–45, 62–63
  effects on offspring, 53–54
  epidemiology of, 37–38
  evaluation and treatment of, 47–53
  insanity defense based on, 140–141
  missed opportunities for identification of, 171–172
  nosology of, 38–39
  organizations dedicated to, 243, 249–250
  plasticity of, 136
  pregnancy denial and, 94
  prevalence of, 36
  prevention of, 252
  risk of recurrence for, 62, 63
  undiagnosed and untreated, 61, 64

Postpartum Support International (PSI), 250

Postpartum syndromes. *See also* Neonaticide syndrome
  insurance and disability claims for, 181
  recognition of, medical and legal dilemmas in, 180–182
  use in civil cases, 177–180
  use in criminal cases, 173–177

Posttraumatic stress disorder (PTSD)
  pregnancy denial and, 92, 94
  rape and, 156, 205

Poverty, and risk for child abuse, 216

Pregnancy
  adjustment to, psychological
      requirements of, 216–217
  cognitive styles during, 87
  denial of. *See* Pregnancy denial
  as developmental state, 237
  emotional reactions to, 82–83
  hormones during, 45, 72
  hysterical (pseudocyesis), 114–115
  mother-infant bonding during, 237
  risk assessment in, 216–219, 228,
      237–238, **241**
  woman's attitude toward, and
      mother-infant attachment, 219
Pregnancy denial, 81–102
  biological model of, 114–115
  cognitive models of, 87–88
  consequences of, 93–95, 102
  dissociation/trauma paradigm of,
      113–114
  emotional stressors related to,
      88–90
  family dynamics with, 107, 111,
      114, 204–206
  fathers and, 244
  identification of, 96, 242
  interventions for, 96–101
  medicolegal issues in, 100–101
  mothers' accounts of, 203–204,
      218
  and neonaticide, 12, 81, 93, 94,
      105, 108–109, 136, 152, 189
      risk for, 242–243
  parenting after, 94–95, 98
  and postpartum psychiatric
      problems, 94
  psychotherapy for, 96–97
  reasons for, 87–90
  recurrence of, 95
  risk factors for, 90–93
  sociocultural factors and, 83,
      92–93, 101
  types of, 82–86
Premenstrual period, postpartum
  disorder symptoms in, 63

Prenatal care. *See also* Obstetric
  services
  delayed, and pregnancy denial, 93
  lack of, and risk for infanticide, 25
Preoccupied attachment, 214
Prevalence
  of infanticide
      underestimation of, 25, 27–28
      in U.S., 19
  of postpartum psychological
      disorders, 36
Prevention. *See also* Identification
  of infanticide, 54, 252
      in Britain, 192–195
      education as method of, 171
      missed opportunities for,
          244–246
      need for training in, 43
      psychotherapy for, 210
      recommendations for, 28
  of neonaticide, 242–243
  of postpartum depression, 50–51,
      240
      estrogen therapy for, 73–74
  of postpartum psychosis, 51–52
Probation, for infanticide, in Britain,
  16, 192
Progesterone
  effects on brain chemicals, 72
  in postpartum psychosis, 46
  in pregnancy, 72
  and regulation of neurotransmitter
      activity, 66, 68
Projections, maternal, 224–225
Pseudocyesis (hysterical pregnancy),
  114–115
PSI. *See* Postpartum Support
  International
Psychiatric disorders. *See* Mental
  illness; Postpartum psychiatric
  disorders
Psychoanalytic theories
  of infancy, 210–211
  of mother-infant relationship,
      211–212

Psychosis
  dissociative, in neonaticide, 110
  hysterical, 115
  postpartum, 9, 169
    acute onset as bipolar disorder,
      42–43
    alternative diagnoses for use in
      legal defense, 148
    and criminal justice system,
      9–10, 140
    diagnosis of, 41, 44–45
    evaluation for, 47
    hormonal factors in, 46
    hospitalization for, 240
    identification and initial
      management of, need for
      training in, 43
    insufficient understanding of,
      xvi, xvii
    lack of full recognition of, 147
    mood disorders and, 39
    vs. non-childbearing-related
      psychoses, 41–42
    plasticity of, 9–10, 238
    pregnancy denial and, 94
    prevention of, 51–52
    as psychiatric emergency, 246
    recurrence rate for, 51, 54
    rehabilitation of mothers
      recovering from, 243
    symptoms of, 41
    treatment of, 51–53
    vulnerability to, 36
Psychotic denial of pregnancy, 85–86,
  88, 89
  dissociation/trauma paradigm and,
    113
  interventions with, 99, 100
  schizophrenia and, 91–92
PTSD. *See* Posttraumatic stress disorder
Punishment. *See also* Sentencing
  justifications for, 14–16
  for neonaticide/infanticide, 137
    court vs. personal, 191
    in seventeenth century, 170

Rape, neonaticide following, 202, 205
Rape trauma syndrome (RTS),
  155–156
Recognition. *See* Identification
Recurrence
  of neonaticide, 95
  of postpartum psychosis, 51
  of pregnancy denial, 95
  risk of, in postpartum disorders, 54,
    62, 63
Reflective self-functioning, 214
Rehabilitation. *See also* Treatment
  after postpartum psychosis, 243
  as rationale for punishment, 15–16
Reilly, Bernadette, 140
Reporting of infanticide, 20–23
Repressive cognitive style, during
  pregnancy, 87
Resistant attachment, 213
Retribution
  fear of, in neonaticide perpetrators,
    191
  as rationale for punishment, 15,
    208
Right and wrong test. *See M'Naghten*
  test
Risk(s)
  for child abuse
    assessment of, 216, 248–249
    postpartum disorders and, 240
  for infanticide, assessment of, 195
  to mother-infant relations,
    209–210
    early identification of, 228
    transactional model of,
      215–216
  for neonaticide, pregnancy denial
    and, 242–243
  in pregnancy, assessment of,
    216–219, 228, 237–238,
    241
  of recurrence, in postpartum
    disorders, 54, 62, 63
  women at, identification of,
    213–214, 238–243

Risk factors
for infanticide, 23, 24–25, 28,
251–252
identification of, 44
reduction of, 54
for pregnancy denial, 90–93
Rome, ancient, 4
RTS. *See* Rape trauma syndrome
Ruddick, Sara, 123–124
Rush, Bobby, 251

Sacrifice
child death as, 127
infant, 4
Sargent, Carolyn, 126
Satcher, David, 55
Schizophrenia
and infanticide, 172–173
in postpartum period, 38
and pregnancy denial, 92
use in legal defense, 149–150
SCID-D. *See* Structured Clinical
Interview for Dissociative
Disorders
Scotland
homicide rates and legislation in,
187–188
infanticide legislation in, 192
Screening tools, 54, 248–249
Secure attachment
adult, 214
mother-infant, 213
Sedatives, postpartum depression, 49
Sensitizing cognitive style, during
pregnancy, 87
Sentencing
of fathers vs. mothers, 192
inconsistencies in, in United States,
174, 179, 247
of infanticide perpetrators
in Britain, 16, 192
in United States, 140–141
of neonaticide perpetrators
in Britain, 189, 190
in United States, 138–140

Serotonin
chemical precursor of, 66
dysfunction, in postpartum period,
41
in "fight or flight" response, 70
neurotransmitters, 65
role in depression, 66
Serotonin selective reuptake
inhibitors (SSRIs)
for postpartum depression, 48, **48,**
49
use during breast-feeding, 49–50
Sertraline
for postpartum depression, 48, **48**
use during breast-feeding, 49–50
Sex-selective infanticide, 5–6
Sexual abuse
and pregnancy denial, 112, 114
and reproductive conflicts, 237
Sexuality, conflicts related to, and
pregnancy denial, 88
Skeoch, Dorothy, 140–141
Sleep deprivation, and cognitive
disorganization, 42
Smith, Susan, 208
Social isolation
and pregnancy denial, 93
and risk for child abuse, 216
and risk for infanticide, 245
Social support, inadequate, and
pregnancy denial, 99
Sociocultural factors
for infanticide, 4, 125–126, 187, 188
for neonaticide, 92, 101, 208
for pregnancy denial, 83, 92–93,
101
Specific deterrence, as rationale for
punishment, 14–15
Spitz, Renee, 212, 215
SSRIs. *See* Serotonin selective
reuptake inhibitors
Stern, Daniel, 214, 215, 217
Stigma
of birth defects, 125–126
of mental illness, 239

Stokes, Melanie, 251
Stress axis, 70–71
Structured Clinical Interview for Dissociative Disorders (SCID-D), 116
Substance addiction, and pregnancy denial, 83, 91
Sudden infant death syndrome (SIDS)
deaths caused by, 22
infanticides attributed to, 27
Suffocation/strangulation, infant deaths caused by, 21, **22**
Suicide, postpartum illness and, 251
Support organizations, 243, 249–250
Synaptic space, events in, **67**
Syndrome(s)
DSM-IV definition of, 155
postpartum. *See also* Neonaticide syndrome
insurance and disability claims for, 181
recognition of, medical and legal dilemmas in, 180–182
use in civil cases, 177–180
use in criminal cases, 173–177
rape trauma, 155–156
Syndrome evidence, 155, 156–157

Tarahumara Indians, infanticide practiced by, 126
TCAs. *See* Tricyclic antidepressants
Temperament
dimensions of, 219
and mother-infant relationship, 219–221
Therapy
in Britain, 190, 193
cognitive-behavioral, 47–48
countertransference in, 202, 247
couple/family, 243
for infanticide perpetrators, 247
interpersonal, 47, **48**
interpretive, 228
for neonaticide perpetrators, 190
case study of, 201–208

parent-infant, 210, 226–229
effectiveness of, research on, 227–229
groundwork for, 212
success of, 216, 219
for postpartum depression, 47–48
for pregnancy denial, 96–97
as protective factor, 216
Thyroid disorders
and mood, 68–69
and postpartum depression, 47, 69–70
Traumatic deaths, 21
Treatment. *See also* Pharmacological treatment; Therapy
of family units, 243
of mothers at risk, 240
of postpartum depression, 47–51, **48**
of postpartum psychosis, 51–53
of pregnancy denial, 243
Trial. *See also* Civil cases; Criminal cases
impending, and therapy, 206–207
Tricyclic antidepressants (TCAs)
for postpartum depression, 47, **48**
use during breast-feeding, 49
Tryptophan, 66
Typology
of infanticide, 10–13, **11**
of pregnancy denial, 82–86
Tyrosine, 66

Ultrasound examinations, with pregnancy denial, 98
Unintentional injury, infanticides attributed to, 27
United States
contemporary responses to infanticide in, 10–13
legal treatment of infanticide in, xvi, 9, 14–16, 134, 137–138, 192
infanticide court cases, 140–141
injustices in, 207–208
neonaticide court cases, 138–140

United States *(continued)*
    legislative initiatives in, 250–251
    prevalence of infanticide in, 19
Unknown causes, infant deaths from,
    22–23

Valproate
    for postpartum psychosis, 51
    use during breast-feeding, 52–53
Vaughan, Hester, 105
Venis, Joyce, 250
Victim, mother as, xv

Welfare policy, and infanticide, 10
Wernick, Stephanie, 151–154
Winnicott, D. W., 209, 211

Witchcraft inquisition, infanticide
    during, 7
Women. *See also* Mother(s)
    depression in, 65
    hormonal relationships in, **69**
    mood disorders in, 63–64
    at risk, identification of, 44,
        213–214, 238–243
    thyroid disorders in, 68

Yates, Andrea, case of, xvi–xvii,
    174–177
    American Psychiatric Association
        response to, 246–247
    missed opportunities for
        prevention, 244–246